E. MANSELL PATTISON is Professor of Psychiatry and Human Behavior, Social Science, and Social Ecology, and is Vice-Chairman, Department of Psychiatry and Human Behavior, University of California, Irvine.

THE
EXPERIENCE
OF
DYING

E. Mansell Pattison

A SPECTRUM BOOK

PRENTICE-HALL, INC., Englewood Cliffs, N.J. 07632

Library of Congress Cataloging in Publication Data

Pattison, E.   Mansell, date
The experience of dying.

(A Spectrum Book)
Bibliography: p.
Includes index.
1.   Terminal care.   2.   Death—Psychological aspects.
I.   Title.
R726.8F37   362.1   76-44542
ISBN 0-13-294629-7
ISBN 0-13-294611-4 pbk.

©1977 by Prentice-Hall, Inc., Englewood Cliffs, New Jersey 07632

A Spectrum Book

10   9   8   7   6   5   4   3   2   1

Printed in the United States of America

Prentice-Hall International, Inc., *London*
Prentice-Hall of Australia Pty. Limited, *Sydney*
Prentice-Hall of Canada, Ltd., *Toronto*
Prentice-Hall of India Private Limited, *New Delhi*
Prentice-Hall of Japan, Inc., *Tokyo*
Prentice-Hall of Southeast Asia Pte. Ltd., *Singapore*
Whitehall Books Limited, Wellington, *New Zealand*

Contents

IV

ADOLESCENCE

V

YOUNG ADULTS

IV

MIDDLE AGE

VII

THE ELDERLY

Contributors

Bruce II. Beard, M.D.
Professor and Associate Chairman
Department of Psychiatry
Texas Tech University School of Medicine

Martin A. Berezin, M.D.
Associate Clinical Professor
Department of Psychiatry
Harvard Medical School

Jean E. Carlin, Ph.D., M.D.
Associate Dean, College of Medicine
Assistant Clinical Professor
Department of Psychiatry and Human Behavior
University of California, Irvine

Henry P. Coppolillo, M.D.
Professor and Director
Division of Child Psychiatry
University of Colorado School of Medicine

Don DeFrancisco, M.D.
Clinical Instructor
Department of Psychiatry and Human Behavior
University of California, Irvine

William M. Easson, M.D.
Professor and Head
Department od Psychiatry and Behavioral Sciences
Louisiana State University Medical Center

Roy G. Fitzgerald, M.D.
Assistant Clinical Professor
Department of Psychiatry
University of Pennsylvania Medical School

David B. Friedman, M.D.
Associate Professor
Department of Psychiatry
New York University School of Medicine

Richard Galdston, M.D.
Assistant Professor
Department of Psychiatry
Harvard Medical School

Leonard J. Hertzberg, M.D.
Private Practice of Psychiatry
Baltimore, Maryland

Maurice Levine, M.D.
deceased
Professor and Head
Department of Psychiatry
University of Cincinnati

Ake Mattson, M.D.
Professor of Psychiatry and Pediatrics
Director, Division of Child and Adolescent Psychiatry
University of Virginia Medical Center

Caroline E. Preston, M.A.
Associate Professor
Department of Psychiatry and Behavioral Sciences
University of Washington

John E. Schowalter, M.D.
Associate Professor of Pediatrics and Psychiatry
Child Study Center
Yale University

Roslyn Seligman, M.D.
Assistant Professor of Child Psychiatry
Department of Psychiatry
University of Cincinnati

Herbert G. Steger, Ph.D.
Assistant Professor
Department of Physical Medicine and Rehabilitation
University of California, Irvine

Marcia J. Swanson, R.N.
Clinical Staff Nurse
Orange County Medical Center
Orange, California

Thomas R. Swanson, M.D.
Clinical Instructor
Department of Psychiatry and Human Behavior
University of California, Irvine

Rudolph Toch, M.D.
Clinical Instructor
Department of Pediatrics
Harvard Medical School

Brenda D. Townes, Ph.D.
Assistant Professor
Department of Psychiatry and Behavioral Sciences
University of Washington

Stanley van den Noort, M.D.
Dean, College of Medicine
Professor of Neurology
University of California, Irvine

Donald E. Watson, M.D.
Clinical Instructor
Department of Psychiatry and Human Behavior
University of California, Irvine

David A. Wold, M.D.
Private Practice
Coeur d'Arlene, Idaho

Paul E. Wood, M.D.
Assistant Clinical Professor
Department of Psychiatry and Human Behavior
University of California, Irvine

Acknowledgements

Chapter 25. *Partial Grief for the Aged and their Families* is an abridged form of the article, *The Psychiatrist and the Geriatric Patient,* by Martin A. Berezin. The original article was published in *Journal of Geriatric Psychiatry,* Vol. 4, No. 1, pp. 53-64, Fall 1970. It is reprinted here by permission of International Universities Press.

Chapter 27. *A Memo from ML,* by Maurice Levine was originally published as a chapter in *Psychiatry and Ethics* by Maurice Levine, George Braziller, Inc. New York, 1972, publisher. Reprinted with the permission of the publisher. Copyright (c) 1972 by Diana Bailen Levine.

INTRODUCTION

As recently as ten years ago the topic of death and dying was taboo for both the general public and the scientific community. In the past decade American society has awakened to the fact that death had been dismissed from our culture. In the process of dismissing death, we dismissed the dying. In part due to public concern and in part due to an outpouring of professional research, we are now aware of the fact that the care of the dying has been badly neglected.

This is a clinical book. My goal is to provide a broader, in-depth, portrait of the dying process in its many personal forms. My hope is that the book will provide a framework within which the general processes of dying can be understood, and at the same time the unique individuality of each dying person will be recognized. The result, I trust, will be a humane, dignified, and personal approach to the care of the dying.

This book has evolved out of ten years of experience in death and dying education for professional and lay persons. This experience has shown me that despite the plethora of literature in which "dying has been worked to death," there is still a lack of simple, clear guidelines for the care of the dying. Furthermore, there are a number of issues that have not been carefully examined. Therefore, in organizing this book I have given specific attention to some issues that make this book unique.

First, in my opinion there have been drawn from a few cases some hasty overgeneralizations that are used to draw global conclusions about the dying process. Often clinical observations of dying behavior have been overpsychologized. Dying behavior is observed and interpreted within the framework of psychopathology, thus ignoring the normal, the

1

adaptive, the necessary, the functional, and the relevant styles of dying. Therefore, I shall seek to call attention to adaptive styles in the dying process, rather than looking for normal or abnormal styles of dying.

Second, although there are general processes that obtain in perhaps most dying experiences, we have neglected the variations in the dying process exhibited in different contexts. Thus I have deliberately included descriptions of accidents, infections, malformations, metabolic diseases, different types of cancers, organ transplants, and so on where the illness influences the process of dying.

Third, in our attempt to construct the "right way to die," we may overlook the many ways in which a person copes with dying. Too often I have observed family, friends, and professional staff expecting and demanding that a person cope with dying in a preconceived rigid fashion. Sometimes the dying person is approached with the assumption that we know how he should cope with dying, and we attempt to force the dying person to behave according to our expectations. I shall suggest an alternative approach—namely, to ask how this person copes with his dying and seek to adapt ourselves to his style.

Fourth, little attention has been given to the dying process throughout the life cycle. In this book I shall examine both the meaning of death and coping styles of dying in each of the major eras of the life cycle. Because of the importance of the life cycle, I have organized the clinical reports along this line to highlight the significant differences in each epoch of life.

Fifth, the dying process is not organized in the same time and expectation frame for all people. I shall introduce the concept of the living-dying interval, *within which there are different* dying trajectories. *That is, some people face dying with a certain expectation of death, whereas others are faced with uncertain expectations. Similarly, some people experience an acute trajectory toward death, while others face a chronic trajectory. These two dimensions, certain versus uncertain and acute versus chronic, directly influence the process of dying. Therefore, I have specifically labeled each clinical case report in terms of these dying trajectories to highlight their influence on all the people involved.*

Sixth, there has been widespread use of the concept of stages of dying. In this book I specifically look at the evidence for stages and conclude that the concept of stages of dying is not accurate. I shall propose, however, that there are phases *in the dying process that have some clinical utility.*

Seventh, much of the literature has focused on the dying person per se. This ignores the dying process as a social interaction. The dying person does not die alone, but dies in relationship with others—family, friends, and professional staff. To observe only the dying person is to ignore the impact of the dying process on others and ignores the impact of significant others on the dying person. So I have asked each author to specifically comment on the entire social system of the dying. I particularly wish to call attention to the family involvement in the dying process. I must confess dissatisfaction in not having more to offer on the family in this book, but we have much to learn about family participation in the dying process.

Eighth, the dying process is personal. Much of the scientific work on dying has omitted the personal variable. I have taken the liberty to include and describe my own experiences. I have asked the authors to include their own personal views and reactions. Many have done so, often in a most intimate fashion. However, I believe that the care of the dying must first start with our own appreciation for death in our own lives. Thus, I wish to underscore the fact that it is not only the dying or their families who must cope with dying, but that we too, as helpers, are intimately affected in our own lives as we live with the dying.

ORGANIZATION OF THE BOOK

This book is addressed to those who care for the dying. This includes physicians, psychiatrists, nurses, medical technicians and aides, psychologists, social workers, mental health workers, health educators, clergy men, and morticians. Therefore, I have tried to eliminate technical jargon and the language of professional specialties, so that both students and members of these various disciplines may find a common language of discussion.

For the specialist I have cited the relevant professional literature in the introductory chapters, although I have avoided a professional style of presentation.

For the student who may use this book as a text, the introductory chapters are intended to give an accurate survey of the clinical field of death and dying. Further specialized readings can be found in the topical bibliography at the end, where I have collected the major current works in the field. As a quick glance at the bibliography will reveal, the topic of death can lead quickly into a wide panorama of related topics. In this book I have chosen to keep the focus rather narrowly on the dying process.

In Part I, then, I shall present an overview of the major themes in the clinical care of the dying. This will provide a synthetic view of the general process of dying.

Parts II through VII present specific and individual portraits of the dying process, in each stage of the life cycle, with different dying trajectories, with different illness contexts. These are the variations on the general theme.

In Part VIII I shall present my syntheses of all of the original work presented in the clinical reports. I shall offer some conclusions about the issues raised in this introduction. And I shall offer some guidelines for the care of the dying.

Part IX is a topical bibliography.

It is my hope that this analysis of the process of dying will provide stimulation for further questions, for more clinical innovation, and an understanding of not one way to die, but many styles of appropriate dying.

1

Attitudes toward Death

E. Mansell Pattison

When I was ten years old I lived on a farm. One day I found a bird with a broken wing. I took the bird home, nursed it, fed it, gave it care and attention for three days. Then it died. I cried. I put the bird in a shoe box and buried it in the garden. The grave was marked with a stick, covered with flowers. For a day or so I mourned and then the bird was forgotten. Except that *I* remember.

When I was twenty years old, I went to work as an orderly in a hospital. My first night at work I was summoned to assist another orderly on a "man's job." The two of us walked briskly onto the ward. All the doors were shut, visitors gone, the nurses standing hushed at their station. They nodded silently toward a closed door. My colleague and I stepped inside the room. There lay the emaciated corpse of an old man. We pulled the tubes and needles. Taped the eyes and mouth. Stuffed the orifices. Tied the limbs to body. Placed the corpse on a stretcher. We peered out the door. The nurse nodded—no one in sight. We whisked down the hall to a waiting elevator, held for us to arrive. Down to the basement, into the morgue. Then back to the ward. Everyone was moving about—lively, animated, busy at the job of healing people. The vile threat had been removed.

Two years later, I was working in a mortuary. It was time to move a casket from the "preparation" room. We adjusted the clothes. Coiffured the hair. Added some touches of cosmetic. Folded the hands. "Ah, so lifelike," we said. Up to the "slumber" room. We adjusted the lights, the piped-in music, and the temperature. Sprayed the room with subtle perfume. And drew a "slumber veil" across the casket so the "loved one" was not seen too clearly, nor touched. Perfect.

A decade later. Grandfather died. He lay in the mortuary. We arrived with the children, all small and not acculturated to civilized ways. As we walked in the entrance, they loudly pointed to the pretty flowers, stained glass windows, and marble statuary. What a nice place! The receptionist frowned at our entrance. We found the right room with relatives already there. "Where's Grandpa?" the kids asked. There were silent nods toward the casket. "Oh, here he is!" Curious childish fingers pulled away the "slumber" veil. They patted his chest. Pulled his nose. Felt his whiskers. "It's Grandpa, alright. But it's just his body—he isn't here." And with that, the little cousins fell to childish chatter and games.

In these personal vignettes I have tried to capture the contradictory attitudes that we face in our culture: the inevitable experience of death, loss, and grief; the avoidance and seclusion of death; the denial of the reality of death through almost macabre rituals; and finally the profound simplicity that death is.

Why are we concerned about issues of death and dying? There are two reasons.

First, death is a major life event that stresses our human existence. The failure to cope appropriately with death and to resolve the subsequent loss and grief process is likely to lead to emotional maladaptation (Bowlby 1960). The loss of a parent when one is a child is a severe stress that may profoundly compromise healthy development (Furman, 1974; Moriarty, 1967). The loss of important people in adulthood may precipitate not only depression but other neurotic and psychotic reactions (Carr et al. 1970). The loss of a spouse in old age is likely to precipitate illness and death in the surviving spouse (Parkes 1972). In his book, *Death and Neurosis*, Meyer (1975) summarizes the cumulative evidence that failure to cope with death is the seedbed of neurosis. It is not that death per se is neurotogenic. In his classic article on the importance of grief, Lindemann (1944) reported that it was the *failure* to mourn appropriately that precipitated neurotic reactions. But we cannot appropriately cope with death unless we can face death.

Second, just as death has been ignored, so have the dying. "There's nothing more I can do for you. You're going to die." So said the doctor, leaving the patient, family, nurses, and friends in a dilemma of confusion. Our culture has made the process of dying a medical problem, yet no one takes responsibility. A general practitioner, Dr. Merrill Shaw (1956) who was himself dying of rectal cancer, pinpoints the problem:

The period of inactivity after a patient learns that there is no hope for his condition can be a period of great productivity. I regard myself as fortunate to have had this opportunity for a "planned exit." Patients who have been told there is no hope need help with their apprehension. Any doctor forfeits his priesthood of medicine, if, when he knows his patient is beyond help, he discharges his patient to his own services. Then the patient needs his physician more than anyone else does. The doctor who says merely, "I'll drop in to see you once in awhile, there's nothing more I can do," is of no use to the patient. For the patient goes through a period of unnecessary apprehension and anxiety.

The problem is this: death has been taboo in our culture.

CULTURAL ANTECEDENTS

Death has not always been tabo in Western culture. Even a casual visit to Europe reveals death in paintings, statues, carvings, graves and monuments—a historical litany of Western civilization's preoccupation with death throughout our cultural history. Aries (1974) has recounted this history, rooted in the Judeo-Christian heritage, in which the mortality of the human being stood center stage in the life of the culture. But as Feifel (1963) has documented, since about 1900 there was increasing denial of mortality and the reality of death. So by midcentury, death was no longer admitted into the thought of civilized people. Death had become taboo.

What factors may account for this process? Parsons and Lidz (1967) point out that after 1900, in America at least, there were no more wars fought on our soil We did not immediately observe and experience violent death. Public executions were banned. Medical science conquered the infectious diseases of childhood, so the threat of infant mortality was largely removed. We expect that all of our children will live to be adults, and we do not need to sire 10 children that two might survive. Trauma of childhood and the fatal dangers of frontier life have vanished. Whereas in 1900 people died at age 40 and many children were orphaned, parents now live to age 70 or more and usually see their grandchildren. Yet our aged and feeble no longer live in the family home or neighborhood but are sequestered in retirement colonies, decaying neighborhoods, or nursing homes. We are a culture of youth; the aged and dying do not exist. Thus, there is much in our culture that removes death and dying from the midst of our everyday life.

But that which is taboo and repressed re-emerges in perverse forms to create neurosis. In Victorian times, cultural denials and taboos centered on sexuality. As Freud so aptly observed, sexuality then emerged in perverse form and became the nidus for the generation of psychopathology. Sexuality has been readmitted into human discourse, but death has become the taboo. As a result we see preoccupation with death in its perverse forms. The lurid desecration of death in pornographic form that dehumanizes dying is seen in movies such as *The Loved One, Straw Dogs*, and *Clockwork Orange*. The intimate close-up gore of brutal killing is the nightly fare on television prime time. Thus, we do not escape death, but it returns as a preoccupation of our culture, which both denies death and is obsessed by its observation. It is not surprising then to find much scientific data to support the notion that death is neurotogenic in our time. The problem is succinctly put by anthropologist Sir Geoffrey Gorer (1965):

> Pornography would appear to be a concomitant of prudery . . . pornography has been concerned with sexuality . . . copulation and birth were the unmentionables . . . in the twentieth century, however, death has become more and more unmentionable *as a natural process* . . . preoccupation with such processes is morbid and unhealthy, to be discouraged by all and punished in the young . . . If we dislike the modern pornography of death, then we must give back to death—natural death—its parade and publicity, readmit grief and mourning.

Beside the return of the repressed, other factors bring death back into our attention. First, medical technology has prolonged the process of dying. For the first time in history we have made it possible for people to live on borrowed time. Cancer can be suppressed with drugs, hearts transplanted, kidneys supplanted by dialysis machines. The dying process can be weeks, months, or even many years (Crane 1975; Ford 1970).

Second, man is faced with the threat of massive nuclear annihilation. As Robert Lifton (1964) notes:

> In every age man faces a pervasive theme which defies his engagement and yet must be engaged. In Freud's day it was sexuality and moralism. Now it is technological violence and absurd death. We do well to name the threat and analyze its components.

Third is the crisis of meaning. The challenge of traditional values and their religious supports has left many facing an existential dilemma of providing purpose to keep on living. The towering existential philosophers of our time, Camus and Sartre, have labeled life absurd. The challenge they throw down to modern man is stark: the only important question is whether there is reason to live.

Without an ultimate justification for life, the only value becomes living itself. Thus, we see an almost panicky tenacity to hold onto one's life. It is no longer fashionable to give one's life for family, friend, neighbor, or country. Life is all I have, so I had better hang on to it.

As a result, modern medicine has become servant of the culture, devoted to the preservation of life at all cost, and death is viewed as an intrusion into the medical scientific quest for eternal existence. The maintenance of life per se as our ultimate value is reflected in science fiction, in movies such as *2001*, and the cryogenic societies that would hope to preserve life through freezing and then the wait to thaw! The denial of death is inadvertently well stated by an eminent medical scientist (Goldfarb, 1965) as follows:

> I, myself tend to adhere to the concept of death as an accident, and therefore find it difficult to reconcile myself to it for myself or for others . . . people do not forgive themselves easily for having failed to save their own or other's lives.

CULTURAL ATTITUDES

Our behavior throughout life is determined by our culture, and the same is no less true of our behavior toward death. Primitive cultures do not perceive death as a final biological state. The worlds of the gods, both in heaven and hell, exist in a continuum with the middle world of mortals. Life and death are part of an eternal process. Mortal man is part of the larger ongoing continuity of existence. Consider this African poem:

> Listen more often
> To things than to beings;
> The fire's voice is heard
> Hear the voice of water.
> Hear in the wind
> The bush sob
> It is the ancestor's breath.
> Those who have died have never left,
> They are in the woman's breast
> They are in the wailing child
> And in the kindling firebrand
> The dead are not under the earth.
> They are in the forest, they are in the home
> The dead are not dead.

In contrast, Western culture holds death to be an inevitable termination and destruction of existence.

At present we may observe four distinct different cultural attitudes toward death: death denying, death defying, death desiring, and death accepting.

The *death-denying* attitude has been most common and pervasive in our time. I have already noted many manifestations of death denial in our culture. It is curious to note that the care of the dying has been handed over to the medical profession and to hospitals. Yet Feifel (1965) reports that physicians deny death more vigorously than the general populace. Even psychiatrists, who are trained for sensitivity to human emotion, avoid death . . . they just use more abstruse mechanisms. Thus, Wahl (1958) notes:

> It is interesting also to note that anxiety about death, when it is noted in the psychiatric literature, is usually described solely as a derivative and secondary phenomenon, often as a more easily endurable form of the "castration fear" . . . it is important to consider if these formulations also subserve a defensive need on the part of psychiatrists, themselves.

We can observe the threat of death in many psychotherapy settings: how a patient's threat of suicide cows the therapist; how the psychiatrist puts him- or herself in physical danger with a violent patient; the therapist's reluctance to allow a patient to expose the deepest threatening fantasies and psychotic thoughts that intimate the annihilation of the self. How often as a young psychiatrist I despaired in my work in prison, facing men with life sentences or worse, sentenced to death. How did one, did I, relate to dead lives?

The denial of death is seen in hospitals—in the apprehension and avoidance of the dying patient. Often hospital staff suggest that it is unwise to talk to dying patients about their dying because the patients will become nervous, upset, hurt, anxious, or injured. Kübler-Ross (1970) reports that only two percent of dying patients rejected the opportunity to discuss their dying, but that many staff became emotionally upset. Similarly, I have found that most dying patients are not only willing but want to share their dying experience with others. It is rare that such discussions upset the dying person. But I have seen many nurses, physicians, and mental health personnel become nervous, anxious, upset, and distraught. At times they angrily denounce my inhumaneness for frank discussions with the dying. May it be that the fear and anger is not concern for the patient, but a projection of the anxieties that professional persons experience about their own feelings of death?

The *death-defying* attitude is rooted in our traditional Judeo-Christian heritage. St. Paul sounds the keynote: "Death is swallowed up in victory.

O death, where is thy sting? O grave, where is thy victory?'' (I Corinthians 15:54). The poet Dylan Thomas is more poignant in his themes like "Death, Be Not Proud" or "Rage, rage against the dying of the light." We can all recall many instances of people who have fought for causes, ideologies, families, or countries in defiance of the fact that they die in the doing.

The *death-desiring* attitude is much more common in our culture than we admit, for it is not considered acceptable to desire death either for oneself or for others.

A desire for death may be a means to resolve life conflicts, or to kill onself for revenge or retaliation. We are now aware that there are multiple overlapping motivations for suicide and degrees of death desiring (Wolman, 1976). Along a related line there are neurotic and psychotic fantasies of a different life in death. For example, one may seek reunion with loved ones in the magical union of death. In Othello and in Aida, the lovers will be reunited eternally in death.

Still a different death-desiring attitude is found in those who are severely debilitated, disabled, and the unhappy elderly, who seek release and escape from the misery of their lives. And there are those happy people who have reached fulfillment and look toward death as the satisfying and acceptable end of their lives.

We also must be aware that there are many circumstances where we may desire the death of others. We may have a humane desire to see the end of suffering and misery. We may desire relief from personal, emotional, and financial responsibilities and burdens. There may be people who are a source of anger, frustration, or resentment, whose death may be a welcome termination of relation. Death-desiring attitudes and emotions may be neither neurotic nor abnormal. Yet this may still remain the most taboo attitude toward death.

Death-accepting attitudes place death in perspective as a part of life and integral to existence. Death as the concluding episode of one's life plan is eloquently described by Bertrand Russell (1956):

> An individual's human existence should be like a river—small at first, narrowly contained within its banks, and rushing passionately past boulders and over waterfalls. Gradually, the river grows wider, the banks recede, the waters flow more quietly, and in the end, without any visible break, they become merged in the sea, and painlessly lose their individual being.

This might be termed "death as conclusion." But this is a romantic view. for as Schneidman (1971) points out, this view makes accidental death or early death a tragic and nonnatural event—the romantic progress of life has been interrupted!

A very different death-accepting attitude might be called *death integrating*. Existential thought has placed death at the center stage of life. Death is not physiological termination. It is our frail mortality. It is not the threat of body stoppage. It is threat of one's own nonbeing. Heidegger (1974) puts it that we are faced with a basic anxiety about our authentic potentiality for-being-in-the world. If we do not face and come to terms with the existential frailty of our existence—the fact that we plan life trajectories that will lead us to old age . . . when our life may be snuffed out at any moment—if we deny this fragile life, we become vulnerable to all the neurotic processes of denial. In *Life Against Death*, Norman O. Brown (1959) argues that neurosis arises from our incapacity to die. Once freed from avoiding our own nonbeing in death we can joyously embrace life. In his book *Denial of Death*, Ernest Becker (1973) states that it is the resignation to and acceptance of our limited existence that is the central task for achieiving maturity. Jacques Choron (1964) notes: "Postponement of death is not a solution to the problem of the fear of death . . . there still will remain the fear of dying prematurely." So it is not the integration of death, of which we speak, but the integration of a sense of being-meaning that is at issue. As Becker (1973) says:

> Fear of death is not the only motive of life; heroic transcendence, victory over evil for mankind as a whole, for unborn generations, consecration of one's existence to higher meanings—these motives are just as vital and they are what give the human animal his nobility even in the face of his animal fears.

Becker suggests what has been a traditional religious solution, and one that finds its expression in the Judeo-Christian heritage: "For whosoever will save his life shall lose it; and whosoever will lose his life for my sake shall find it." (Matthew 16:25) Death integration is perhaps then not an individual psychological solution, but can be integrated only within a transcendent belief.

In summary, cultural attitudes toward death rarely exist in pure form, any more than personal attitudes exist in pure form. Indeed, since the mid-1960s we have moved from a rather death-denying culture toward a more open death-integrating one. Perhaps it is the complexity and constant shift of many attitudes toward death of which we must be aware.

DEATH DENIAL AND DEATH ACCEPTANCE—A DIALECTIC

Who is afraid to die? What is it we fear? We are asked to understand and respond to the dying person. Yet to understand another person in his or her life requires that we understand that same conflict, same feeling, same situation, located within ourselves—for all humans partake of universal feelings and reactions. To understand dying in others demands that we deal with dying within ourselves.

Freud (1915) suggested that the unconscious does not recognize its own death, but regards itself as immortal: "It is indeed impossible to imagine our own death; and whenever we attempt to do so, we can perceive that we are, in fact, still present as spectators." In this Freudian view, we fear the unknownness of death. On the other hand, more recent observations suggest that death anxiety does not pertain to physical death but is the primordial feeling of helplessness and abandonment. The fear of the unknown of death is the unknown of annihilation of self, of being, of identity. Leveton (1965) describes this sense of "ego chill" as "a shudder which comes from the sudden awareness that our nonexistence is entirely possible."

This unknown threat cannot be processed within the self. Robert Jay Lifton (1964) has graphically described his personal reactions while interviewing the survivors of the Hiroshima atomic bomb. At first he was profoundly shocked and emotionally spent as he sensed his own human frail mortality, but as the interviews went on he found himself becoming detached as a scientific observer. He did not become insensitive but found himself inexorably developing a sense of "psychic closing off"—the development of a distance between the experiencers of death and his own personal relationship to death—for him to function effectively as a physician and as a scientist.

This personal account from Lifton is a critical observation: *we cannot for long look at our own nonbeing.* In fact, the central theme of Becker in *Denial of Death* is that life is an unordered chaos in which there is no predictability or sense. To survive, says Becker, the human organism *must repress* his or her sense of frailty, must submerge his or her awareness of mortality, and must construct a mythology of existence—which we call our mature sense of reality. Reality is *not* out there to be rationally comprehended. Reality is the construction we make to exist. To sense our own nonbeing is perhaps vital, but we cannot for long look directly at it. It is like the sun. We can only look directly at the sun for a few fleeting blinding moments at one time. For the most part, we look at the sun indirectly. In the same fashion, we look at our own nonbeing indirectly.

What is the practical import here? To talk to, work with, and understand the dying person evokes intense personal feelings. As Weisman (1970) notes, the care of the dying arouses some of the most pervasive fears of all people—extinction, helplessness, abandonment, disfigurement, and loss of self-esteem. We could not long survive, much less serve our fellow beings if we had to struggle continuously at the raw edge of our own existence.

Too often we have encouraged the denial of death—but the remedy is not a defenseless wallowing in the blinding acuteness of our own mortality. Rather, there is that psychic distance to be achieved—*compassionate detachment. Appropriate repression* of our death anxieties is a necessary prelude to effective professional care. Here I mean the capacity to bring into consciousness the fundamental awareness of death anxiety, feeling acceptably comfortable about one's own finite mortality, and thus able to allow the fundamental concerns to lie out of conscious sight most of the time. When necessary, or when evoked by life circumstance, one can then respond without conflict to the stirrings of one's own concerns about death.

PROFESSIONAL DISTORTIONS

A posture of compassionate detachment is difficult to attain and maintain. Over the past decade of professional interest in the problems of the dying, two major distortions of compassionate detachment have emerged.

The first is *exaggerated detachment*. Instead of denial of death in a gross and crass manner, emotional distance is achieved through professionalization. Dying is made an object of scientific inquiry. Death is made a disease—a thing. Death is no longer a threat because it can be therapized. So we can now turn to the "right treatment of dying." Dying is no longer a subjective experience of persons but an impersonal objective external problem. Such people often demand that specific regimens be set up for dying persons. People are now supposed to die in the "right way." They look for logical and rigid patterns of progression of dying so that they can rigorously follow the scientific course of action. I have had such professional people seek my consultation because dying persons were not in the right stage, not reacting the right way, or otherwise failing to respond to the professional and scientific treatment of the dying. In a word, dying is made acceptable through professional *objectification*.

The second distortion is *exaggerated compassion*. Here, instead of separation from the dying there is fusion with the dying. Such professionals not only identify with the dying person but may seek in their work to undo past guilts, relieve past shame, restore personal self-esteem, rework their own prior death experiences, anticipate their own death anxieties. They live, die, and are reborn with each dying person. Such vicarious identification is also a defense. The dying person is me . . . but then the miraculous occurs, for when the dying is dead, I am still alive. I have beaten death after all. Such professionals often become personally and professionally overinvolved in the life of the dying person. I have seen these persons angrily denounce any distance or detachment they see in others who work with the dying. How can you have compassion if you are not totally involved? Here, dying is made acceptable through professional *subjectification.*

LOVE AND HATE: THE AMBIVALENCE TOWARD DYING

In the recent past we have hated and despised death—and now at least some would have us welcome, embrace, even love death! I am reminded of those who hate or love the fact that they were born. But birth *is*, we had no say. Even so, death *is*, we have no say. Feelings of love or hate are irrelevant. Life *is.*

However, feelings of love and hate are most relevant to people. All important relationships are a mixture of love and hate. No important person fails to disappoint and frustrate us. The very depth of loving importance increases the probability of disappointment. For the most part we accept and tolerate the negative hateful emotions and tend to experience in our consciousness only the positive ones. But it is clear that all of us harbor love and hate together. Our capacity to accept, tolerate, and even utilize the ambivalence of our feelings is one major hallmark of emotional maturity.

The importance of universal ambivalence is central to our attitude toward the dying. The dying person who is important to us evokes not only feelings of tender loving compassion but also feelings of anger, despair, frustration, disappointment, even hatred. If we expect that loving feelings are the only dimension of caring for the dying, we shall delude ourselves and fail to cope appropriately with the arousal of hateful feelings.

The process of appropriate grief and mourning revolves around the successful recognition and integration of our love and hatred toward the dead person we mourn. Thus, our attitudes toward dying are rooted in our attitudes toward ourselves and toward others; an integration of the likeable and the despicable. So it turns out that the process of dying is a part of our life that can be best understood as we understand the nature of human nature.

REFERENCES

ARIES, P., *Western Attitudes Toward Death: From the Middle Ages to the Present.* Baltimore: Johns Hopkins Press, 1974.

BECKER, E., *The Denial of Death.* New York: Macmillan, 1973.

BOWLBY, J., Separation anxiety: a critical review of the literature. *Journal of Child Psychology and Psychiatry* 1: 251-275, 1960.

BROWN, N.O., *Life Against Death.* Middletown, Conn.: Wesleyan University Press, 1959.

CARR, A., D. PERETZ, B. SCHOENBERG, and A. KUTSCHER, eds. *Loss and Grief: Psychological Management in Medical Practice.* New York: Columbia University Press, 1970.

CHORON, J., *Modern Man and Mortality.* New York: Macmillan, 1964.

CRANE, D., Decisions to treat critically ill patients. A comparison of social versus medical considerations. *Health and Society* 53: 1-34, 1975.

FEIFEL, H., The function of attitudes towards death, in *Death and Dying: Attitudes of Patient and Doctor.* New York: Group for the Advancement of Psychiatry, 1965.

———— , The taboo on death. *American Behavioral Scientist* 6:66-67, 1963.

FORD, A.M., Casualties of our time. *Science* 167: 256-263, 1970.

FREUD, S., Thoughts for the times on war and death. Collected papers, Vol. 4. London: Hogarth, 1915.

FURMAN, E., *A Child's Parent Dies.* New Haven: Yale University Press, 1974.

GATCH, M., *Death: Meaning and Mortality in Christian Thought and Contemporary* Culture. New York: Seabury Press, 1969.

GOLDFARB, I.A., Discussion, in *Death and Dying: Attitudes of Patient and Doctor.* New York: Group for the Advancement of Psychiatry, 1965.

GORER, G., The Pornography of death, in *Encounters,* eds. S. Spender, I. Kristol, M. Lasky. New York: Simon & Schuster, 1965.

GROTJAHN, M., Ego identity and the fear of death and dying. *Journal of the Hillside Hospital* 9: 147-155, 1960.

HEILBRUUN, G., The basic fear. *Journal of the American Psychoanalytic Association* 3:447-466, 1955.

KÜBLER-ROSS, E., *On Death and Dying.* New York: Macmillan, 1970.

LEVETON, A., Time, death, and the ego-chill. *Journal of Existentialism* 6:69-80, 1965.

LIFTON, R.J., On death and death symbolism: the Hiroshima disaster. *Psychiatry* 27: 191-210, 1964.

LINDEMANN, E., Symptomatology and the management of acute grief. *American Journal of Psychiatry* 101: 141-148, 1944.

MEYER J.E., *Death and Neurosis.* New York: International Universities Press, 1975.

MORIARTY, D.M., *The Loss of Loved Ones.* Springfield, Ill.: C.C. Thomas, 1967.

PARKES, C.M., *Bereavement: Studies of Grief in Adult Life.* New York: International Universities Press, 1972.

PARSONS, T., and V. LIDZ, Death in American society, in: *Essays in Self-Destruction*, ed. E. S. Scheidman. New York: Science House, 1967.

RUSSELL, B., *Portraits from Memory.* New York: Simon & Schuster, 1956.

SCHNEIDMAN, E.S., On the deromanticization of death. *American Journal of Psychotherapy* 25: 4-17, 1971.

SHAW, M., Dying of cancer. Horror attitudes most harmful. *Seattle Times,* March 24, 1956.

WAHL, C.W., The fear of death. *Bulletin of the Menninger Clinic* 22: 214-223, 1958.

WEISMAN, A.D., Misgivings and misconceptions in the psychiatric care of the terminal patient. *Psychiatry* 33: 67-81, 1970.

WOLMAN, B.B., *Between Survival and Suicide.* New York: Gardner Press, 1976.

2

Death throughout the Life Cycle

E. Mansell Pattison

In the first chapter we examined general attitudes toward death. Now we must turn toward a developmental view of death throughout the life cycle. In comparison to the many studies of generalized adult attitudes, there are few studies on the development of concepts of death through childhood, or on the variation in attitudes toward death in each stage of the life cycle (Anthony 1940; Cook 1974; Spinotta 1975). The child's concept of death is intimately involved with his or her concept of identity, such that as the child grasps the meaning of identity, so does he or she grasp the concept of death (Maurer 1966; McConville, Boag, Purchit 1970; Pertz 1972). So there is a maturation of the notion of death as the child matures into adulthood. However, the matter does not end there, for with each epoch of adulthood our view of personal identity shifts—and along with it our perception of death.

DEATH AND DYING AS A PART OF IDENTITY

So far as our experience of human mortality is being alive; then we may say that nonbeing is death. Hence, concepts of death and how we cope with dying are intimately entwined with our concepts of life and being, and how we cope with life. So the study of death throughout life is grounded in our study of the development of identity, the sense of self, and manner by which we live out our lives.

For the person who has little sense of personal being, there can be little sense of nonbeing—that is, death. Thus, the small infant, the severely mentally retarded, and the person whose consciousness has been impaired will have little appreciation of the cessation of their existence. Somewhere in the middle ground of everday existence we maintain a steady background awareness of our self-existence; we might call it normal self-consciousness. In this everyday state of affairs we focus on the necessities, pleasures, and pains of daily realities. Here we do not constantly focus on our being and the possibility of nonbeing. We act and live within an *experience* being who we are. We neither particularly question who we are, nor do we concern ourselves much with being different or facing our nonbeing. Yet at the far end of this spectrum there are times and circumstances when our self-awareness is heightened, when our consciousness is acute, and when the issue of our being and nonbeing stands central to our existence. One example is during normal child development as the child moves toward definition of self, reaching its apogee in adolescence. In adolescence there is the "crisis of identity," as the young person questions his or her values or life styles, and seeks to define the person he or she wishes to be. It is not surprising that the teenager also is concerned about his or her nonbeing, as reflected in teen-age reflections and concern about death. And, unfortunately, this struggle for identity sometimes leads to death, with suicide a major cause of death in adolescents. Another example of identity consciousness with heightened death awareness occurs during a variety of altered states of consciousness. Psychotomimetic drugs, such as LSD, produce an intense state of awareness of self. Persons report that in such heightened awareness they become excruciatingly aware of their possible nonbeing, and may then experience intense fear of death. Still another example is the occurrence of a life-threatening event—a robbery, a disaster, or an acute illness. Again the normal flow of life is interrupted. One is faced with one's immediate existence and the threat of extinction.

In summary, we see death as we see ourselves. When we see ourselves dimly we see death, nonbeing dimly. When we see ourself, our being, in sharp clear light, we see our nonbeing, our death, in the same hard etched light.

DEATH AND IDENTITY IN THE YOUNG PRESCHOOL CHILD

At birth the child emerges into the world with more potentiality than actuality. He or she is a being that will become a person. From this point the child will move slowly toward an awareness of his or her body as him- or herself. The child is fingers, the child is toes, the child is tummy and mouth. The sense of self is primarily lodged in body perception and body awareness. Says the small child, "Here I am" as he or she pats his or her body and points to him- or herself.

The small child has an identity that is also tied to parents and family. He or she is part of them and they are part of him or her. The child does not have a clear line of demarcation between him- or herself and others. Thus, the small child maintains a self sense of being by virtue of being with others. When mother or father or family are absent—in the other room—the small child may experience anxiety and difficulty in function. In a sense, part of him- or herself is missing and he or she cannot act as a person. The distance grows that can be tolerated, but the need for the intimate others as part of oneself remains. Watch a group of three-year-olds play in the yard, while mother watches from the window. She says, "Go on playing while I go to the store." Does the child play on? No! He or she wails in anguish. The child can only play while mother is near to maintain his or her sense of self.

These two aspects of identity—the bodily self and self as part of others can be seen as dominant dynamics in relation to death and dying. This young child has no appreciation of the intellectual notions of death and dying. Here the issues of death and dying are not intellectual but exper-iential. The young child does experience pain, discomfort, bodily dysfuntion if ill. Therefore, coping with dying in the young child is to help him or her feel comfortable and relieve bodily distress. The second aspect deals with presence and separation. Separation from mother and father is loss of the security and sense of self. To be with one's family is to be oneself. To be alone is to experience annihilation of oneself. Therefore, the care of the dying young child centers around maintaining the young child with his or her family if possible. If hospital care is necessary, then a stable and reliable parent substitute must meet the child's need for someone to love him or her and maintain his or her sense of being (Easson 1970).

DEATH AND IDENTITY IN THE OLDER PRESCHOOL CHILD

As the child grows into the years of three to six, he or she acquires a more unique sense of him-or herself. The capacity to think, to reflect, to inquire begins to emerge. He or she acquires a sense of self-control and self-direction. He or she feels a sense of action and result. This is the age of fantasy and daydream, of dreams and nightmares, of magic and mystery in the world. In the world of fairy tales there are manifold possibilities.

The dawning intellectual appreciation of death appears. But death is still separation, death is not-being-here-anymore. A neighbor child moves away across the continent. The child crys. Mother says, "Yes, it is sad we won't see your friend anymore because she is far away." The child questions, "If my friend is gone and not coming back, that means she's dead?" The question is appropriate, for we often speak of dead as not coming back, of going away. In another way, in the world of magic fairy tales, death is not permanent nor irreversible. We play cowboys and Indians. "Bang! You're dead." You promptly drop dead! But then you come alive, to fight the next war. A psychiatrist friend of mine dropped in on a friendly frontier war one night as he came home. "Bang! You're dead," cried his son. The psychiatrist compliantly dropped to the grass. But then lay immobile beyond the prescribed dead period. "Come alive, come alive," screamed the terrified son. So death is not pretend. It is real—but not permanent.

Again we have two motifs—magical fantasy and real but impermanent death (Nagy 1948). The lively play of fantasy, not yet modified into tested reality, leave this age child vulnerable to misinterpretation and misunderstanding of sickness and death. The child may view illness and disability as punishment for real or imagined actions. He or she may experience treatment procedures in magnified fantasies and may see hospitalization as abandonment and rejection by parents. He or she may interpret the grief, sorrow, and unhappiness of his or her parents as anger or disappointment in the child. Thus, dealing with dying calls for carcful explanation of the causes of illness, the need for procedures and treatment. The child needs to understand the emotional reactions of parents so that he or she docs not feel guilty, does not feel rejected, does not feel unwanted or unloved.

Just as separation is important for the younger nonverbal child, separation is still a major anxiety for the verbal preschool child. Death is separation, death is being alone. The preschool child does not live in an experiential world of years but of minutes and hours. Eternity is the time between breakfast and supper. Death is sleep and sleep is death. And with death there is resurrection. The little nursery rhyme is perhaps not so dreadful and morbid as it might seem: "Now I lay me down to sleep, I pray the Lord my soul to keep, If I die before I wake, I pray the Lord my soul to take." Note the fusion of death and sleep. Note the fusion of human parent and godly parent. It is a fairy tale world of continuity between the mortal and immortal. That is reassurance of continuity the child needs. A little girl came into the hospital one night puffed up with leukemia. She looked up at me and said, "Will I die?" "Yes," I said. "Will you keep me company?" she asked. "Yes, I'll sit here and hold your hand and you can go to sleep." She smiled and cuddled on the pillow. She clutched my hand in relief and drifted to sleep. I held her hand until she lapsed into a coma and died as the sun rose in the window.

DEATH AND IDENTITY IN THE GRADE SCHOOL CHILD

The school-age child is a doer. Life and being consist in the acting. "Look, Ma, I can ride the bike—no hands." "I can run faster than you can." There is pride in achievement, affirmation of self in accomplishments, the definition of who I am by what I can do. As before, there is the social reinforcement of self by others as well. "Us boys can do it." "Don't bother us girls." The clique and gang of best friends are a circle of mirrors that reflect the image of oneself as seen in others. My identity as a human, and more specifically as a boy or a girl, is supported by the fact that my friends like me and that they are like me. They like the games I like, the records I like, the friends I like. They are okay, so I am okay. Fantasy is replaced by action, and there is little time for reflection.

The school-age child now begins to see the distant horizon of a life to be lived. Fantasies now relate to a possible reality. There are heroes and idols and great deeds be done. There is death in this world, but it is distant, not personal. It is the end of the play, the interruption of the game. "Aw, do we have to quit now, we're just in the middle. I don't want to come home for supper." But if I must come home I will, and I will live with that frustration and disappointment, for life is here and now and i can dream about tomorrow.

As we turn to death and dying then, we can see that the child here must cope with bodily disability and dysfunction as an interference with his or her capacity to be a person. He or she needs to be able to do, to do what he or she can, to do what gives him or her satisfaction, to continue his or her involvement in his or her activities. Further, the child needs his or her friends, the daily concourse of interchange that tells the child that he or she is okay. The child can appreciate the intellectual notion of his or her death, but his or her experience is still rooted in the life of today. He or she can and will dream of tomorrow, even if that tomorrow will not come, for at this age who knows what tomorrow there will be? Thus, the issue in coping with dying lies in the life of the present where life and identity are squarely placed. And let us dream of the possibility of a tomorrow (Zeligs 1973).

DEATH AND IDENTITY IN ADOLESCENCE

One might think that the adolescent had a strong identity indeed. It is time for Bringing Up Father and Putting Mother in Line. Parents are a reflection of exquisite self-consciousness. To be sure, most adolescents move along in fairly unruffled vein, even in this age of youth consciousness. On the one hand, the adolescent is iconoclast and skeptic, and on the other hand, devoutly religious, looking for a sure faith in life that will command steadfast commitment. Who am I? is the central question. As the typical adolescent stares earnestly in the mirror, both learning to love and appreciate oneself as a unique person, while hoping that if the mirror does not answer back "you are the fairest of them all," at least it might give back some inkling of what sort of creature I really am. Adolescence is a time of intense intellectual and emotional preoccupation with oneself. It is the time to grasp oneself firmly, to shout "I am." The doing is surordinated to being. There is a subtle but critical transformation from what I do makes me important to being what I am makes what I do important. The sense of respect for the integrity of my unique self is paramount.

Here, the concept of death acquires an intellectual importance that meets the emotional experience of oneself. The adolescent now has a sense of being, a sense of person, a sense of me. Characteristically, the adolescent does *not* have a sense of longevity. The length of life is not at issue, but the quality is. Thus, we see many romantic notions of death in the thoughts of adolescents. Who cares how long one lives, so long as one lives and dies as the real me. So, adolescents make brave soldiers because they do not fear annihilation so much as whether they are brave and glorious. The image of oneself is important, the life of oneself much less so (Kastenbaum 1959; Maurer 1964; Sarwer-Forner 1972).

So, in coping with dying in the adolescent, we are faced with the youth who may fear the loss of his or her newly gained sense of true being. Am I strong, am I beautiful? Am I a decent human being? Am I really me? Or will I die before I know who I am? Will I die before I have a chance to show others who I am? The affirmation, confirmation, and clarification of the adolescent as a unique and real human being may be the most important task in coping with dying at this age. For example, a 15-year-old boy with rapidly growing sarcoma in his pelvis was now unable to walk. He readily agreed to talk with a group of doctors about his malignancy. He was not much worried about death, he said. He had resolved his religious doubts and had become a full member of his church. He was proud that he could come to tell the doctors about the importance of his faith and share what he had learned about the meaning of life. He was peaceful, the doctors were crying. In another instance, a 19-year-old All-American football player developed acute leukemia just before the season. He was worried that the team would be ashamed of him and his weakness. The coach and team and cheerleaders visited him, to inform him of their concern and respect. I noted how strong his bones were; I kept bending my bone biopsy needles. He was pleased that I admired his physical build and his reputation. He didn't mind being sick so much as long as he could keep track of the team. He died watching their first game on television in his room.

DEATH AND IDENTITY IN THE YOUNG ADULT

The young adult is on the threshold. All has been preparation for life, and now here it is. It is the beginning of a career, of a home, or a marriage, of children. There are hopes and aspirations. Goals now set are to be tested by experience. How will it go? I can hardly wait. There is intensity, fervor, impatience, excitement, new ideas and places waiting.

The issue of death in the young adult is one of frustration and disappointment. To reconcile what might have been with what is. There may be sense of being cheated, of unfairness, not getting one's fair share of life. Why me? Perhaps the sense of frustration is more central than any other. A 22-year-old young woman with chronic leukemia wanted to be an artist. She had talent and drive. She would erupt in angry hatred at her weak body that did not allow her to go to school when she wanted. A 30-year-old architect became depressed because his emerging creative ability was just now beginning to bloom, yet his leukemia was fulminating and he was rapidly dying.

To cope with dying in the young adult is to deal with disappointment, with rage and frustration, with anger at the world and at oneself. Perhaps more than at any other age, one faces the tenacity of holding onto one's existence. I am here now, ready and able to live. A young woman of 25 with leukemia, another of 30 with carcinoma, both wanted to live with vitality, read, talk, keep their homes so long as they could. They wanted to maintain the integrity of their adult mandate to live their lives. Perhaps this sustenance of the active, striving, coping, able adult is good. Dying with the harness on is where the young adult is.

DEATH AND IDENTITY IN MIDDLE AGE

The middle years of adulthood are a neglected time. Certainly adulthood is not a plateau. Each decade of life brings new challenges and new perspectives. The impetuous drive of youth mellows to the steady pull of maturity. A growing sense of the surety and familiarity of oneself, one's marriage, one's spouse leads toward a possible appreciation of the more subtle and muted rewards of life. It is striking to interview couples at different decades of their lives. Each couple claims to like the decade they are living in the best. But they appreciate the value and perspective of each decade gone before. For the man, he will likely come to a more realistic appraisal of his goals and abilities. For the woman, a greater freedom and opportunity for expanded self-hood. As one moves from one decade to another, there is usually more security, more time for reflection, the opportunity to gather some fruits from the labors of life.

The issue of death in the middle years is more likely to take on an interpersonal tone. The middle years have usually seen the development of meaningful ongoing relations with family, spouse, children, friends, relatives, and neighbors. Hence, death is a disruption of the involvement with others. It is not that you cannot leave the ones you love, it is that you do not want to go. They fill your life. There are responsibilities and obligations. Who will fulfill them? Thus, coping with dying involves coping with the involvements you have with others. This may then become the focal issue in our response to dying at this age (Jaques 1965). For example, a 45-year-old housewife with breast cancer called me in a state of great agitation one afternoon. We had discussed her death on several occasions, and I was quite surprised that she should be so upset. When I arrived at her room, the situation became immediately clear. The intern had ambiguously suggested that she might not leave the hospital. Actually this referred to treatment that was suggested rather than her immediate death. She quickly assured me that she had no concern about death, but she did not want to die before she returned home and got the house set in order, arranged for housekeeping for her husband, and care for her teen-age children. Above all, she wanted to be able to sit down with her family and plan how they would manage together after she died.

DEATH AND IDENTITY IN OLD AGE

More and more people now live longer in our society. To be old does not mean that death is perceived as just around the corner. A man of 70 told me recently, "Just because I am retired doesn't mean I don't enjoy life every bit as much as you do." Retirement and old age do not mean that one has come to peace with life and is now ready to accept death. In *Death of a Salesman,* Willy Loman wryfully says, "A man can't go out just the way he came into it. He's got to amount to something."

Old age brings one to a reflection upon the entirety of one's life. Identity is still at issue. Was I a real person and am I a person still? Can I respect myself and love myself in the face of what my life has been? Robert Butler (1963) has pointed out that many old people engage in a type of perseverative reminiscence of their lives. They go over and over their lives. Did it make sense? Was it worthwhile? Are they okay? In my conversations with old people, I find many who are not yet ready to die. They have not made peace with themselves. They still question and doubt their existence. Death will be an intrusion, unless and until they can affirm that their life was a unique existence to them, that allowed of no other existence. So again, coping with dying turns to an affirmation of the real personhood of the aged persons (Jeffers, Nichols, Eisdorfer 1961; Kalish 1970; Preston, Williams 1971; Swenson 1961).

REFERENCES

ANTHONY, S., *The Child's Discovery of Death.* New York: Harcourt Brace, 1940.

BUTLER, R. N., The Life Review: an interpretation of reminiscence in the aged. *Psychiatry* 26: 65–76, 1963.

COOK, S. S., *Children and Dying: An Exploration and Selective Bibliographies.* New York: Health Sciences Publications, 1974.

EASSON, W., *The Dying Child.* Springfield, Ill.: C. C. Thomas, 1970.

JAQUES, E., Death and the mid-life crisis. *International Journal of Psychoanalysis* 46: 502–514, 1965.

JEFFERS, F. C., C. R. NICHOLS, and C. EISDORFER, Attitudes of older persons toward death: A preliminary study. *Journal of Gerontology* 16: 53–56, 1961.

KALISH, R. A., The aged and the dying process: the inevitable decisions. *J. Soc. Issues* 21: 87-96, 1970.

KASTENBAUM, R., Time and death in adolescence, in *The Meaning of Death,* ed. H. Feifel. New York: McGraw-Hill, 1959.

MCCONVILLE, B. J., L. C. BOAG, and A. P. PURCHIT, Mourning processes in children of varying ages. *Canadian Psychiatric Association Journal* 15: 253-255, 1970.

MAURER, A., Adolescent attitudes toward death. *Journal of Genetic Psychology* 105: 75-90, 1964.

_____, Maturation of concepts of death. *British Journal of Medical Psychology* 39: 35-41, 1966.

NAGY, M. The child's theories concerning death. *Journal of Genetic Psychology* 73: 3-27, 1948.

PERTZ, A., The child's sense of death. Stages in affective organization and notional development, in *Death and Presence,* ed. A. Godin. Brussels: Lumen Vitae, 1972.

PRESTON, C. E., and R. H. WILLIAMS, Views of the aged on the timing of death. *Journal of Gerontology* 11: 360-394, 1971.

SARWER-FORNER, G., Denial of death and the unconscious longing for indestructibility and immortality in the terminal phase of adolescence. *Canadian Psychiatric Association Journal* 17: 51-57, 1972.

SPINOTTA, J. J., The dying child's awareness of death: a review, in *Annual Progress in Child Psychiatry and Child Development,* eds. S. Chess and A. Thomas. New York: Basic Books, 1975.

SWENSON, W. M., Attitudes toward death in an aged population. *Journal of Gerontology* 16: 49-52, 1961.

ZELIGS, R., *Children's Experience with Death.* Springfield, Ill.: C.C. Thomas, 1973.

3

The Family Matrix of Dying and Death

E. Mansell Pattison

As we have seen, the meaning of dying is embedded in the life cycle and our relationships with others. Thus, we must turn to the family to examine how we learn about death, dying, and mourning. For it is in our family experience that we learn how to face death. I shall illustrate this process with a clinical case study, but first let us examine some preliminary issues.

DEATH PREVENTION IN THE FAMILY

As we noted in Chapter 1, the dying person has been removed from the home and family context in modern Western society. As a result children are not exposed to death and dying as part of the natural process of life. In fact, the taboos about death have been so strong that people have suggested it is harmful for children to see corpses and attend funerals. Yet this antiseptic approach to death may have proved more harmful than helpful, for we then deprive children of the opportunity to incorporate a meaningful concept of death into their concept of life. I am constantly struck by the number of middle-aged people who tell me they have never seen a corpse or attended a funeral. Then a death occurs; they are shocked and have no idea of how to react. How do we expect people to cope appropriately with death and dying, if in their childhood and adolescence they have never learned about death and dying? Our culture is perhaps the first in history to insulate our children from death. It is no wonder that these children become adults who react to death with dysfunctional and pathological reactions. We have not provided death preparation. The great interest in courses and classes on death and dying may well attest to a growing cultural awareness of our need to become acquainted with death.

In the 1950s, in his pioneering study of dying, psychoanalyst Kurt Eissler (1955) suggested that we should practice "orthonasia," that is, to teach children about death as part of life, so that children will learn how to incorporate healthy attitudes toward death into their coping repertoire and be adequately prepared to deal with death events in their own life cycle. It is encouraging to note a number of children's books being written specifically for children about death (Grollman 1967; Jackson 1966; Vogel 1974). It is a beginning.

Later in this chapter we will examine some basic learning experiences within the family that serve as the matrix for learning about death in a nonverbal level of behavior between parents and children. In addition, I should like to suggest that death is a timely topic for conversation at the dinner table, where the most important conversations in a family usually occur. We will discuss this further at the end of the chapter.

DEATH INTERVENTION IN THE FAMILY

Dying is not just an individual experience; it involves the whole family. A great deal of attention has focused on the dying person, but little attention has been paid to the impact of dying on the systemic function of the family (Hamovitch 1964; Wahl 1960). Dying is not just a stress for the individual members of the family, but it also impacts on the family as a system. The death of a family member involves a shifting of tasks, roles, affection, discipline, resources, and the like. It is not just that a member is lost, but the whole family must go through a period of readjustment and re-equilibration of the family system to achieve a new balance among the remaining members (Goldberg 1973; Troup, Greene 1974).

Clinical studies illustrate how emotionally vulnerable the family system is to the experience of dying (Gordon, Kutner 1965; Krieger, Bascue 1975; Welldon 1971). So we need to be concerned not only for the dying person but also for his or her family. The importance of the family is given specific attention in this book, and the reader is invited to note the many clinical descriptions of family involvement in the clinical studies that follow.

In brief, there are three concerns for the family. The first is to assist the family in coping with the dying person during the living-dying interval. Second is to assist the family to achieve a new functional equilibrium after the death. Third is to assist the family to proceed through an appropriate mourning as a family. It is not enough that individual members mourn, but the entire family system must be able to work through its grief (Jensen, Wallace 1967; Pincus 1974).

What I have just described is not *treatment* of the family, for we are not talking about pathology, but *preventive intervention* that may assist the family in coping successfully with a major stress in the family's life.

One type of family death that is of particular significance in terms of prevention is the death of a parent when the children are young. Because early parental death has been linked to later psychopathology, there has been much concern about what can be done for such child survivors (Kliman 1968; Rheingold 1967).

Psychiatric opinion is divided on the questions of: 1) how traumatic the death of a parent is to a child, 2) how irreversible is the effect of such loss, and 3) how the effects of death may be meliorated for the child.

At the pessimistic pole of opinion are those who view parental death as a major irreversible trauma. Moriarty (1967) states: "Those who suffer from exposure to death in early childhood may be haunted for the rest of their lives by these memories. . . . many children who lose a loved one remain thereafter more or less morbidly preoccupied and discontented."

A more mediating position holds that death experiences are a severe childhood stress but not necessarily a dire trauma. Laufer (1966) says: "While itself not pathogenic, object loss can become the nucleus around which earlier conflicts and the latent pathogenic elements are organized." Similarly, Furman (1974) concludes: "When a child's parent dies, each surviving member of the family faces so complex and difficult a situation that no form of assistance may seem adequate to the task . . . yet, many children and parents . . . can master the stress."

At the optimistic pole, I would suggest that much of the problem lies with the attitudes toward death that have made death experiences pathogenic. Later I shall present evidence for the following propositions: 1) much of the observed psychopathology of childhood death experiences results from the sociocultural failure to integrate death appropriately as part of natural life experience; 2) the family system incorporates and embodies the cultural denial of death; 3) the family management of death is dysfunctional for both the family and the child because the family system fails to integrate death appropriately within the family; 4) the family deals with death through avoidance mechanisms of family myth and family mystification; and 5) the family myth and mystification processes are the pathogenic elements rather than death events per se.

The optimistic point of view is summed up by Eliot (1955) who concluded that death is inevitable but not insurmountable in the family.

THE POSTVENTION OF DEATH IN THE FAMILY

By the term "postvention," I refer to means of assistance to avoid the deleterious consequences of death upon survivors. As noted, in the family system this is of great importance, for a death in the family may permanently disrupt the effective equilibrium of family adjustment if the members do not achieve a new family style of operation. The result may be a chronic dysfunctional family (Berman 1973).

For parents who have lost a spouse, there may be major problems of adaptation. The widow or widower is no longer invited to couples' functions. There may be major problems of coping with children, finances, new job, and so on. Many a survivor parent finds no one available to help cope with these new stresses of being a single parent. For this reason voluntary community groups such as Parents Without Partners have developed out of mutual need. Such a community resource may be invaluable and of more importance than counseling and other formal mental health aids.

Similarly, the loss of a parent may mean that younger children no longer have a parent model available. The recruitment of other adult relatives to fulfill some parent surrogate roles can be of real assistance to the child. Again, community groups such as Big Brothers and Big Sisters have evolved to meet the needs of children who no longer have a parent available for them. Such groups can fill a major need for survivor children.

Finally, there is a neglected group—the aged survivor spouses. The role of widow or widower is a lonely one in our society (Langer 1957). There is the old folktale that the aged widow soon dies after her husband because of a broken heart. As it turns out, Parkes (1964) has shown that it is no fable, but that the aged survivor is highly likely to become ill and shortly die. He calls this the "morbidity of bereavement." Here again community groups have emerged as a resource, in widow-to-widow programs. Typically in such programs an effort is made to reach out to the widow or widower and establish new contacts and social support (Hiltz 1975; Silverman 1969).

In summary, the family must receive its due recognition in our concern for death and dying, if we are to effect programs of prevention, intervention, and postvention. This leads us now to an in-depth study of the meaning of death in the family.

A CLINICAL STUDY

A 40-year old doctor named Harry came to me for psychotherapy. He complained of alcoholism for the past four years since the sudden death of his wife, Florence. She had undiagnosed leukemia, which erupted in fulminating symptoms with sudden death following four days of initial illness. He expressed profound and unrelating guilt for her death, which he drowned out in the silence of booze. His marriage with Florence had been happy and idyllic. She had been the perfect woman for him as well as the acclaimed epitome of feminine motherhood by all who knew her.

Three months of therapy relieved his intense guilt, resolved his reactive depression, and his drinking was controlled. Harry was able to return to his medical practice and function at a socially competent level. He was an intelligent, articulate, psychologically sophisticated and introspective man. He readily recognized that his neurotic grief reaction and alcoholism were the symptoms of long-standing life conflicts. The next period of psychotherapy unfolded the story of Harry.

Harry was an orphan. He had no knowledge of his biological parents; he had been a deserted infant, left on the doorstep of two maiden sisters. These two spinster ladies, Aunt Millie and Aunt Mary, reared him to adolescence. The younger sister, Aunt Millie, was kind, sweet, and gentle. He lived with her until he started kindergarten. Then, for reasons unclear to him then and now, he had been moved to live with the older sister, Aunt Mary, who was stern, severe, and businesslike. He still mourned his separation from kind Aunt Millie, who had been like a mother to him. Although he saw Aunt Millie at holidays, he was never again allowed to live with her. Still he had affection for both women; they were his aunts, his only relatives. He saw them on several occasions each year, which were to him a family reunion.

Kind Aunt Millie had had a boyfriend for many years by name of Mr. Brown. He had always taken a kind, even fatherly interest in Harry, and had provided some financial support. Harry was always told that Aunt Millie and Mr. Brown planned to get married after the death of the man's sickly wife. When Aunt Millie and Mr. Brown did get married they would legally adopt him, and Harry would inherit the business of Mr. Brown. But sickly Mrs. Brown remained sickly and did not die. It was Mr. Brown who died, when Harry was 14 and ready for high school. So Aunt Millie and Mr. Brown were never married, Harry was not adopted, and Harry did not inherit a business. When Mr. Brown died, it seemed that Harry was even less welcome in the home of severe Aunt

Mary. He felt dejected, rejected, alone. So he ran away. He lived in a series of homes of his boyfriends until he could work full time and live alone. He was an able student with a winsome personality. Through scholarships and his own gutty persistence, he worked his way through college and medical school. He met his wife in college, she helped him through medical school, they had three children, and he embarked on a successful medical career for 10 years until the sudden death of his wife.

At this point it became clear that Harry had not developed his severe guilt, depression, and alcoholism immediately after the death of his wife. After an initial period of mourning he had seemingly made a good adaptation. Within six months he married his second wife, Sarah. It was after the second marriage that his disturbing emotions and symptoms began to develop. Since the second marriage was also happy, mutually rewarding, and a success, Harry could not account for his increasing inability to function.

Sarah, the second wife, was not a newcomer in Harry's life. Florence and Sarah had been roommates in college. They were contrasts in personality. Florence, the first wife, was kind, sweet, gentle, and unassuming. She had been a contented and loving wife and mother. Sarah was rather brusque, businesslike, and capable. She had never married but pursued a successful career as a psychiatric social worker. She had continued to remain friends with Florence and Harry during the years. Most curiously, Harry and Sarah had intermittent sexual liaisons during the 15 years of the first marriage. Neither considered this a threat to their respective relationships with Florence, who ostensibly was unaware of the liaisons. After the death of Florence, Sarah immediately volunteered to come help with the children. Shortly thereafter, Harry and Sarah were married.

During this period of psychotherapy, Harry continued to function well in his medical practice, his social life, and in his marriage, and he remained abstinent from alcohol. Yet as the history of his life unfolded, Harry began to experience new and disturbing affects. He reported a sense of foreboding as if his existence were to be snuffed out. There was an inchoate deep stirring in his stomach as if his insides were being wrenched. Then a sense of panic and dark anxiety as if he must jump up and run, run, run. He could not locate himself. It was bewilderment, confusion, diffuse ennui. This amorphous state of profound panic was more than Harry could endure. He remembered that he had felt this way when he left Aunt Millie. The memory swept him and he shuddered. But he had endured. He felt this way when Mr. Brown died. But he had endured. He felt this way just after marrying Florence. But he had endured.

He had felt this way when Florence, his first wife, died. But he had endured.

The only times that he could now endure, when he could emerge from this engulfing lostness, was when he talked to me. I was here. He was here with me. But there was no one else, it seemed. His wives were an attempt to create a mother. But they were not his mother. "Where, oh where is my mother!" he sobbed.

"If my mother is dead, then let her be dead. But maybe she is alive. Sometimes I think Aunt Millie is my mother, and I think Mr. Brown was my father. I know it's not true, but I wish it were so. It wouldn't have to make any difference to them. But just to know that I came from some-where, that I belong to somebody, that I'm just not a nothing. God! How can I be. I'm nothing, nothing, nothing. Mother, mother, mother where are you? Dead? Dead? All right. Give me your grave. Let me put flowers on it. But be! Dammit! Be! You know, Mansell, sometimes I know Millie is my mother. I don't want anything from her. I just want to know. I have to have a mother! God! Oh God! Have mercy upon me."

The next day Harry went to see Aunt Millie and Aunt Mary. He was armed with resolute conviction that they held some knowledge of his parentage. He would brook no evasion—only the stark truth whatever it was. He returned crestfallen to report that there was nothing to report. Aunt Millie and Aunt Mary knew nothing about his origins, and he was certainly not the son of Millie and Brown. What can I say of Harry? For he said very little that day.

At 2:00 A.M. in the morning my telephone rang. "Hello?" "Mansell, this is Sarah." "Yes?" "*Harry is dead.*"

EPILOGUE AND EPITAPH

The epitaph is not a night of whiskey drinking that failed to drown out his senses and needed just a few barbituates to bring a bit of sleep. Nor is it the will that Harry left, that his ashes, himself, be strewn over the sea. Rather it is a prosaic bit of historical fact. Sarah went to visit Aunt Millie and Aunt Mary after two weeks, to offer her condolences to these two old ladies. Shaken by the death of Harry, they said they now could say what could not be said. For Aunt Millie was, indeed, his mother and Mr. Brown his father. Harry, the out-of-wedlock son. The shame of Millie's family and the protection of Brown's family led to a pact between Millie, Mary, and Brown that Harry should never be told. And when Millie and Brown later returned to their former relationship, they protected themselves from Harry by shipping him off to Aunt Mary.

So Harry was right all along. He knew he could not know what was known.

THE PSYCHODYNAMICS OF DEATH IN THE FAMILY

The story of Harry is the story of the several families of Harry. To begin with, Harry is never provided an unambiguous mother object. He is first reared by two sisters, neither of whom assumes primary responsibility for the child. Although he lives with Millie, she does not claim him as her own child, as a foster child, or as an adopted child. The basic infant ambivalence toward mother is reinforced by his ambiguous status with mother. The splitting of the mother object into good mother and bad mother is reinforced in reality by the presence of two mother objects, who in turn assume a good-accepting and bad-rejecting role with the boy. He is given no opportunity to resolve his ambivalence and attain an object constant mother. In turn he has no basic nurturant mother object to internalize, upon which to build his own constant object self.

A second step in object identification is also blocked. He is offered a tentative identification with Mr. Brown. However, when Brown re-enters the scene, it is just as the onset of the oedipal stage. The desexualized good mother object, Aunt Millie, is transformed into a sexualized wife role with Brown. The boy is not offered identification with Mr. Brown nor allowed to retain a desexualized relationship with good mother. Rather he is extruded and sent to bad mother, Aunt Mary. Why? For his oedipal sexualization of good mother? For being competitive with Mr. Brown? Which one does not want him for what reason? He is not told. Bad mother is better than no mother at all at this point. And he is still given hope of adoption by Mr. Brown and the inheritance of his business. The opportunity for identification with Mr. Brown makes life with bad mother tolerable. But Brown dies, and with that death the tentative identification with father is lost. Harry cannot tolerate the threat of life with bad mother, so his only alternative is to run away and attempt to make life on his own.

As Harry reaches adulthood, he recapitulates his search for mother. He marries a desexualized good mother object, but at the same time the sexual bad mother is present from the beginning of courtship, throughout his first marriage, and bad mother eventually becomes the woman he is left with. Just as the two sisters collude in their mother relationship, so too, do the two roommate women collude in the wife relationship. The death of first wife, good mother, evokes bewilderment and guilt, just as the loss of first mother, good mother, evoked bewilderment. The sudden mysterious leukemia of the wife is the mysterious loss of first mother, both unexpected, both unpredicted, both unexplained. It is noteworthy that Harry's depressive and alcoholic symptoms emerge only after his marriage to second wife, bad mother. In this case, Harry again found temporary hope in identification with a male father object—the psychotherapist. The threat from bad mother was attenuated, and Harry was able to attain symptom relief. The psychodynamic analysis in therapy uncovered the projections into his current life, thus releasing his wives and myself at least partially from the transference roles. Yet on the other hand, this placed Harry right back at the earliest stage of object relations—a search for the mother object and a profound primordial panic in himself. He could not be a person without the mother object upon which he could ground his sense of self. A dead mother would release him from the search and he could recathect living objects. A rejecting mother would give him a reality to work with. But the third alternative was unbearable; a mother who gave cues recognizable in preconscious form that declared he was her son and verbal cues that declared he was not. The family myth declared he had no known parent. But the mystification of the myth subtly implied that the myth was myth. Psychotherapy dispelled the clouds of mystification. Harry attacked the myth. When the myth was thrown again flat in his face, Harry knew he had lost. He could not have the truth about himself. If mother does not acknowledge your existence, how then do you exist? Harry could not.

OBJECT CONSTANCY AND LOSS IN THE FAMILY

The family matrix provides the basic critical objects for the infant. The young child must have constant objects to accept, love, and nurture him or her. It is this matrix of constant love objects that provides the young child with a sense of identity. John Framo (1970) comments:

> The power of life-sustaining family relationship ties is much greater than instinctual or autonomous strivings . . . because abandonment has such disastrous consequences, the child will sacrifice whatever ego integrity is called for in order to survive . . . to be alone or pushed out of the family either physically or psychologically is too unthinkable.

On a similar note, Edith Weigert (1967) says: "The child needs, before all, the constancy of being accepted . . . he often sacrifices the inferior value of pleasure gain or pain avoidance for the high value of object constancy and ego identity."

A major task of the family is to provide the young child with constant objects of nurturance. The loss of a parent object can be tolerated *if the family* provides unambiguous definitions of the loss and unambiguous object replacements. (In the case of Harry, there was ambiguous definition of the loss and ambiguous replacement of the parental object.)

Failure to deal with psychological separations and losses in the family of origin give rise to subsequent family pathology. Norman Paul, (1967) for example, finds family pathology not only in loss by death, but in the failure to deal with the loss of the primary parent object. Children fail to resolve their symbiotic dependence on the family matrix of objects. They then fail to work through the grief of loss of the symbiotic dependence, and therefore fail to achieve mature individuation.

The process of maturation requires a movement from object constancy provided by the loving accepting parent object to object constancy built upon the internalized parent object, transformed into the self, so that one can love oneself and maintain one's own object constancy. This can only occur through the gradual severance of the symbiotic object relationship, in which the parent rejects the dependence of the child. Again Weigert (1967) observes: "The child loves himself not only when he feels loved by his family, in growing independence he loves himself in spite of rejection by others." To this I would add that the child learns to love him- or herself *because* of rejection by the symbiotic parent object. And the child must suffer this loss, and recathect him- or herself in lieu of the parent. It seems to me that the family management of this parental loss is critical to the family nurturance of both self-individuation and the management of the physical losses of death. *Thus, the family management of death is grounded in the family management of object separation and object loss.*

We may consider object separation and loss as a necessary growth and individuation experience. Heretofore we have considered object loss as an undesirable stress, whereas it may be a necessary precursor to self object development. Hofling and Joy (1974) have reported such favorable growth consequences of loss. *Object separation and object loss is a necessary growth experience that provides the anlage for later successful management of death experiences.*

This thesis is consonant with the theoretical work on object splitting by Roland Fairbairn (1952). The exciting-frustrating symbiotic object can be split by the child into the good object and the bad object. Where the child is unable to reconcile this ambivalence, he or she may retain the good-bad internal object split. Indeed, people may exist in reality as good-bad counterparts to the internal dichotomy. And a person may continue in life to make active unconscious attempts to force and change close relationships to fit the internal role models.

Thus, if the child does *not* resolve the basic object ambivalence and achieve separation and autonomy apart from the symbiotic object parent, he or she may continue into adulthood striving to prevent the loss of the ambivalent symbiotic object.

John Framo (1970) summarizes the dynamics well:

> Projective transferences, externalizations, vindicative phantasies, vicarious participations, all serve the function of recapturing the symbolically retained old love objects who have their representation in current real family members, thus delaying the pain of loss and mourning . . . object possession . . . helps prevent individuation which can result in the catastrophy of separation, the old dread of abandonment, and facing of the fact that one has irretrievably lost one's mother and father.

The loss of the parent is necessary to individuation, and physical death of the parent may well be considered as a varient in the normal process of loss of the parent that every family must work through.

The concept that the physical death of a parent is a pathological trauma is a myth that precludes awareness of the necessary and inevitable loss of the infantile symbiotic parent object. (In the case of Harry, there was no opportunity to work through the ambivalent symbiotic relationship with his two wives. Harry could not grieve the loss of the mother object because there was no defined object to lose. Harry could not achieve individual existence because he did not have a concrete mother object to internalize and from which he could then separate.)

THE ROLE OF MYTH AND MYSTIFICATION

It is now clear from family therapy experience that family psychopathology often centers around family myths. Ferreira (1967) defines the family myth as:

> . . . a series of well-integrated beliefs, myth-like, which members of a family entertain about each other and their relationship . . . the family myth is to the family what the defense is to the individual . . . the family myth is a group defense against disturbances or changes in the relationship.

So the family myth is a neurotic mechanism for family coping and homeostasis around an unresolvable conflict.

The process of mystification is the secondary mechanism that maintains the myth. Mystification, as Laing (1965) explains it: "is to befuddle, cloud, obscure, mask whatever is going on, whether this is be experience, action, or process . . . the state of mystification is a feeling of being muddled or confused." Mystification is described by Wynne, et al. (1958) as "pseudomutuality," and by Searles (1959) as the mode of driving the other person crazy by techniques that tend: "to undermine the other person's confidence in his own emotional reactions and his own sense of reality."

Our culture has developed enormous myths about death, and as a culture we engage in massive mystification mechanisms about our myths of death. I have selected the case of Harry to discuss because it so clearly demonstrates the process of family myth and family mystification in regard to the death of the parent. It was the myth and mystification of his mother's existence or death that drove Harry to *his* death. *The death of a family member is not pathogenic, but myth and mystification of death is pathogenic.*

THE FAMILY AS MEDIATOR
OF MYTHS OF DEATH

The family is the bridge and mediator between the social matrix and the individual. It is through the medium of the family that the child learns to participate in the larger social perceptions and constructions of reality (Boszormenyi-Nagy 1965). At present, in regard to the issues of death, we live in a social matrix that defines death as unnatural, pathological, and even pornographic. Our society has elaborated myths and mystifications about death. In turn, it is not unexpected that families transmit and participate in myths and mystification of death in the family. It should not be surprising to us that we find our clinical data to reveal that children (as well as adults) have difficulty copying with death. *Children can cope with death but will have difficulty coping with family myths and mystification of death.*

Two conceptual distinctions must be noted here. I am not suggesting that the death of a parent is not stressful. The distinction here is that successful family copying may enable the child to cope with *stress* so that it is *not converted into trauma.* The other distinction is between levels of death anxiety. The first level is the experiental relationship with an object. We might term this "psychological death anxiety." The second level is the relationship of self with world. We might term this "existential death anxiety." Ernest Becker (1973) has brilliantly shown that we confuse these two levels. He suggests that only when we come to grips with the existential dilemma of death do we equip ourselves to deal with psychological loss. I concur with Becker. In this book, I suggest that we engage in mystification of psychological loss as a maneuver to deal with the existential dilemma of death.

Our existential view of death is also our view of life. If we cannot admit death is part of life, may it be that we cannot face the fundamental psychological issues of separation and individuation that contains the kernels of loss? Therefore, I suggest that *the management of death in the family is rooted in the basic management of object relation separation and loss in the family, which in turn is a reflection of the existential death position of the family.*

Perhaps a personal vignette can best summarize this last point. When my children were young, my wife and I sat down one night at supper with them where our talk led to the death of an elderly neighbor. After some speculative questions about death, the children got right to the gut of it: "Mom, Dad, are you going to die?" Our answer was something like this:

> Yes, we will. We are in good health and do not expect to die while you are young and need our help. You can do some things for yourself now, and when you grow older you will not need us to help you. Even if we die when we are old, we will miss each other. It will be sad, but it will be all right because you will be able to take care of yourself. And if we should happen to die while you are growing up, we have made arrangements with Aunt and Uncle for them to become your parents in our place. They cannot replace us, but they can help you as we would want to help you. We would be sorry to die now and not be here to help you and enjoy you. But you will always have our love and that is the most important thing. And because we love you, we have made plans with Aunt and Uncle, who love you too. We cannot predict or prevent our death. We will die someday in your lives. But we can enjoy our family now. And when we die you will have these good days to remember, which always will be a part of your lives.

REFERENCES

BECKER, E., *The Denial of Death.* New York: Free Press, 1973.

BERMAN, E., *Scapegoat: The Impact of Death-Fear on an American Family.* Ann Arbor: University of Michigan Press, 1973.

BOSZORMENYI-NAGY, I., A theory of relationships: experience and transaction, *Intensive Family Therapy*, eds. I. Boszormenyi-Nagy and J.L. Framo. New York: Hoeber, 1965.

EISSLER, K.R., *The Psychiatrist and the Dying Patient.* New York: International Universities Press, 1955.

ELIOT, J.D., Bereavement: inevitable but not insurmountable, in *Family, Marriage, Parenthood,* eds. H. Becker and R. Hill. Boston: Heath, 1955.

FAIRBAIRN, W.R.D., *An Object-Relations Theory of the Personality.* New York: Basic Books, 1952.

FERREIRA, A.J., Psychosis and family myth. *American Journal of Psychotherapy* 21: 186-197, 1967.

FRAMO, J.L., Symptoms from a family transactional viewpoint, in *Family Therapy in Transition,* ed. N. Ackerman. Boston: Little, Brown, 1970.

FURMAN, E., *A Child's Parent Dies.* New Haven: Yale University Press, 1974.

GOLDBERG, S., Family tasks and reactions in the crisis of death. *Social Casework* 54: 406-411, 1973.

GORDON, N.B. and B. KUTNER, Long term and fatal illness and the family. *Journal of Health and Human Behavior* 6: 190-196, 1965.

GROLLMAN, E.A., ed., *Explaining Death to Children.* Boston: Beacon Press, 1967.

HAMOVITCH, M.B., *The Parent and the Fatally Ill Child.* Los Angeles: Delmar, 1964.

HILTZ, S.R., Helping widows: group discussions as a therapeutic technique. *Family Coordinator* 24: 331-336, 1975.

HOFLING, C.K., and M. JOY, Favorable response to the loss of a significant figure: a preliminary report. *Bulletin of the Menniger Clinic* 38: 527-537, 1974.

JACKSON, E.N., *Telling a Child about Death.* Des Moines: Meredith, 1966.

JENSEN, G.D., and J.G. WALLACE, Family mourning process. *Family Process* 6: 55-76, 1967.

KLIMAN, G., *Psychological Emergencies of Childhood.* New York: Grune & Stratton, 1968.

KRIEGER, G.W., and L.O. BASCUE, Terminal illness: counseling with a family perspective. *Family Coordinator* 24: 351-356, 1975.

LAING, R.D., Mystification, confusion, and conflict, in *Intensive Family Therapy,* eds. I. Boszormenyi-Nagy and J.L. Framo. New York: Hoever, 1965.

LANGER, M., *Learning to Live as a Widow.* New York: Messner, 1957.

———, Object loss and mourning during adolescence. *Psycholanalytic Study of the Child* 21: 269-293, 1966.

MORIARTY, D.M., *The Loss of Loved Ones.* Springfield, Ill.: C.C. Thomas, 1967.

PARKES, C.M., Effects of bereavement on physical and mental health—a study of the medical records of widows. *British Journal of Medicine* 2: 274-279, 1964.

PAUL, N.L., The role of mourning and empathy in conjoint marital therapy, in *Family Therapy and Disturbed Families,* eds. G.H. Zuk and I. Boszormenyi-Nagy. Palo Alto: Science and Behavior Books, 1967.

PINCUS, L., *Death and the Family: The Importance of Mourning.* New York: Pantheon, 1974.

RHEINGOLD, J., *The Mother, Anxiety, and Death: The Catastrophic Death Complex*. Boston: Little, Brown, 1967.

SEARLES, H.F., The effort to drive the other person crazy—an element in the etiology and psychotherapy of schizophrenia. *British Journal of Medical Psychology* 32: 1-18, 1959.

SILVERMAN, P.R., The widow-to-widow program. *Mental Hygiene* 53: 333-337, 1969.

TROUP, S.B., and W.A. GREENE, eds., *The Patient, Death, and the Family*. New York: Scribner's, 1974.

VOGEL, L., *Helping a Child Understand Death*. Philadelphia: Fortress Press, 1974.

WAHL, C.W., *Helping the Dying Patient and His Family*. New York: Family Service Association of America, 1960.

WEIGERT, E., Narcissism: benign and malignant forms, in *Cross-Currents in Psychiatry and Psychoanalysis*, ed. R.E. Gibson. Philadelphia: Lippincott, 1967.

WELLDON, R., The shadow of death and its implications in four families, each with a hospitalized schizophrenic member. *Family Process* 10: 281-302, 1971.

WYNNE, L.C., I.M. RYCKOFF, J. DAY, and S.I. HIRSCH, Pseudomutuality in the family relations of schizophrenics. *Psychiatry* 21: 205-220, 1958.

4

The Experience of Dying

E. Mansell Pattison

Death itself is not a problem of life, for death is not amenable to treatment or intervention. We may consider death only as an issue between man and God. But the process of dying is very much a part of a person's life. As noted before, advances in medical technology now make it possible to prolong the period of dying, so that dying may stretch over days, weeks, months, and even many years. For perhaps the first time in history, we have many people who experience a new phase of life—*the living-dying interval*.

The human dilemma of this living-dying process was first illuminated for me personally by a letter from a lady unknown to me:

> Dear Dr. Pattison: Quite by accident I read your treatise on dying. Because I am so grateful for your guidance I am writing not only to thank you but to suggest that the article be made available to relatives who care for patients . . . My husband has been treated for chronic glomeruli nephritis for nine years. For the past five years, he has had biweekly dialysis, which equates to a living-dying stage of long duration. In these times, when there is no doctor-patient relationship in this type of indirect care, the entire burden of sharing the responsibility of death falls to the member of the family. . . . Your listing of the fears was so apparent when I read your paper, yet when my husband experienced them I was unprepared to see them or even acknowledge them. When a patient is accepted on a kidney program, he knows he is dying. Would it not be a kindness to the person caring for him to know his fears and how to help?

As said so clearly by this wife, the period of living-dying is most important to the patient, family, friends, relatives, and professional staff.

THE LIVING-DYING INTERVAL

All of us live with the potential for death at any moment. All of us project ahead a *trajectory* of our life. That is, we anticipate a certain lifespan within which we arrange our activities and plan our lives. And then abruptly we may be confronted with a crisis—*the crisis of knowledge of death.* Whether by illness or accident, our potential trajectory is suddenly changed. We find that we shall die in days, weeks, months, or several years. Our life has been foreshortened. Our activities must be rearranged. We cannot plan for the potential, we must deal with the actual. It is then the period between the "crisis knowledge of death" and the "point of death" that is the living-dying interval (see Figure 1).

Figure 1

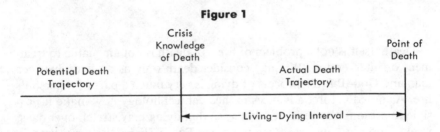

The period of living-dying can be divided into three clinical phases: 1) the acute crisis phase, 2) the chronic living-dying phase, and 3) the terminal phase. We cannot intervene with the ultimate problem of death. However, we can respond to the acute crisis, so that it does not result in a chaotic disintegration of the person's life during the process of dying. Thus, our first task is to deal appropriately with the crisis of knowledge of death, so that the dying person can move into an appropriate trajectory that integrates his or her dying into his or her life-style and life cir-

Figure 2

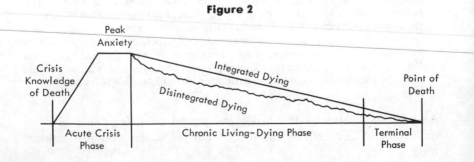

cumstances. The second task is to respond to the adaptive issues of the chronic phase. And, finally, the third task is to assist the patient to move ineluctably into the terminal phase when it becomes appropriate. (See Figure 2.)

DYING TRAJECTORIES

The phases of dying are related to several different types of trajectories or "death expectations" that are set up by the crisis of knowledge of death. Glaser and Straus (1966, 1968) suggest four different trajectories: 1) *Certain death at a known time.* In this trajectory it is possible to move rapidly from the acute phase to the chronic phase, because the time frame for resolving dying issues is quite clear. In very rapid trajectories, such as in acute leukemias or accidents, the dying process may remain only within the acute phase. 2) *Certain death at an unknown time.* This is the typical trajectory of chronic fatal illness. Here the problems tend to center on the maintenance of effective living in an ambiguous and uncertain time frame. 3) *Uncertain death but a known time when the question will be resolved.* One example here is the radical surgery, where a successful outcome will be known. Thus, the patient and family must live through a continuing period of acute crisis. On the other hand, there are long-term problems, such as possible arrest of cancer, where ambiguity may remain for years. 4) *Uncertain death and an unknown time when the question will be resolved.* Examples are multiple sclerosis and genetic diseases, which leave the person beset with a life of ambiguity.

The effect of these different trajectories upon the living-dying process will be examined throughout this book, and we shall return in the final chapter to some clinical observations about the influence of these trajectories.

DENIAL AND OPENNESS

Before we examine the phases of living-dying, we must clarify our approach to the dying patient. About 10 years ago a common question was: Should we tell the patient or keep it a secret? The question is false. The care of the dying does not revolve around telling or not telling but rather the whole panorama of human interactions that surround the dying person.

Further, there are many levels of communication between people, and many degrees of awareness. For example, the acutely ill patient who is barely conscious should not be subjected to long discussions about the severity of his or her illness. He or she knows that he or she is ill and may well die. Care and comfort are foremost. On the other hand, a patient who is experiencing progressive physical deterioration and is told there is nothing to worry about may say nothing but wonder much.

It is difficult to keep secrets. The problem is when our actions say one thing and our words another. This is what is termed "closed awareness" of dying. You know and I know, but we both know we cannot let each other know. This blockage of communication does nothing but set up trouble for all involved.

The questions a patient has are many. "Am I going to die?" is only the first of many questions that the patient may need to pose and receive specific answers to, not only from the physician but from many people around him or her. To avoid questions about death means that one also must avoid all other questions about his or her life that the patient has. Kalish (1970) has listed a variety of information inputs that come to the patient:

1. Direct statements from the physician.
2. Overheard comments of the physician to others.
3. Direct statements from other personnel, including aides, nurses, technologists.
4. Overheard comments by staff to each other.
5. Direct statements from family, friends, clergy, lawyer.
6. Changes in the behavior of others toward the patient.
7. Changes in the medical care routines, procedures, medications.
8. Changes in physical location.
9. Self-diagnosis, including reading of medical books, records, and charts.
10. Signals from the body and changes in physical status.
11. Altered responses by others toward the future.

It is evident that the dying person is engaged in multiple communications with many people. If the messages are congruent, the dying person can make sense out of the experience. But if the messages are confused, ambiguous, contradictory, the result is needless apprehension, anxiety, and the blockage of appropriate actions on the part of both the dying person and those around him or her.

On some fronts we have seen a frontal attack on denial, as if it were a terrible pathology. As a result we sometimes see brutal, blunt, and tactless confrontations in the name of openness.

What do we mean by denial? I suggest four levels of denial. The first is *existential denial*, the fundamental approach to mortality and place of death in one's life. As suggested in Chapter 1, we engage in degrees of existential denial as a necessary mechanism for existence. Second is *psychological denial*, an unconscious defense mechanism by which we repress that which is known. As will be evident from subsequent chapters, both staff and patients use denial mechanisms rather frequently. It is doubtful that we could eradicate denial mechanisms, and they often fulfill useful purposes. It is only when denial is pervasive, and the sole or predominant defense, that it becomes a major problem. Third is *nonattention denial*. We engage our attention elsewhere, and for the moment we are unaware of the undesirable.

We should not expect that at all times we always look at ourselves in the stark cold light of reality. There is an interplay of levels of denial and levels of awareness. Human communication is full of nuances. Thus, it seems absurd to expect that suddenly when it comes to discussions with the dying, all of our patterns of human communication should change. If we are able to talk with people about their lives in many ways that are comfortable and acceptable to both of us, then we should be able to talk about dying in many ways that are acceptable and comfortable. Thus, I am not concerned with the issue of how much denial or openness there is. But I am concerned that there be *opportunity, availability*, and *possibility* for open communication with the dying.

THE ACUTE PHASE

The crisis of knowledge of death can be seen as a crisis in the life of the person. During the period of acute crisis, there is an increasing anxiety that will reach a peak of tolerance. No one can continue to function long at peak anxiety, and, therefore, the patient will call upon whatever psychological mechanisms are available to reduce the anxiety. If ineffective mechanisms are used, a disintegrative dying style will follow.

The knowledge of death as a crisis event can be analyzed in terms of five aspects of crisis (Parad 1965):

1. This stressful event poses a problem that by definition is insolvable in the immediate future. In this sense, dying is the most stressful crisis because it is a crisis to which we bow but do not solve.
2. The problem taxes one's psychological resources since it is beyond one's traditional problem-solving methods. One is faced with a new experience with no prior experience to fall back on, for although one has lived amidst death, that is far different from one's own death.
3. The situation is perceived as a threat or danger to the life goals of the person. Dying interrupts a person in the midst of life, and even in old age it abruptly confronts one with the goals one set in life.

4. The crisis period is characterized by a tension that mounts to a peak, then falls. As one faces the crisis of death knowledge, there is mobilization of either integrative or disintegrative mechanisms. The peak of anxiety usually occurs considerably before death.

5. The crisis situation awakens unresolved key problems from both the near distant past. Problems of dependency, passivity, narcissism, identity, and more may be activated during the dying process. Hence, one is faced not only with the immediate dying process but also the unresolved feelings from one's own lifetime and its inevitable conflicts.

The first response to this state may be one of immobilization. It is as if life is standing still. One's life flashes before one. There may be no panic, no anxiety, no trace of despair, no pain, but rather an altered state of consciousness. Noyes and Kletti (1976) term this a "depersonalization" phenomenon—"This is not really happening to me, I'm just watching."

Then may come an overwhelming, insuperable feeling of inadequacy—a potential dissolution of the self. There is bewilderment, confusion, indefinable anxiety, and unspecified fear (Montefiore 1973). There is seemingly no answer, and the anxiety makes it difficult to look at what needs to be done.

As part of this process in the acute phase, we may see many pathologically appearing defenses, such as Kubler-Ross (1970) describes as the stages of denial, anger, and bargaining. Yet Kubler-Ross described patients mostly seen in the hospital in the acute phase, where we might expect to see initial mobilization of pathological defenses.

We should not be surprised to see many pathological defenses in this acute stage, nor perhaps react too vigorously to them. For if we focus on the reduction of anxiety through a focus on reality issues and appropriate emotional support, it is likely that the dying person will move on toward appropriate emotional responses to his or her living-dying.

THE CHRONIC LIVING-DYING PHASE

During the chronic phase the dying patient faces a number of fears. It is important at this time to specify the precise issues the dying person faces so that he or she can resolve each specific issue in an appropriate manner. One cannot deal with all issues of dying simultaneously. Rather, our task is to separate each issue, take one at a time as it occurs. Then the dying person can resolve the issues of dying in a rewarding fashion that enhances self-esteem, dignity, and integrity. The dying person can take pride then in having faced his or her crisis of dying with hope and courage, and come away having dealt successfully with his or her dying. One might call this "healthy dying."

Now let us consider the specific fears of the living-dying interval.

FEAR OF THE UNKNOWN. The initial phase of crisis may involve a bewildering array of concerns. However, as the dying person looks forward on his or her dying trajectory, he or she may fear the fact that he or she does not know what lies ahead. It is important to separate those things that can be known from those for which there is no answer. Diggory and Rothman (1961) suggest the following fears of the unknown:

1. What life experiences will I not be able to have?
2. What is my fate in the hereafter?
3. What will happen to my body after death?
4. What will happen to my survivors?
5. How will my family and friends respond to my dying?
6. What will happen to my life plans and projects?
7. What changes will occur in my body?
8. What will be my emotional reactions?

It is evident that some of the above questions can be answered rather well immediately, some answers will be found in the process of time, and some cannot be answered. The issue is summed up rather well in the ancient prayer of serenity: "Grant me the courage to accept the things I cannot change, the strength to change the things I can, and the wisdom to know the difference."

FEAR OF LONELINESS. When one is sick, there is a sense of isolation from oneself and from others. This is reinforced by the fact that others tend naturally to avoid a sick person and leave him or her alone.

This mutual process of withdrawal is even more evident when a person is dying. The isolation attendant to dying is not only a psychological phenomenon but is also a reflection of our social management of dying. No longer does our culture afford us the luxury of dying amidst our family, friends, and belongings, for over 60 percent of deaths now occur in impersonal, isolated hospital rooms. We have given medicine and hospitals the social responsibility of caring for the dying, yet the hospital is not geared to care for the dying (Krant 1974).

There have been many critiques of the depersonalized and mechanized care of the dying in general hospitals. Yet our criticism of hospitals and their staff may be misplaced. Most hospitals are socially constructed to provide acute remedial care. To then ask the same social institution to provide chronic supportive care is to place the hospital staff in a double bind. Which priorities do they respond to? In fact, recent studies show that hospital staff do not necessarily ignore dying patients, but that they give priority to patients for whom they can provide life-saving measures. This is not unreasonable.

The dilemma is that acute care hospitals are not well equipped to care for the dying. As a result, the dying are isolated, ignored, and left with little human contact, although perhaps given good technical care. The solution, to my mind, does not lie in depreciation of acute care hospital staff, but rather in the provision of chronic care facilities that are devoted to the appropriate care of the dying. An example is St. Christopher's Hospice in London, directed by Cicely Saunders, which is a hospital for the dying.

The acute care hospital is necessarily geared toward *curative* functions; the dying require *caring* functions. Oliver Wendell Holmes stated the difference well: "Our task is to cure rarely, relieve sometimes, and comfort always."

The fear of loneliness is perhaps sensed by the dying from the beginning. The necessary withdrawal from work or recreational activities may begin to accentuate the loss of everyday contacts. It may become difficult to maintain social relations. The dying person may not know what to say to others, and others don't know what to say in return. This social awkwardness is revealed in the autobiography of a dying woman (Kelly 1970). An insurance salesman came to the door. When asked if she was interested in life insurance, she replied: "Yes, I'm dying and need the insurance right away!"

Increasing physical debilitation and confinement to bed further may limit social contacts with family and friends. Hospitalization may do so even more. In the hospital the dying person may be placed in a private room, which isolates him or her to a greater degree. Where only supportive technical care is provided, the dying person may be left essentially alone most of the time.

The impact of this social isolation is a sense of human deprivation. As shown in many experiments of sensory deprivation, the human deprived of contact with other humans quickly disintegrates and loses a sense of ego integrity. For the human who is dying, human isolation and deprivation sets the stage for what may be termed "anaclitic depression." This depression is not due to loss but to *separation*—the sense of being away from those we love and depend upon (Schoenberg et al. 1970).

Without human interaction the dying person is vulnerable to the confusional syndrome of human deprivation that we call *loneliness*. It is one thing to choose to be alone at times—as we all desire—it is another to be left alone. It seems that the fear of loneliness is paramount when the person first faces the prospect of death and fears that he or she will be deserted in dying.

FEAR OF SORROW.   We do not like to face situations of grief and sorrow; if possible we would like to avoid them. Yet the dying person is faced with many losses, which he or she may fear to face. "Can I stand thinking about what I am losing?" There is the fear that one cannot tolerate the painful experience of sorrow. There is the loss of job, of future plans, of strength and ability, of the ongoing pleasure of relationships and activities (Fulton, Fulton 1971).

The task that faces the dying person may seem formidable. Yet not all of these losses are likely to occur simultaneously; some joys and pleasures may be taken from some aspects of life during the living-dying interval. This requires that we help the dying person to avoid *premature* sorrow that cuts the person off from available satisfactions (Aldrich, 1963).

On the other hand, it is also necessary to help the dying person engage in *anticipatory grief.* That is, to handle each episode of grief as it occurs, so that one can work through the grief and set it aside. Thus, one is not beset by constant grief and sorrow but may have interludes of satisfaction and accomplishment. One may grieve over that given up, but then proceed to engage in what is present in life now (Schoenberg et al. 1970).

FEAR OF LOSS OF FAMILY AND FRIENDS.   The process of dying confronts the person with the reality of losing one's family and friends through one's death, just as much as if they were dying. This is a real loss to be mourned and worked through (Glaser, Straus 1966). Rather than denying this real separation and preventing the grief work, it is possible for both the person and his or her family to engage in anticipatory grief work. The completion of such grief work may allow the person and the family to work through the emotions of separation and part in peace (Gordon, Kutner 1965; Vollman et al. 1971).

The grief of separation before death is akin to the Eskimo custom of having a ritual feast of separation before the old person steps onto an ice floe, waves goodbye, and drifts off into the sea. Similarly, in the Auca tribe of South America, after a farewell ceremony, the old person leaves the village and climbs into a hammock to lie alone until death.

Failure to recognize this real loss ahead of time may block the normal and healthy process of grief. This makes it difficult for the dying person to distinguish between his or her own problem of death and the problem of grief and separation from those he or she is leaving. Thus, the grief of separation should be accomplished *before* death.

FEAR OF LOSS OF BODY.   Our bodies are not just appendages but a vital part of our self-concept. When illness distorts our bodies, there is not only physical loss but a loss of self-image and self-integrity (Szasz 1957). This narcissistic blow to the integrity of self may result in shame, feelings of disgrace and inadequacy, and loss of self-esteem. As before, we may help the dying person to grieve these losses of body without incurring a loss of integrity or esteem.

Since we humans do not tolerate ambiguity well, it is more difficult to tolerate ambiguous distortions of the body. External disfiguring disease may be more acceptable because one can see what is wrong, whereas an internal silent process, such as a failing heart or brain, may be more dismaying.

On the other hand, external disfigurement may provoke a sense of being ugly and unacceptable. The dying person may despise his or her distorted body image and may feel like rejecting his or her ugly body. Then the dying person may try to hide his or her unlovely self from loved ones, for fear that the family will also despise the ugly body, reject him, or her and leave him or her alone.

FEAR OF LOSS OF SELF-CONTROL.   As debilitating disease progresses, one is less capable of self-control. There is less energy, less vitality, less strength, less responsiveness. These all are part of one organism. We think less quickly, less accurately, and we may fear this loss of body and mind.

This problem is particularly acute in our society, which has placed strong emphasis on self-control, self-determination, and rationality. As a result, most people in our culture become anxious and feel threatened by experiential states that pose loss of control or obtundation (dulling) of consciousness. This is reflected in our cultural ambivalence over the use of psychedelic drugs and alcohol, which produce diminished states of self-control and altered states of consciousness. In contrast to Eastern mystical experiential states that many participate in, it is unusual in Western culture to experience any acceptable loss of self-control. Even alcoholic "highs" are viewed with ambivalence. Thus, we come ill-prepared to times of life when we must give up some degrees of control over ourselves (Tart 1969).

When we come to the experience of dying, the loss of control over body and mind, with a diminished sense of consciousness, may then create anxiety and fear about the integrity of ourselves. One is placed in a position of dependency and inadequacy so that in a sense the ego is no longer master of its fate nor captain of the self.

Therefore, it is important to encourage and allow the dying person to retain whatever authority he or she can, to sustain him or her in retaining control of daily tasks and decisions, avoiding shaming for failure of control, and help the person to find rewarding experience in the self-determination yet available.

FEAR OF SUFFERING AND PAIN.   Our social and cultural experience pre-condition us in our response to pain. Some ethnic groups are pain accen-tuators; others are pain minimizers (Petrie 1967). But, more importantly, we learn the *meaning* to give to pain. Thus, pain is not the issue per se but our response to pain makes it either *sufferable* or *suffering*.

A certain level of awareness of one's body and one's consciousness is necessary to engage in the experience of suffering. Suffering does not occur when we are unaware. This self-awareness may either diminish or exacerbate pain and transform it into suffering (Shontz, Fink 1959).

We may deal with the problem of pain by using medical means of pain relief and thus diminish suffering. This is all to the good, and those who say that pain is not a problem have likely not felt much pain nor had to live with it. But the mere diminution of pain does not eradicate suffering, nor is oblivion the answer.

Another alternative is to diminish suffering through awareness and understanding. David Bakan (1968) suggests that a humanistic approach to pain and suffering lies in our understanding of and awareness of pain. The patient who fears pain is more likely expressing a fear of suffering. And what is suffering? It is pain that has no meaning, no location, no explanation. Clinically, studies of pain in the dying bear this out: pain relief is not closely related to the dosage of pain-killing drugs, but rather relief is closely tied to the person's attitude toward pain.

The fear is not just a physical fear, but a fear of the unknown and unmanageable. Senseless pain is perhaps intolerable. On the other hand, pain may be accepted and dealt with if that pain does not mean punish-ment, or being ignored, or not being cared for. People will not suffer long, but they will endure pain.

FEAR OF LOSS OF IDENTITY.   The loss of human contact, the loss of family and friends, the loss of body structure and function, the loss of self-control and total consciousness all threaten the sense of one's identity. Human contacts affirm who we are, family contacts affirm who we have been, and contact with our own body and mind affirms our own being-self.

We can see that the dying process faces the person with many threats to self-identity. How does one maintain identity and integrity in the face of these forces of dissolution? Bowers (1964) concluded: "When life cannot be restored, then one can accept the fact with a meaning that gives dignity to his life, and purpose even to the process that is encroaching on his own vitality."

Willie Loman, the salesman in *Death of a Salesman*, says of his own death: "A man must not be allowed to fall into his grave as an old dog."

It is not *that* we die but *how* we die. The tasks are to retain self-esteem and respect for the self until death, to retain the dignity and integrity of the self throughout the process of living we call dying. There are three major mechanisms for this:

The first mechanism is most important. We maintain our identity through contact with those who have been and are part of our life. We do not become a number, a case, an object, if others continue to see us, react to us, talk to us, relate to us, *as the unique person I am*. Here again is the familiar theme of dying; maintaining contact with the familiar that keeps on reaffirming to the dying person that he or she is the person he or she has been always.

A second mechanism is reinforcement of identity through the continuity of one's life in family and friends. One sees one's self in one's children, life work, and in the bequeathing of one's possessions to others. One cannot only leave a will but can leave parts of one's body in bone banks and eye banks. This personal sense of continuity was illustrated by a middle-aged man who was dying of lung cancer. I had spent much time talking with him about his life as he lay dying on my ward. He was transferred to another ward where the surgeons wanted to perform a biopsy. He refused until he could talk to me. I explained to him that the biopsy would not change his disease, but it would help my understanding of it. Then he was pleased to comply, for he felt he was giving me something, his diseased tissue, that in a sense I would carry with me in my professional life. He had given me a part of himself to be with me after his death.

A third mechanism maintains identity through a desire for reunion with loved ones who have died before or who will die and join one. These reunion fantasies include the sense of return to the primordial mother figure as well as reunion with specific loved ones (Brodsky 1959; Greenberg 1954). There will be reunion with one's parentage and one's progeny. Hence, one can place oneself at one point in the continuum of ongoing human relationships, of which my death is merely one point in the more universal span of existence.

FEAR OF REGRESSION.   Finally, there is fear of those internal instincts that pull one into retreat from the outer world of reality, into a primordial sense of being where there is no sense of time or space, no boundaries of self and others. We have all had this sense of pull toward regression into self when we awaken in the morning. As the alarm rings, we drowsily douse the noise, turn over, feel the immense weight of our sleep pulling us back into slumber. We luxuriate in the indefinite sense of our boundaries, the relaxation of our awareness, the freedom from the demands and constrictions of the real world that await our awakening. With exquisite pleasure we allow ourselves to float back off into a timeless, spaceless, self-less state of nonbeing (Needleman 1966). Certain religious mystical experiences, psychedelic experiences, and body aware-ness exercises produce similar altered states of consciousness.

In most of life the ego fights against this instinctual regression into self-lessness. In our culture we have difficulty regarding such states as acceptable. We fear such states.

For the dying person, especially as he or she approaches and enters the terminal phase of living-dying, the fear of regression begins to loom. With the diminution of physical capacity and the clouding of conscious-ness, the sense of regression may be frightening. The dying person may fight against the regression, trying to hold onto concrete, hard, reality bound, consciousness of him or herself (Montefiore 1973). This may produce the so-called death agonies, the struggle against regression of the self.

It is here that we must help the person shift away from reality and turn inward toward the self, to allow regression and withdrawal to occur. With such support the dying person may then accept the surrender to the internal self, allow oneself to turn away from life, seek reunion with the world out of which he or she has sprung. Then psychic death is accept-able, desirable, and at hand.

THE TERMINAL PHASE

The onset of the terminal phase of living-dying is not precise. However, we can roughly state that it begins when the dying person begins to withdraw into him or herself in response to internal body signals that say he or she must now conserve energies unto him- or herself (Rioch 1961; Shontz, Fink 1959). Perhaps it is like the experience we may have with a bad case of the flu. We feel terribly sick, lose interest in food, activities, and friends. All we want to do is curl up in a warm bed and be left alone in quietness. The onset of this withdrawal is the onset of the terminal phase.

Lieberman (1965), has found that the terminal phase is marked by both physical withdrawal and subtle signs of emotional disorganization. Hinton (1963) has observed that there is a decrease in anxiety and an increase in depressive involution. Davies et al. (1973) have found that this psychological withdrawal is a type of "apathetic giving up," which accompanies a deterioration of the physical state of the person.

This turning from the outside world to the internal self is clearly described in this case report by Janice Norton (1963):

> She told me her only remaining fear was that dying was strange and unknown to her, that she had never done it before. Like birth, it was something that only happened once to any individual, and similarly one might not remember what it was really . . . She no longer worried about what was to happen to her after death . . . she felt that she might be unnecessarily concerned with the actual process of death itself.

CHANGES OF HOPE.   At the outset of the living-dying interval, the dying patient has an *expectational hope*. That is, a set of expectations that have some possibility for fulfillment. There may be remissions, arrests, sometimes possible cures. There may be weeks, months, years of some rewarding life yet to be fulfilled. And it well may be that the dying person will cling to this expectational hope in a useful sense throughout the living-dying interval.

However, as a person enters the terminal phase, it may be signaled by a change in hope. Stotland (1969) has clarified the point that expectational hope now changes to *desirable hope*. That is, I may still hope that I might not die, that is a desirable thought but no longer expectable as a hope. This transformation from expectancy to desire may herald the psychological process of "giving up." It is for this reason, as Cappon (1959) notes, that hope should not cease until shortly before psychic death. However, we should also attend to the fact that we may aid the dying person in making the necessary transition from expectancy hope to desirability hope as he or she enters the terminal phase.

TYPES OF DEATH.   When we consider the terminal phase, we must take into account the four definitions of death: 1) *Sociological death,* the withdrawal and separation from the patient by others. This may occur days or weeks before terminus if the patient if left alone to die. The person is treated as if dead. Some families desert the aged in nursing homes, where they may live as if dead for several years. 2) *Psychic death,* the person accepts death and regresses into him- or herself. Such psychic death may accompany the appropriate diminution of the physical body status. But anomalies can occur; psychic death can precede terminus as in voodoo death (Cannon 1942) or in patients who predict their own deaths and refuse to continue living (Barber 1961; Vollman et al. 1971; Weisman, Hackett 1961). 3) *Biological death*, organism as a human entity no longer exists. There is no consciousness nor awareness, such as in irreversible coma. The heart and lungs may function with artificial support, but the biological organism as a self-sustaining mind-body is dead. 4) *Physiological death*, where vital organs such as lungs, heart, and brain no longer function.

The importance of these four types of death is that they can occur out of phase with each other. And that becomes a major source of ethical and personal confusion. As shown in Figure 3, as the person enters the

Figure 3

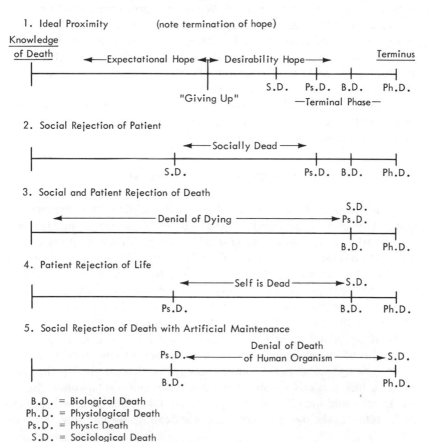

B.D. = Biological Death
Ph.D. = Physiological Death
Ps.D. = Physic Death
S.D. = Sociological Death

terminal phase, this can be considered as the onset of giving up and withdrawal. Social death would be allowing the dying person to withdraw, leading to psychic death, which is usually shortly followed by biological and then physiological death.

However, there are distortions of this process also shown in Figure 3. Where there is social rejection of the patient, he or she may become socially dead long before the other aspects of death occur. On the other hand, where there is social and personal rejection of the dying process, we have the problem of precipitous death that is not anticipated nor dealt with. This also can occur when a patient suddenly deteriorates and dies contrary to expectation. It may precipitate a shocked reaction to all involved, because the anticipated trajectory has been upset. Another pattern is where the patient rejects life. This is usually met with social disapproval. For example, old people are not supposed to say they are ready to die, nor is the acutely ill person. We want people to want to live. In so doing, we may interfere with their own dying trajectories. And, finally, there is the case of death of mind and body—the artificial preservation of life—in which there is social denial of the fact that both psychic death and biological death have occurred. This is currently a source of much medical-ethical controversy in our culture.

In summary, our task is to synchronize each type of death dimension so that optimally they will converge together in a appropriate fashion, rather than being disjointed and out of phase with each other.

THE SEQUENCE OF DYING

In this chapter I have sketched a rough outline of the sequence of dying. However, I must caution that this is not a format but rather a framework that may guide our clinical thinking. Always we must keep in mind that human life is unique for each person. Our generalizations are just that. Therefore, we must beware of fitting a dying person into a procrustean bed (a doctrine of conformity) of "scientific facts." Human life does not fit into neat categories and sequences. Thus, our charge is to understand the specific experience of dying for each person.

To recapitulate; at first the person is faced with the seeming impossible crisis of knowledge of death, which threatens to overwhelm the self. Human beings seem always to have recognized that no one has the capability to face this crisis alone, for we develop cultural customs whereby we actually and literally help people to die. Given our interest, support, and guidance, the dying person can face death as an unknown with the realization that he or she cannot know, and instead he or she can turn to deal with living-dying.

In the chronic living-dying phase, if not deprived of human contact, the person can learn to endure the inevitable degrees of separation without loneliness. He or she can face the loss of relatives, friends, and activities if he or she can actively mourn their loss where grief is defined and accepted. He or she can tolerate loss of body and structure if others accept that loss too. He or she can tolerate the loss of self-control if it is not perceived by him or herself and others as a shameful experience and if he or she can exercise control where feasible. The dying person can tolerate pain if he or she can see the source of pain and its meaning so that it is not transformed into suffering. He or she can retain dignity and self-respect in the face of the termination of the life cycle if he or she can place his or her life in perspective within his or her own personal history, family, and human tradition.

It is then possible to enter the terminal phase, in which expectational hope is transformed into desirability hope, where it is possible to give up one's grappling with life, and an acceptable regression occurs where the self gradually returns to the state of nonself.

REFERENCES

ALDRICH, C.K., The dying patient's grief. *Journal of the American Medical Association* 184: 329-331, 1963.

BAKAN, D., *Disease, Pain, and Sacrifice: Toward a Psychology of Suffering.* Chicago: University of Chicago press, 1968.

BARBER, T.X., Death by suggestion: a critical note. *Psychosomatic Medicine* 23: 153-155, 1961.

BOWERS, M., ed., *Counseling the Dying.* New York: Nelson, 1964.

BRODSKY, B., Liebestod fantasies in a patient faced with a fatal illness. *International Journal of Psychoanalysis* 40: 13-16, 1959.

CANNON, W., Voodoo death. *Amer. Anthropol.* 44: 169-181, 1942.

CAPPON, D., The dying. *Psychiatric Quarterly* 33: 466-489, 1959.

DAVIES, R.K., D.M. QUINLAND, F.P. MCKEGNEY, and C.P. KIMBALL, Organic factors and psychological adjustment in advanced cancer patients. *Psychosomatic Medicine* 35: 464-471, 1973.

DIGGORY, J.C., and D.Z. ROTHMAN, Values destroyed by death. *Journal of Abnormal and Social Psychology* 63: 205-210, 1961.

FULTON, R., and J. FULTON, A psychosocial aspect of terminal care: anticipatory grief. *Omega* 2: 91-100, 1971.

GLASER, B.G., and A.L. STRAUS, *Awareness of Dying.* Chicago: Aldine, 1966.

———, *Time for Dying.* Chicago: Aldine, 1968.

GORDON, N.B., and B. KUTNER, Long term and fatal illness and the family. *Journal of Health and Human Behavior* 6: 190-196, 1965.

GREENBERG, I.M., An exploratory study of reunion fantasies. *Journal of the Hillside Hospital* 13: 49-59, 1954.

HINTON, J. The physiological and mental distress of dying. *Quarterly Journal of Medicine* 32: 1-21, 1963.

JENSEN, G.D., and J.G. WALLACE, Family mourning process. *Family Process* 6: 55-66, 1967.

KALISH, R.A., The onset of the dying process. *Omega* 1: 57-69, 1970.

KELLY, J., *Free Fall.* Valley Forge, Pa.: Judson Press, 1975.

KRANT, M. J., *Dying and Dignity: The Meaning and Control of a Personal Death.* Springfield, Ill.: C.C. Thomas, 1974.

KÜBLER-ROSS, E., *On Death and Dying.* New York: Macmillan, 1970.

LIEBERMAN, M.A., Psychological correlates of impending death. *Journal of Gerontology* 20: 181-190, 1965.

MONTEFIORE, H. W., ed., *Death Anxiety.* New York: MSS Information Corporation, 1973.

NEEDLEMAN, J., Imagining absence, nonexistence, and death: a sketch. *Review of Existential Psychology Psychiatry* 6: 230-236, 1966.

NORTON, J., Treatment of a dying patient. *Psychoanalytic Study of the Child* 18: 541-560, 1963.

NOYES, R., JR., and R. KLETTI, Depersonalization in the face of life-threatening danger: a description. *Psychiatry* 39: 19-27, 1976.

PARAD, H.J., ed., *Crisis Intervention: Selected Readings.* New York: Family Service Association of America, 1965.

PETRIE, A., *Individuality in Pain and Suffering.* Chicago: University of Chicago Press, 1967.

RIOCH, D., The psychopathology of death, in *The Physiology of Emotions,* ed. A. Simon. Springfield, Ill.: C.C. Thomas, 1961.

SCHOENBERG, B. et al., eds. *Anticipatory Grief.* New York: Columbia University Press, 1974.

_____ , *Loss and Grief: Psychological Management in Medical Practice.* New York: Columbia University Press, 1970.

SHONTZ, F.C., and S.L. FINK, A psychobiological analysis of discomfort, pain, and death. *Journal of General Psychology* 60: 275-287, 1959.

STOTLAND, E., *The Psychology of Hope.* San Francisco: Jossey-Bass, 1969.

SZASZ, T., *Pain and Pleasure: A Study of Bodily Feelings.* London: Tavistock, 1957.

TART C.T., ed. *Altered States of Consciousness.* New York: Wiley, 1969.

VOLLMAN, R.R., A. GANZERT, L. PICHER, and W.V. WILLIAMS, The reactions of family systems to sudden and unexpected death. *Omega* 2: 101-106, 1971.

WALTERS, M.J., Psychic death: report of a possible case. *Archives of Neurology and Psychiatry* 52: 84-85, 1944.

WEISMAN, A.D., and T. HACKETT, Predilection for death: death and dying as a psychiatric problem. *Psychosomatic Medicine* 23: 232-256, 1961.

5

The Will to Live and the Expectation of Death

E. Mansell Pattison

Throughout history and across many cultures, people have held to the view that human beings can influence their own times of death.* This is reflected in the popular notion that we have a "will to live." Therefore, we often encourage dying persons to "want to live" and "fight for their lives." Conversely, there is the notion that people "give up" and "allow themselves to die." Put simply, can the dying influence their prognosis; can they predict their lives or deaths in some fashion?

In terms of long-term contingencies that influence death, Lasagna (1970) has shown that our cultural lives, such as stress and environment, influence our life-spans; our social relations do also—for example, married persons tend to live longer than single persons—and medical technical advances have certainly prolonged the lives of many.

But these long-term issues really do not address the issue at hand for the dying person. Unfortunately, there have been few scientific studies on either the will to live or the expectation of death. But there are a handful of provocative observations that suggest that the ancient folklore may not be misguided. Although it is obvious that the biological processes of disease ultimately override all psychological and social influences, there may be significant psychosocial processes that do influence the immediate prognosis of the dying person.

To illustrate some of these possible processes, I shall briefly present a clinical study in which we followed a group of severely ill patients over a

*I acknowledge with appreciation the assistance of Donald L. Dudley, M.D., and Robert J. Rhodes, Ph.D., who were coinvestigators in a larger series of studies from which these data were drawn.

period of time to determine what psychosocial factors might influence their lives or deaths. Then I shall review some of the most pertinent studies that point us toward an understanding of how we may influence our dying.

A CLINICAL STUDY

The Patient Population

The subjects were patients with DOPS (diffuse obstructive pulmonary syndrome, or clinical emphysema, a disease marked by lung, and sometimes heart, impairment). Patients with severe advanced DOPS pose a difficult management problem, for they exist in such precarious cardiopulmonary balance that death is always a real possibility.

Psychophysiological studies on these patients have demonstrated an intimate interdependence between the emotional state of the patient and his or her cardiopulmonary function (Dudley et al. 1969). Emotional states of action-activation, such as anger, anxiety, or fear, increases both cardiac and respiratory activities. Conversely, emotional states of action-inhibition, such as depression or apathy, decrease both cardiac and respiratory functions. In normal subjects or minimally diseased persons, such shifts in affect and behavior with the concomitant shift in cardiopulmonary function may be uncomfortable and result in dyspnea, or distressful shortness of breath, but there is adequate physiological reserve for the person to maintain cardiopulmonary compensation.

However, the patient with severe DOPS has such reduced pulmonary adjustment capacity that there is only a very narrow range within which he or she can maintain cardiopulmonary and metabolic balance. A rapid shift to either action-activation or action-inhibition immediately influences cardiopulmonary function, and it sets the stage for cardiopulmonary embarrassment.

Dyspnea is the hallmark of cardiopulmonary embarrassment, and it is dependent on the subjective judgment of the patient, not blood gas levels or ventilatory abnormalities. Further, dyspnea has been found to relate to emotional variables independent of cardiopulmonary disease. For the patient with severe DOPS, dyspnea is a danger signal to be avoided at all costs. The patient learns to avoid affects that influence his or her cardiopulmonary function, and literally develops an emotional "straitjacket." Thus, the DOPS patient learns that he or she cannot face or admit the existence of emotional issues or conflicts.

This protective emotional straitjacketing develops at a point where the disease state is producing major changes in the patient's self-image and life-styles. The physiological-psychological bind that faces the patient also faces the ward staff. Treatment and nursing procedures may be met by resistance. When the staff attempts to override this resistance, the patient may respond with increased passivity as a defense against entering into over conflict with the staff, or the patient may be mobilized into open conflict, which may then precipitate a cardiopulmonary crisis. At times, this results in an almost explicit blackmail, with the patient warning the nurse or doctor not to enforce treatment lest they antagonize the patient and thereby kill him or her. The end result is a stalemate and immobilization of the treatment program and personnel.

The seriousness of the disease is illustrated by a 5-year survival rate of under 50 percent and a 10-year survival rate of 10 percent. This was dramatically borne out in this study, where 5 of 12 patients died during the 18-months observation period (Dudley et al. 1969).

Method

Twelve male subjects from a ward designed for the long-term intensive care of DOPS patients were selected for the study. Subjects were excluded if imminent death, discharge, or transfer might make them unavailable for study.

At the outset we assessed the characteristics of the sample, which turned out to be relatively homogenous in these terms—they were "early aged," with a grade school education, holding a variety of semiskilled jobs during their lives, now severely incapacitated by disease. They closely approximate the description of the chronic tubercular given by Holmes (1956): ". . . sensitive, anxious, rigid, and emotionally labile . . . marginal people with disintegration of a precarious psychosocial adjustment in the years preceding the onset of relapse of disease."

At the beginning of the observational period, physiological, psychological, and sociological assessments were made. These initial measures were treated as independent variables, with clinical outcome as the dependent variable.

Eighteen months later, the clinical status of each patient was assessed. During the first six months an intervention program in group therapy was undertaken. However, this did not prove to be a successful intervention for most patients, and participation in group therapy was found not to be a predictive variable (Pattison, Rhodes, Dudley 1971).

Instruments

Physiological measures consisted of blood gas and ventilatory measurements. All physiologic studies were conducted while the patients were in a clinically steady state. This battery of studies was repeated at the end of six months observation.

Psychological measures were used to assess gross psychiatric symptomatology (or symptoms of the disease). The Inpatient Multidimensional Psychiatric Scale (IMPS) describes disorders of thought, feeling, and behavior characteristics of hospitalized psychiatric patients. The Cornell Medical Index Health Questionnaire (CMI) describes self-reported physical and emotional symptoms. A total symptom score and a neurotic index score were used. Ratings were obtained at the study outset and not repeated.

Sociological measures focused on functional capacity. The Nurses' Observations Scale for Inpatient Evaluation (NOSIE-30) is a 30-item ward behavior rating scale, which yields six scores and a composite score, based on the ward nurse's observations of the immediate behavior of the patient in social interaction. The scale was designed specifically to measure changes in interpersonal behavior in chronic ward patients, who are relatively asymptomatic in terms of overt psychiatric symptoms but are characterized by apathy and indifference. All patients were rated at the outset and at monthly intervals for six months.

At the outset of the study, we also conducted a clinical assessment of the social relations of each patient. Each chart was reviewed for data on family relations. The ward nursing staff were interviewed and asked to review their knowledge and observations on the visitors for each patient. Finally, each patient was interviewed specifically in regard to his family and friendship relationships. The summation of this data was then reduced to simple categories of psychosocial resources as independent variables.

RESULTS

Clinical outcome, as the dependent variable, was assessed at the end of 18 months. Outcome was divided into three categories: 1) discharged improved, 2) continued hospitalization, and 3) deceased.

The physiological variables, neither on initial or six-month measurement, were predictive of clinical outcome.

The psychological measurements used in this study were not very helpful. The initial scores on both the IMPS and CMI were uniformly flat with no significant differences between individuals. The degree of denial and repression manifest in these test scores was so great that repeat measurements were not conducted. These psychological measures were not predictive. Neither were demographic variables predictive. The striking characteristics of the entire population was the relative psychological uniformity.

The sociological measurements did turn out to be predictive, from both a statistical and a clinical correlational view.

Table 1 lists clinical outcome for each patient with his mean NOSIE-30 scores for a six-month period. As illustrated, low scores are related to death, intermediate scores to hospitalization, and high scores to clinical improvement and discharge. As a rough clinical guide, the data suggest a high probability of death for patients with mean NOSIE-30 scores of less than 100, continued hospitalization with scores of 100-150, and improvement in patients with scores over 150. This conclusion also is supported by the fact that although there were individual fluctuations in NOSIE-30 scores over time, each patient's scores consistently remained within the score range of his ultimate clinical outcome group.

Table 1   Clinical Outcome and Individual Mean
NOSIE-30 Scores

Clinical Outcome	Patient	Mean NOSIE-30 Score
Dead	HA	65
	RH	115
	SW	135
	WA	50
	GI	120
Hospitalized	LE	100
	ST	160
	OR	125
	PO	150
Discharged	BR	180
	CH	190
	DI	195

Table 2 presents the group mean scores for each clinical outcome category. As indicated, each clinical outcome group differs at a statistically significant level from each other.

In Table 3 we see the comparison of clinical outcome with the initial assessment of psychosocial assets. Although one cannot make a strong

Table 2   Clinical Outcome and NOSIE-30
Group Mean Scores

Outcome	Group NOSIE Mean Score
Dead (5)	97
Hospitalized (4)	140
Discharged (3)	188

$p = 0.01$ (2-tailed)

TABLE 3   Comparison of Psychosocial Assets
with Clinical Outcome

Clinical Outcome	Psychosocial Assets
Discharged N = 3	Attentive wife and family. Divorced with attentive family. Attentive wife and family.
Hospitalized N = 4	Rejecting wife. Widowed with no close family. Widowed with poverty stricken family. Widowed with no close family.
Dead N = 5	Divorced with no close family. Widowed with attentive family. Widowed with attentive niece. Rejecting wife. Divorced with no close family.

case from such inferential data, it is striking that clinical improvement is correlated with intact and positive family relations, whereas death is correlated with both disruption and negative family relations.

In summary, these patients had severe physiological debilitation—in fact, 40 percent died during our 18-month observational period. Yet the base rates of cardiopulmonary function did not predict death.

In similar fashion, these patients had severely crippling psychological characteristics, with a background of precarious psychosocial adaptation. Yet neither their demographic background nor the characteristic psychological coping style was predictive of death.

Yet the NOSIE-30 scores were predictive of each type of clinical outcome. In essence, the behavior measured here is the patient's observed ability to engage in effective and appropriate interpersonal behavior. *Thus, clinical outcome in part may reflect the ability to use available social resources.* On the other hand, our data on psychosocial resources indicate the potential importance of an *intact and positive network of social resources.*

Past and Present Factors

There are two hypotheses that can be advanced concerning the severe psychophysical straitjacket that characterized these patients. The first hypothesis suggests that these men had reasonably adequate coping mechanisms for dealing with affect prior to their disease, and that the emotional crippling is an adaptive response to the severe physiologic crippling. In support of this hypothesis is the fact that these men had been self-sufficent, albeit marginal, males through their lives without manifest psychiatric symptoms or complaints. However, they also had a history of unsuccessful marital relations, suggesting difficulties in interpersonal relations.

The second hypothesis suggests that these men had not developed adequate coping mechanisms for dealing with affect and interpersonal conflict. Hence, when faced with a disease state where affect expression brought rapid psychologic change, they were severely restricted in their capacity to handle this affect without precipitating a physiologic crisis.

In either case, the end result is that the only psychological mechanisms for handling affect and interpersonal conflict are gross denial, suppression, and repression of all affect and conflictual cues. This, or course, becomes a vicious cycle, for as they face the realistically severe problems associated with an incapacitative disease and chronic hospitalization, they cannot face their feelings or deal with the interpersonal conflicts without literally endangering their lives. The rigid avoidance of affect and conflict only perpetuates the problems and increases frustration, anger, and despair, which in turn cannot be dealt with, and they cannot resolve it.

The patients quickly stated, and it is clinically obvious, that emotionally charged issues were difficult if not impossible for them to face directly. We repeatedly noted that when a patient began to discuss an emotionally charged topic, it would usually stir immediate manifestations of anxiety, fear, anger, or depression in him as well as in other group members. The physiological concomitants of these emotions rapidly upset their precarious cardiopulmonary balance and led to cardio-respiratory embarrassment as exhibited by marked dyspnea and cyanosis (bluish skin color). It was not uncommon to note patients begin to approach an emotional topic, then start to develop acute physiologic distress, and in response immediately return to mundane topics. The perceived threat to their lives was manifest in their only half-facetious comment that the purpose of the group was to kill them through group discussions! Elsewhere I have discussed necessary modifications of group methodology that are required for patients with various physiological-psychological limitations.

In terms of clinical outcome, the physiologic data illustrate that in patients with this level of severe lung disease, the basic level of physiologic disease as reflected in blood gas levels and ventilatory capacities does not predict clinical outcome on a short-term basis.

The psychological data are not predictive. The IMPS and CMI reflect a gross degree of denial and the inhibition of manifest psychiatric symptomatology. Yet, the NOSIE-30 scores, which reflect ability to use social resources, turn out to be an accurate predictor of clinical outcome. Further, the social resources available to the patient appear to be determinants of clinical outcome.

Those patients who had intact and positive social resources came to their illness and the hospital with some emotional capacity to respond to the frustrations of that illness and hospitalization without upsetting their cardiorespiratory balance. These patients also were able to participate in group discussions and profit from them. Finally, they were afforded an avenue of support, sustenance, and recourse for return to the community.

In conclusion, the data suggest the importance of physiological, psychological, and psychosocial factors in patient adaptation and rehabilitation. The physiological limitations of these patients posed specific limitations on the psychological defense mechanisms available to the patient and the nature of psychological treatment that might be employed. Yet the psychosocial competence of the patient and the psychosocial resources available to him proved to be more significant variables in the short-term prognosis of the illness.

Biological Factors

The importance of biological factors in the dying process seems obvious. Yet it is tempting for mental health personnel to overpsychologize the coping responses of the dying person. We cannot understand the psychology of a person without taking into account his or her present biological state. For there is a reciprocal interaction between our psychological state and our biological state, which together produce the observed state of the human organism. This process is clearly illustrated by the patients in the clinical study. Their biological state made it impossible for them to tolerate intense emotion, while emotional changes immediately compromised their biological state and brought them near to death. So we can readily see how the emotional-biological relationship bears directly on the possible death of the dying person.

Along these lines, Duff and Hollingshead (1968) note that the chronically ill patient: "focuses on his physical state which is seen as life-threatening, even though his psychosocial problems may be most crucial." In a word, the dying person's interest is going to be drawn inexhorably to his or her physical state, which demands his or her attention. For this reason, severely ill patients tend to "flatten out" emotionally (Olin, Fischer, Huddell 1968; Kimball 1969). The lack of emotional response and psychological withdrawal is often misinterpreted as denial, repression, suppression, rationalization, depression, or some other psychopathological defense. This overlooks the necessary conservation of energy, interest, and attention that every sick person experiences. Thus, an alternative explanation is that severely ill persons cannot maintain their investment and involvement with others, and must psychologically and biologically withdraw into themselves to have enough energy to continue living. This emotional withdrawal, then, is a necessary protective maneuver for the sick organism. Emotional and physical demands on the person at this stage of illness may tax the organism beyond its capacity, and may hasten death.

Psychological Factors

What are important psychological attitudes for the dying person? We may be tempted to answer in terms of past coping styles effective in other situations. But Lipowski (1970) points out that what worked before may not work now, in the novel role of being a sick patient. What, for example, does it really mean to "fight for one's life?" Stavraki et al. (1968) reported that hostile aggressive attitudes favorably influence the short-term prognosis of cancer patients. But Achte and Vauhkonen (1971) found just the opposite, that hostility was used to defend against personal closeness and awareness of the seriousness of illness. Perhaps we confuse *aggression* as a life-driving force and *hostility* as a defensive anger. In the patient sample in my study, I observed one very aggressive patient who wanted to take care of himself in a self-reliant fashion. He was pushy and assertive. He improved and went home. Whereas a second patient was equally aggressive but in a hostile attacking manner. He remained clinically unchanged and stayed in the hospital.

Perhaps aggressiveness does play a role in short-term survival. But then we must note that the sick patient is typically expected to be docile, passive, compliant, accepting, and nonquestioning. Thus, we tacitly encourage patients to submit to their fate. I know of no conclusive answers here, but it is worth pondering as we care for dying people.

Social Factors

In the clinical study, I highlighted the importance of both the *availability* of positive social relations and the *ability* to use human resources. This observation is consistent with clinical reports that indicate that the availability and utilization of close positive human relations does influence short-term survival (Ellison 1969; Hamburg and Adams 1967). Beard (1969) sums up these impressions nicely:

> . . . the patients who had the greatest abilities to relate satisfactorily with others, who had a strong deep relationship with a significant person, and who had the ability to draw upon that relationship in a sharing way during the times of stress, discouragement, and loneliness, made the best initial adjustment to their disease and the uncertainty of their future.

The importance of intact positive human relations is underscored by the work of Parkes (1972) and of Marris (1958), who have shown that loss of the important love-object—typically a spouse—is associated with increased mortality. Carr and Schoenberg (1970) conclude that the correlation evidence is strong that loss or absence of loving relationships may precipitate physical illness or deterioration in the sick person. In my study it is intriguing to note that those who died had suffered major object loss or a deterioration in their important human relations; those who survived and improved had not sustained loss and had maintained strong positive loving relations.

THE WILL TO LIVE

Kastenbaum and Kastenbaum (1971) have been working on a "Will to Live" scale in an attempt to measure this salient but subtle aspect of human life. LeShan (1969) has conducted many studies on cancer patients, from which he has concluded that hope and the associated will to live does influence the life-span of such patients. But the word "hope" is just as elusive in human terms as the will to live (Pruyser 1963; Stotland 1969). The one really solid study I have found to date is by Ikemi et al. (1975) in Japan. They report a careful study of five cancer patients who had spontaneous and total remission of the cancer. They found several common factors. First, all had severe existential crises in their lives at the time of development of the cancer. All took responsibility for resolving their own life crisis. Second, all reacted to their fatal illness without anxiety or depression. Third, all the patients had a passionate religious faith and committed their lives to the will of God. Fourth, in all there was a dramatic change in their outlook in life. It was if their impending death pushed them into a sudden "existential shift" or enlightenment toward the meaning and purpose of their lives.

In summary, the will to live seems to be associated with having *something or someone to live for*.

THE EXPECTATION OF DEATH

Factors that promote hastened death seem more clear than the above factors. Ever since the pioneering report by Walter Cannon (1942) on "voodoo death," there have been intermittent reports on self-induced death (Barber 1961; Walters 1944). Biostatistic surveys indicate that mortality rates cannot be adequately accounted for solely in terms of biological variables, thus giving credence to a "psychogenic" factor (Barrett, Franke 1970). In contrast to those who have something to live for, those who hasten toward death have nothing to live for. Engel and Schmale (1967) describe this as the "giving up" complex. In essence, if one experiences critical object-loss, then there is no will to live, there is no hope to regain living relationships, and, therefore, one gives up the attempt to live (Montefiore 1973).

Weisman and Hackett (1961) report that those who accurately predict their own death had given up: "The prospect for death becomes filled with suffering when defeat and demoralization are added to the deterioration of disease." LeShan (1969) observed: ". . . deep psychological isolation, the loss of ability to relate and to love, lowers the ability to fight for health." Eisendrath (1969) found that: ". . . the patient who died had a sense of abandoment, panic, pessimism, and an immobilization of the will to live." Titchener et al. (1958) compared those who reacted to surgery with depletion versus renewal responses. Those who reacted with depletion and deterioration had lost their accepting and comfortable home, were aware of their physical deterioration, had a decreased ability to handle stress, and exhibited withdrawal of affect from external objects. Those who reacted with renewal had hope for life, a freedom to continue activity, and an ability to invest in other persons.

Thus, those for whom life has no more meaning, may well give up, and in that process affect their own deaths.

THE CONNECTION OF MIND AND BODY

In this chapter we have examined some possible interconnections of mind and body that affect the dying process. In our clinical study we saw the obvious interconnection between the emotional and biological parts of the human organism. Later we observed some influences of attitude that affect our will to live and our expectation of death. Here the interconnections are more subtle and less clearly defined. In an overly simplistic way we have termed these psychosomatic or psychophysiologic relations. But that only acknowledges the obvious interconnection, without showing us the links. C.P. Richter (1959), an early pioneer in experimental work, demonstrated how anxiety, fear, and giving up may precipitate death. There are now new provocative research studies that show various correlations between dying experience and bodily reactions (Frederick 1971; Hofer et al. 1972; Miller 1969). It is not my intent to delve into that complex realm here but to call attention to the fact that the dying experience encompasses the mind-body totality of the whole person.

REFERENCES

ACHTE, K.A., and M. L. VAUHKONEN, Cancer and the psyche. *Omega* 2:45-56, 1971.

BARBER, T.X., Death by suggestion: a critical note. *Psychosomatic Medicine* 23: 153-155, 1961.

BARRETT, G. V., and R. H. FRANKE, Psychogenic death: a reappraisal. *Science* 167: 304-306, 1970.

BEARD, B. H., Fear of death and fear of life. *Archives of General Psychiatry* 21: 373-380, 1969.

CANNON, W. B., Voodoo death. *American Anthropology* 44:169-181, 1942.

CARR, A.C., and B. SCHOENBERG, Object-loss and somatic symptom formation, in *Loss and Grief: Psychological Management in Medical Practice*. eds. B. Schoenberg, A.C. Carr, D. Peretz, and A.H. Kutscher. New York: Columbia University Press, 1970.

DLIN, B.M., H.K. FISCHER, and B. HUDDELL, Psychological adaptation to pacemaker and open heart surgery. *Archives of General Psychiatry* 19:599-610, 1968.

DUDLEY, D.L., J. W. VERHEY, M. MASUDA, C.J. MARTIN, and T.H. HOLMES, Longterm adjustment, prognosis, and death in irreversible diffuse obstructive pulmonary syndrome. *Psychosomatic Medicine* 31:310-325, 1969.

DUFF, R.S., and A.B. HOLLINGSHEAD, *Sickness and Society*. New York: Harper & Row, 1968.

EISENDRATH, R.M., The role of grief and fear in the death of kidney transplant patients. *American Journal of Psychiatry* 126:387, 1969.

ELLISON, D. L., Will to Live: a link between social structure and health among the elderly. *Sociological Symposium* 2:37-47, 1969.

ENGEL, G. L., and A. H. SCHMALE, Psychoanalytic theory of somatic disorder. *Journal of the American Psychoanalytic Association* 15:344-365, 1967.

FREDERICK, J.F., Physiological reactions induced by grief. *Omega* 2:71-75, 1971.

HAMBURG, D. A. and J. G. ADAMS, A perspective on coping behavior. *Archives of General Psychiatry* 17:277-284, 1967.

HOFER, M.A., C.T. WOLFF, S.B. FRIEDMAN, and J.W. MASON, A psychoendocrine study of bereavement. Part II. Observations on the process of mourning in relation to adrenocortical function. *Psychosomatic Medicine* 34:492-504, 1972.

HOLMES, T.H. Multidiscipline studies of tuberculosis, in *Personality, Stress, and Tuberculosis*, ed. P.J. Sparer. New York: International Universities Press, 1956.

IKEMI Y., S., NAKAGAWA, T. NAKAGAWA, and M. SUGITA, Psychosomatic consideration of cancer patients who have made a narrow escape from death. *Dynamische Psychiatrie* 8:77-92, 1975.

KASTENBAUM, R., and B.K. KASTENBAUM, Hope, survival, and the caring environment, in *Prediction of Life Span*, eds. F. Jeffers and E. Palmore. Lexington, Mass.: Heath, 1971.

KIMBALL, C.P., Psychological response to the experience of open heart surgery. *American Journal of Psychiatry* 126:348-359, 1969.

LASAGNA, L., The prognosis of death, in *The Dying Patient*, eds. O.G. Brim, Jr., H. E. Freeman, S. Levine, and N. A. Scotch. New York: Russell Sage Foundation, 1970.

LESHAN, L., Psychotherapy and the dying patient, in *Death and Dying*, ed. L. Pearson. Cleveland: Press of Case Western Reserve University, 1969.

LIPOWSKI, Z.J., Physical Illness, the individual and the coping processes. *Psychiatry In Medicine* 1:19-102, 1970.

MARRIS, P. *Widows and Their Families.* London: Routledge, 1958.

MILLER, N.E., Learning of visceral and glandular responses. *Science* 163:434-445, 1969.

MONTEFIORE, H. W., ed., *Death Anxiety.* New York: MSS Information Corporation, 1973.

PARKES, C.M., *Bereavement: Studies of Grief in Adult Life.* New York: International Universities Press, 1972.

PATTISON, E.M., R. S. RHODES, and D.L. DUDLEY, Response to group treatment in patients with severe chronic lung disease. *International Journal of Group Psychotherapy* 21:214-225, 1971.

PRUYSER, P.W., Phenomenology and dynamics of hoping. *Journal for the Scientific Study of Religion* 3:86-96, 1963.

RICHTER, C. P., The phenomenon of unexplained sudden death in animals and man, in *The Meaning of Death*, ed. H. Feifel. New York: McGraw-Hill, 1959.

STAVRAKI, K.M., C.W. BUCK, S.J. LOTT, and J.W. WANKLIN, Psychological factors in outcome of human cancer. *Journal of Psychosomatic Research* 12:251-259, 1968.

STOTLAND, E., *The Psychology of Hope.* San Francisco: Jossey-Bass, 1969.

TITCHENER, J., I. ZWERLING, L. A. GOTTSCHALK, and M. LEVINE, Psychological reactions of the aged in surgery. *Archives of Neurology and Psychiatry* 79:63-73, 1958.

WALTERS, M.J. Psychic death; report of a possible case. *Archives of Neurology and Psychiatry* 52:84-85, 1944.

WEISMAN, A.D., and T.P. HACKETT, Predilection to death. *Psychosomatic Medicine* 23:232-256, 1961.

6

Religion, Faith and Healing

E. Mansell Pattison

The role of religious belief in the life of the dying person has been the subject of intense interest to many. What is the function of religion in facing death? There is no simple answer. However, in this chapter we will examine some of the issues. First, I shall briefly review the research on religious beliefs and dying behavior, and then present a synopsis of an in-depth study of faith healing to illuminate the meaning of healing.

RELIGIOUS BELIEFS
AND ATTITUDES TOWARD DEATH

A number of questions can be posed about religion. Does religious belief make people more or less afraid or anxious about death? Does religious belief make people more accepting or more rejecting of death? Does religious belief make it easier or harder to cope with dying?

It would seem simple to test such questions. But the problem is confounded by the complexity of religion, for religion is a polygon of variables. It includes content of belief or theology; it includes intensity of belief; it involves degree of participation in a community of religious life; it includes the personal meaning of religion in the tenor of one's life. In *Clinical Psychiatry and Religion* (Pattison 1969), I have detailed the various ways in which religion in its panoply of forms serves both integrative and disintegrative functions in our lives. Thus, what starts out as a search for simple correlations between religion and dying becomes a complex question, for religion is a complex aspect of human life

(Pattison 1966). In my review of the pertinent literature, I have found that only one aspect of religion is usually measured in a specific study, and other aspects are ignored. Hence, it is difficult to draw any specific research conclusions about the specific questions we posed here.

Turning to the research literature we do have, the confused complexity is readily demonstrated. Where direct tests of relationship have been made, three studies report that religion had a negative influence (Alexander, Alderstein 1960; Fuance, Fulton 1958; Feifel 1973), five studies report a positive influence (Jeffers, Nichols, Eisdorfer 1961; Martin, Wrightsman 1964, 1965; Swenson 1961), and four studies found no religious differences in attitudes and behavior (Kalisch 1963; Lester 1970; Templer 1970, 1972). In separate comprehensive reviews, both Lester (1972) and Spilka, Pelligrini; Dailey (1968) conclude that religion per se is not a critical factor in the person's response to dying or to death. People for whom religion has not been significant usually will not turn to religion when they are dying; people whose lives have been imbedded in a religious context will deal with dying within that religious context. In effect, people will use religion in their dying as they have used religion throughout their lives. They may use religion destructively or constructively. Father Andre Godin (1972) sums up our conclusions: "The anxious person finds new reasons for anxiety in his religion; the more serene person also derives from his religion the means of justifying his serenity."

Finally, we must differentiate between general religious beliefs and convictions, and immediate personal reactions of the dying person. Both Hackett and Weisman (1969) and Berman (1974) have found that philosophical and theological concerns do not appear as significant issues for the typical dying person. Concerns for the afterlife are minimal. Rather, the dying person focuses on the immediacy of everyday practical issues and coping with the reality of their present existence. One reasonable generalization we may draw, then, is that the confrontation with dying does *not* sharpen people's concern with overarching philosophical and theological views of life, but, rather, dying pulls the person down to coping with the immediate exigencies of daily living.

FAITH HEALING

Within the rationalistic scientific milieu of the twentieth century, the concept of faith healing has been generally viewed with skepticism. Until quite recently, little serious attention has been given to the meaning and function of faith healing. Several different lines of inquiry have addressed faith healing.

First, the early medical literature of the twentieth century reported on faith healing as a suspect variant of acceptable healing methods. The person who sought faith healing was seen as a socially deviant person who rejected the ministrations of modern medicine. (Goddard 1899; Paulsen 1926; Podmore 1963).

Second, psychiatric reports on faith healing focused on psychodynamic conflicts of those who sought healing, usually concluding that neurotic mechanisms played a central role in the search for such culturally aberrant sources of healing (Blanton 1940; Galvin, Ludwig 1961; LaBarre 1962; Salzman 1957).

Third, with the beginning rapprochement of psychology and theology in the last several decades, serious consideration was given to the fact that faith healing could be accepted as a viable human experience, to be explained through the psychological processes of hypnosis, persuasion, brain washing, or some type of psychosomatic phenomenon (Doniger 1957; Edmunds, Scorer 1956; Frank 1961; Sargant 1957; Schwarz 1960).

Fourth, the notion of psychosomatic healing gained credence in the light of sophisticated research on human psychophysiology. In Chapter 5 we examined some of the clinical evidence that psychological attitudes and belief states may indeed profoundly influence bodily function. The possible links in the process are revealed in the basic science research of psychologist Neal Miller (1969), who has shown that the functions of major body organs can be conditioned through operant conditioning techniques. Out of this research was spawned the current fad in "biofeedback" techniques, namely, that the person can be trained to monitor his or her psychological functions and consciously modify the function of specific organ systems. Although the faddish elements have gone far beyond the research data, it does seem plausible that attitudes and beliefs may profoundly influence our bodily states. Thus, the concept of faith healing has become scientifically plausible.

Fifth, recent sociocultural research on faith healing has demonstrated that widespread utility of "folk medicine" ranging from witchcraft, to primitive healing rituals, to systematized formal religious methods of healing. These studies support the contention that religious modes of healing are viable and significant dimensions of human life (Kennedy 1967; Kiev 1964; Lubchansky, Egri, Stokes 1970; Parrington 1958).

However, all these lines of research do not address the issue of the meaning and function of faith healing in contemporary American society, where rational scientific medicine has become the norm. To illuminate this understanding of faith healing, the following covers the salient details of my own study of faith healing in America today (Pattison, Lapins, Foerr 1973; Pattison 1975).

Research Method

A sample of persons claiming faith healing experiences was sought from churches in an urban metropolitan area that were known to emphasize and practice faith healing (such as the pentecostal sects, Assemblies of God, Nazarene, Churches of God). The ministers of all churches in the area were contacted, their cooperation elicited, and permission sought to interview persons in their congregations who were publicly identified as "faith healed."

After identification of such persons, an interview was conducted in their own homes, having informed the person that this study was sanctioned by the particular pastor and was being conducted to learn more about faith healing. We examined the following areas: (1) the life pattern of the person in relationship to him- or herself, family, work, and social relations prior to the faith healing; (2) life pattern in the same areas subsequent to faith healing; (3) medical history prior to and subsequent to faith healing; and (4) the perceived importance and function of the faith healing experience in the person's life. In addition, personality status was assessed with the Spitzer Mental Status Schedule, a scaled self-report schedule; the Minnesota Multiphasic Personality Inventory; and the Cornell Medical Index.

With almost no exceptions, the subjects were most cooperative with the interviewer, spoke readily of their faith healing experiences, and superficially appeared willing to discuss their life patterns.

Research Results

DEMOGRAPHIC CHARACTERISTICS OF POPULATION.   43 subjects were studied, 19 men and 24 women. At the time of interview their ages ranged from 16 to 80, an overall mean of 52 years old. All subjects were married or widowed, except 1 man and 3 women. The mean educational level for both men and women was partial high school; however, almost all who had some education beyond high school attended Bible schools or technical-vocational schools rather than colleges or universities. The occupational level was similar. The men were skilled blue collar and white collar workers, the women preponderantly housewives with little outside work experience.

SOCIORELIGIOUS LIFE. For the most part social life is religious life for this population. Their social life centered around the church and its activities. Average church attendance was three times per week. Social relations were for the most part confined to fellow church members and relatives, with few instances of membership in community organizations and activities. Daily home Bible reading and home worship were reported by nearly every respondent. An ascetic style of life was followed, without use of alcohol or tobacco, nor attendance at dances or movies. Most reported watching television, but with the stipulation that they did not watch it very much.

Most of the subjects had been Christians throughout their lives, although a number who had been reared in religious environments had not been "born again" (that is, experienced religious conversion) until adulthood. However, only in two instances were the "rebirths" coincident with their faith healing, and here the healings were subsequent to their conversion, not preceding it. In all other cases of adult conversion, the conversion had preceded the healing by at least one year.

Characteristics of the Healing Experience

A total of 71 healings were reported, with 7 men and 11 women reporting multiple healings, the maximum being a man who reported 5 healings. The mean age at which healing occurred was 38. The mean interval between healing and interview was 15 years, with a range of 2 weeks to 51 years.

The diversity of illnesses reported was considerable, with all body systems represented. Of the 71 healings, 12 were appraised as life threatening, such as leukemia, cancer, terminal tuberculosis; 38 were appraised as moderately disabling, such as peptic ulcer, ruptured disc, heart disease; 21 were appraised as minimal ailments, such as plantar warts, sprained ankles, backaches.

In all but 9 of the 71 healings, the person participated in some kind of formal religious ritual, which was credited with the healing. These rituals included formal prayer for the individual in front of the congregaton of the church, anointing with oil and prayer, laying-on of hands, and bedside prayer by the minister or a member of the congregation. The majority participated in only one such ritual before healing occurred. The small number who did not take part in a formal ritual did participate in prayers for healing by themselves.

The majority reported that although a doctor may have been consulted for diagnosis, no medical treatment was received. However, a substantial number of subjects received occasional or continued medical treatment *subsequent* to their healing ritual. Such treatment was regarded as being of secondary importance, and in fact not contributory to their healing.

Half of the subjects reported instantaneous healing, whereas the other half reported gradual healing. However, in both instances this was not based on the subject's observed disappearance of symptoms. Instead, he or she asserted that he or she had been healed, regardless of the state of the symptoms. Thus, the instantaneous healings often occurred in the face of a history that demonstrated continuing symptoms after the instantaneous healing, while the gradual healings were described in terms of being healed with the persistence of symptoms that were "left over" and would now take some time to disappear. This interesting observation was obtained by asking the subjects to describe carefully the time sequence and changes in symptomatology before inquiring about their faith healing. It became apparent through this device that the subjects' perception of healing was related to their participation in a healing ritual, *not a perception of change in symptomatology.*

In terms of long-term residual symptoms, 57 healings left no residual symptoms, 6 minimal symptoms, 7 moderate symptoms, and 1 with severe symptoms.

No correlation was found between initial severity of illness and severity of residual symptoms; between severity of illness and medical treatment received; between medical treatment received and residual symptoms; or between any of the above and instantaneous or gradual healing.

Attitudes Toward Physicians and Medical Treatment

Subjects were asked about their use of medical treatment and their attitudes toward physicians and scientific medicine. The subjects uniformly voiced no disapproval of physicians or the practice of scientific medicine. As noted above, the majority had consulted physicians for diagnositic purposes, and many had obtained occasional or continuous treatment for the conditions that were "faith healed." These latter subjects continued medical treatment many times *after* they had received their faith healing. Almost all the subjects had consulted physicians for medical treatment for conditions both before and after the faith healing. The subjects viewed physicians as "useful and necessary; given to us by God." A majority stated that if they became ill they would first seek faith healing. However, if that did not result in a cure, they would then, without reluctance, seek the help of a physician and follow the prescribed treatment. Indeed, many had done so since their faith healing.

Development of Alternate Symptoms

Each subject was asked a systematic medical history of illnesses, treatment, and a review of systems. Although there were a number of minor intercurrent complaints, we were unable to elicit any instances of suspected or manifest alternation of either organic or psychological symptoms.

Effects of Faith Healing on Life-style

Each respondent was asked initially to describe his or her own emotional functioning, work functioning, and relationships with people prior to the faith healing. Then each subject was asked to describe his or her life-style in each of the above areas after the faith healing. And, finally, each subject was asked to describe changes in each area after the faith healing.

No change was reported by our subjects, using either the indirect descriptive inquiry or on direct questioning regarding changes in life-style.

The subjects reported that their lives, work, and social relationships had always been serene and comfortable. Rarely were personal or interpersonal conflicts reported. In retrospect, even their illnesses, for which they had sought faith healing, were not seen as seriously disruptive events in their lives. Their faith healing was not seen as particularly significant, nor an eventful occurrence in their lives, but almost an expected event. Thus, their faith healing was no watershed that changed their lives. On the other hand, a number of subjects who had been "born again" in adult life did report that their lives had been disturbed prior to their religious conversion, but subsequent to their religious commitment life had become peaceful and satisfying.

The subjects were also questioned regarding changes in religious behavior subsequent to their faith healing. As before, there was *no change* in church attendance, private devotions, Bible reading, or religious interest.

However, there was one major change noted by all respondents. All reported that their *certainty* in their belief in God and their religious convictions was *markedly increased* after their faith healing experiences.

Personality Status

Personality status was first assessed by the Spitzer Mental Status Schedule and by a clinical rating scale in which the interviewer rated each subject on self-reports of: 1) level of energy, 2) worry, 3) anxiety, 4) restlessness, 5) depression, and 6) anger. The scores on both methods of rating were uniformly very low. The subjects reported themselves as having high energy and rarely experiencing worry, anxiety, restlessness, depression, or anger. The standard attitude expressed was that "God can take care of everything," and since they had placed their trust in God there was little about which to be concerned or to get upset. Adverse emotional experiences were seen as "works of the devil." Hence, devout religious persons, such as themselves, would not experience such adverse feelings so long as they lived in the proper religious manner.

In contradistinction to the self-reports, the interviewer noted manifestations of anger, depression, anxiety, and worry during the course of the interviews. However, the subjects would deny or minimize these emotions when questioned. It appeared that they wished to see themselves and present themselves in a uniformly good light.

On the Cornell Medical Index, the scores fell within normal group norms. But on the psychiatric items checked, both men and women were significantly on the low side of "normal" population norms.

The number of illness symptoms checked can be seen as a measure of personal adjustment reflecting perception of self as a psychological failure or a psychological success. In this instance, the uniformly low scores on the CMI suggest that this population viewed themselves as psychological successes.

It should be noted that three men and six women fell outside the "normal" group norm ranges. These subjects also did *not* deny untoward emotional reactions, and reported disruptive personal and interpersonal experiences. Although these persons had experienced faith healing and perceived faith healing in a fashion similar to the other subjects, they readily acknowledged difficulties in life with which they were unable to cope. In these subjects the same psychological coping mechanisms were being used, but were not as effective as for the majority of the subjects.

On the Minnesota Multiphasic Personality Inventory, a relatively uniform pattern was found, with no statistical difference between male and female scores. After statistical analysis of the MMPI scores, it was found that there was minimal deviation among subjects, thus making it appropriate to construct a composite MMPI profile for the entire group of subjects.

The MMPI results corroborate and extend the prior impressions. There is intent to present a good impression of oneself in a highly socially acceptable manner. Yet there is great *defensiveness* against psychological weakness, a defensiveness that verges upon deliberate distortion in the "good" direction; there is reliance on repression and denial of emotional difficulties. This profile implies "an overcompensating rejection of the possibility that the subject is capable of being neurotic . . . the subject tends to overstate his condition in the direction of saying that he does not tire easily, does not get depressed, that life about him is good, that he is having a good time, and he should be grateful for what the world offers him." This aptly sums up exactly how our subjects described themselves in the clinical interview. Further, it suggests that these subjects rely on specific somatic complaints as a method of expressing discomfort, rather than on emotional complaints that are repressed.

We can summarize the MMPI profile as follows:

They are *affiliative, constrictedly overconventional* people. These individuals show prominently in their relations with others an exaggerated striving to be liked and accepted. Characteristically, they maintain an unassailable optimism and emphasize harmony with others, if necessary at the expense of internal values and principles. They are likely to become extremely uncomfortable in, and therefore to avoid, situations demanding angry responses, independent decisions, or the exercise of power. When such persons do end up in the clinic, which is infrequent, they are most resistant to considering that their difficulties may result from emotional conflict. It is also a remarkable fact that even in the face of catastrophic failure, they often resolutely maintain that "things are going fine;" defeated feelings seem to be intolerable to these people.

Summation of Data

A high degree of congruence has been demonstrated from the history of life-style, religious belief and behavior, clinical interview observations, subjects' self-reports, and psychometric analyses.

These subjects present psychological characteristics indicative of a strong need for social acceptance and social affiliation. This exaggerated need, along with the extensive use of denial and repression as major coping mechanisms, is so pervasive that major disruptive events in their lives are ignored and interpreted as part of a normal, smooth, unruffled existence.

These psychological characteristics are consistent with the fact that these subjects do not perceive of illness as a major disruptive event, nor do they perceive their faith healing as a major life enhancing event. Further, these psychological characteristics explain why the subjects perceive of their faith healing as a definite occurrence regardless of presence or absence of symptoms, and regardless of persisting symptoms, and with concomitant medical treatment.

Further, it is not surprising that no evidence for symptom alternation is found, for the subjects do not perceive of their illnesses as conflictual events. Thus, in a sense, their faith healing does not remove their symptoms. Remission of symptoms does not significantly affect their psychic balance of defenses, and, therefore, emergence of alternate symptoms is not required to maintain psychic equilibrium.

The issue of whether the subject actually achieved symptom relief or remission of organic symptomatology was not investigated, since there is ample evidence from psychophysiologic research to provide explanations for perceived and actual change in illness. From the subjects' point of view, relief of symptoms is really a tangential issue. For them, faith healing reaffirms their belief system and their style of life. Faith healing serves to buttress their psychological life-style. From a scientific medical point of view, the question usually asked of faith healing is "does it cure the disease?" But that is not the question asked by the prospective applicant for faith healing. His or her question is, "Am I living in the right way?" Thus, faith healing is not an exercise in the treatment of organic pathology, but an exercise in the treatment of life-style.

MEDICINE OR FAITH?

From early on in the twentieth century, illness and healing have been seen in America solely from the view of scientific medicine. Therefore, faith healing has been viewed as an anachronistic throwback to a prescientific era of thought. From this position, scientific healing and faith healing would be seen as competitive.

However, in our study we found that these two methods of healing were *not* competitive *but complementary*. The same situation has been shown to occur in various studies on folk healing in societies that are undergoing rapid scientific acculturation (Mischel 1959; Nash 1967). In these social settings, both types of healers are used by the populace but *for different reasons*. When a personal problem is perceived by the patient as due to a condition culturally defined as impersonal, such as a germ or accident, then the patient seeks treatment from a scientific healer. However, when a problem is perceived by the patient as due to a condition culturally defined as due to personal evil or evil intent, then the patient seeks a religious healer. The reason is logical, for the religious healer is a healer not of specific things but of the whole person. Further, such sickness is sin, and, therefore, the problem is religious and the cure is religious.

The problem then is *not the condition* but what caused the condition.

Therefore, one seeks either a scientific healer or a religious healer, not in terms of the condition but the cause.

One might casually assume that all people in contemporary America share a common scientific view of the world and the medical scientific view of the cause of disease. But this is certainly not true for the population of people in our study. Illness and emotional distress are not viewed in scientific terms but in religious terms (Havens 1961; Nunn 1964; Nunn, Kosa, Alpert 1968). Thus, as our respondents told us, depression, anger, emotional imperfections, even memory lapses, and especially physical disease are not expected occurrences in life. Rather, they are "works of the devil," and a reflection of personal error and sin. Therefore, it is quite logical within this world view to not seek the help of a scientific healer, but rather to seek religious healing for being a bad person. This ethos is expressed by various charismatic faith healers, such as Oral Roberts or Kathryn Kuhlman, who inform their audiences that God does not intend for any of his children to be ill. If you are sick, you need to confess your sins and make yourself right with God, and then you will be healed.

The results of this research, if taken in isolation, might lead to the conclusion that our subjects participated in faith healing ritual and experienced faith healing solely because of the life-style, which might be labeled neurotic. Such a view, however, is ethnocentric. Within the world view of our faith healing subjects, their life-style and means of coping with emotions and interpersonal behavior are defined by their religious culture. Faith healing in their world is not aberrant behavior, nor can it be considered psychopathological for existence in their world. Rather, faith healing is a culturally defined and sanctioned method for getting right with oneself and one's world to continue living in a functional manner.

In conclusion, to understand the meaning and function of faith healing in the lives of our subjects, we have been led to understand their view of life, their religious culture, and the manner in which it defines patterns of health and illness. Within this cultural context, faith healing is neither illogical nor irrational. Rather, it is an acceptable and appropriate method of dealing with the perceived causes of their illness.

SUMMARY

In this chapter we have examined the uses of religion in response to illness, dying, and death. Religion may be peripheral in one's life, and, if so, religion will doubtless be peripheral in facing dying and death. On the other hand, if religion is a central dimension of one's life, it may play a critical role in one's approach to death and dying.

When religion is central, it may be positive or negative. I have illustrated some of the positive uses of religion in Chapter 5 and in this chapter. Yet we must not neglect the fact that a religious person may use his or her religion negatively, just as Job was tempted to curse God for his fate. For example, a young mother was confronted with her young child dying of leukemia. She blamed God for this illness. Yet she asked her minister to stay with them when the child lay dying. Just after the child died, she began to scream curses at God, and turned to beat on the hapless pastor who represented God to her.

Finally, we should be aware of "foxhole religion." I have in mind those people who frantically search for some magical solution to the problem of dying. They search out each new cure, each new diet, each new healer, each new faith. In this instance, we do not have faith but merely the disheartening and fruitless search for a remedy that cannot be found.

In conclusion, we have looked at some attributes of our human existence that may seem imponderable. Life is more than cold rationality. We are flesh and blood beings. "And now abideth faith, hope, and love."

REFERENCES

ALEXANDER, I.E., and A.M. ALDERSTEIN, Studies in the psychology of death, in *Perspectives in Personality Research*, eds. H.P. David and J.C. Brengleman. New York: Springer, 1960.

BERMAN, A.L., Belief in afterlife, religion, religiosity, and life-threatening experence. *Omega* 5:127-135, 1974.

BLANTON, S., Analytic study of a cure at Lourdes. *Psychoanalytic Quarterly* 9: 348-362, 1940.

DONIGER, S., ed., *Healing: Human and Divine. Man's Search for Health and Wholeness Through Science, Faith and Prayer*. New York: Association Press, 1957.

EDMUNDS, V., and C.G. SCORER, *Some Thoughts on Faith Healing*. London: Tyndale Press, 1956.

FAUNCE, W.A., and R.L. FULTON, The sociology of death: a neglected area of research. *Social Forces* 36:205-209, 1958.

FEIFEL, H., Religious conviction and fear of death among the healthy and the terminally ill. *Journal for the Scientific Study of Religion* 13:353-360, 1973.

FRANK, J.D., *Persuasion and Healing*. Baltimore: Johns Hopkins Press. 1961.

GALVIN, J., and A. LUDWIG, A case of witchcraft. *Journal of Nervous and Mental Diseases* 133:161-168, 1961.

GODDARD, H.H., The effect of mind on body as evidenced by faith cures. *American Journal of Psychology* 10:431-502, 1899.

GODIN, A., Has death changed? in *Death and Presence*, ed. A. Godin. Brussels: Lumen Vitae, 1972.

HACKETT, T. P., and A. D. WEISMAN, Denial as a factor in patients with heart disease and cancer. *Annals of New York Academy of Science* 164:802-817, 1969.

HAVENS, J., The participants vs. the observer's frame of reference in the psychological study of religion. *Journal for the Scientific Study of Religion* 1:79-87, 1961.

JEFFERS, F.C., C.R. NICHOLS, and C. EISDORFER, Attitudes of older persons toward death: a preliminary study. *Journal of Gerontology* 16:53-56, 1961.

KALISCH, R.A., Some variables in death attitudes. *Journal of Social Psychology* 59:137-145, 1963.

KENNEDY, J.G., Nubian Zar ceremonies as psychotherapy. *Human Organization* 26:185-194, 1967.

KIEV, A., *Curanderismo: Mexican-American Folk Psychiatry.* New York: Free Press, 1968.

_____ ed., *Magic, Faith, and Healing. Studies in Primitive Psychiatry Today.* New York: Free Press, 1964.

LaBARRE, W., *They Shall Take Up Serpents. Psychology of the Southern Snake-Handling Cult.* Minneapolis: University of Minnesota Press, 1962.

LESTER, D., Religious behavior and fear of death. *Omega* 2:181-188, 1970.

_____, Religious Behaviors and attitudes toward death, in *Death and Presence,* ed A. Godin. Brussels: Lumen Vitae, 1972.

LOVELAND, G.G., The effects of bereavement on certain religious attitudes and behavior. *Sociological Symposium* 1:17-27, 1968.

LUBCHANSKY, I, G. EGRI, and J. STOKES, Puerto Rican spiritualists view mental illness: the faith healer as a paraprofessional. *American Journal of Psychiatry* 127:312-321, 1970.

MARTIN, D., and L. WRIGHTSMAN, Religion and fears about death: a critical review of research. *Religious Education* 59: 174-176, 1964.

_____ , The relationship between religious behavior and concern about death. *Journal of Social Psychology* 65:317-323, 1965.

MILLER, N.E., Learning of visceral and glandular responses. *Science* 163:434-445, 1969.

MISCHEL, F., Faith healing and medical practice in the Southern Caribbean. *Southwestern Journal of Anthropology* 15:407-417, 1959.

NASH, J., The logic of behavior: curing in a Maya Indian town. *Human Organization* 26:132-140, 1967.

NUNN, C.Z., Child-control through a "coalition with God." *Child Development* 35:417-432, 1964.

NUNN, C.Z., J. KOSA, and J.J. ALPERT, Causal locus of illness and adaptation to family disruptions. *Journal of the Scientific Study of Religion* 7:210-218, 1968.

PARRINGTON, G., *Witchcraft: European and African.* London: Faber, 1958.

PATTISON, E.M., ed., *Clinical Psychiatry and Religion.* Boston: Little, Brown 1969.

PATTISON, E.M., Ideological support for the marginal middle class: faith healing and glossolalia, in *Pragmatic Religion: Marginal Religious Movements in America Today*, eds., I. Zaretsky and M.P. Leone. Princeton, N.J.: Princeton University Press, 1975.

_____ , Social and psychological aspects of religion in psychotherapy. *Journal of Nervous and Mental Diseases* 141:586-597, 1966.

PATTISON, E.M., N.A. LAPINS, and H.A. DOERR, Faith healing: a study of personality and function. *Journal of Nervous and Mental Diseases* 157:397-409, 1973.

PAULSEN, A.E., Religious healing. *Journal of the American Medical Association* 86:1519-1524, 1926.

PODMORE, F., *From Mesmer to Christian Science: A Short History of Mental Healing.* New York: University Books, 1963.

SALZMAN, L., Spiritual and faith healing. *Journal of Pastoral Care* 11:146-155, 1957.

SARGANT, W., *Battle for the Mind: A Psysiology of Conversion and Brain Washing.* Garden City, N.Y.: Doubleday, 1957.

SCHWARZ, B.E., Ordeal by serpents, fire, and strychnine. A study of some provocative psychosomatic phenomena. *Psychiatric Quarterly* 34:405-429, 1960.

SPILKA, B., R. J. PELLIGRINI, and K. DAILY, Religion: American views and death perspective. *Sociological Symposium 1:57-66, 1968.*

SWENSON, W.M., Attitudes toward death in an aged population. *Journal of Gerontology* 16:49-52, 1961.

TEMPLER, D.I., Death anxiety in religiously very involved persons. *Psychological Reports* 31:361-362, 1972.

TEMPLER, D.I., and E. DOTSON, Religious correlates of death anxiety. *Psycholgical Reports* 26:895-897, 1970.

7

An Interview with a Dying Mother

E. Mansell Pattison

Now that we have taken an overview of the general principles involved in the dying process, it is time to take a closer personal look at specific examples.

To introduce this detailed examination, I shall present a verbatim conversation I had with a dying woman. I invite the reader to examine carefully how the patient is coping with dying, and how I cope with the same. This is not a perfect model of how to talk with a dying person. Rather, I want to share this interview because it clearly reveals how two people actually talk, feel, and interact.

INTERVIEW

D = Dr. Pattison
P = 28-year-old mother
Location: Medical ward of a hospital

D: Hello, I don't think I've met you before. I'm a psychiatrist here in the hospital. I understand your doctor talked with you about my visit.

P: This morning.

D: This morning? He talked with you about the purpose of our interview today?

P: He said something about medical histories.

D: Yes. We're trying to teach medical students how an illness develops in a person; how you deal with an illness; what you do when a sickness hits you.

P: Yes. (flat)

D: You've been, I guess, sick now for what, six months or more?

P: Well, most of the last year.

D: Most of the year?

P: Yeah.

D: How did it start?

P: Ah, with bronchitis, with a bad case of bronchitis.

D: Uh um.

P: In January.

D: In January? That would be January of 69 or 70?

P: Oh just this last year. This is 71 (both laugh)

D: So this has gone on for an entire year, and your symptoms started with bronchitis.

P: Yeah.

D: And what's happened since then?

P: (pause) Oh, I had a lot of chest pain, waking up at night. I can't sleep with the pain. (clears throat) And I came into the hospital in August, and they ran a few tests on me, about 100,000.

D: A hundred thousand tests! (both laugh)

P: At least. (pause) I know it's that many X rays, but (pause 15 seconds) I just kept getting sicker and sicker.

D: Were they doing any treatment, or just running tests?

P: Oh treatment. I had an operation and I had radiation therapy.

D: Uh hum.

P: And a lot more X rays, to see what was happening. I had trouble with my heart.

D: You had trouble with your heart?

P: Uh huh.

D: And this was a heart operation that they did?

P: Yes, it was a pericardial drainage.

D: A pericardial drainage?

P: Yes, cause I had fluid around my heart and the sack.

D: You're getting to learn all the right medical terms, aren't you?

P: I don't know, just what they tell me. (laughs)

D: Right! (both laugh)

D: So they found out what the trouble was with your heart?

P: Well, the technical term, ah, ah, angiosarcoma.

D: Angiosarcoma?

P: Of the heart

D: Uh-hum, it's been a while as a psychiatrist since I've looked all those things up in a textbook.

P: I looked it up in the dictionary to see, it's cancer of the blood vessels of the heart.

D: Cancer of the blood vessels of the heart?

P: That's what the dictionary says.

D: Uh-hum.

P: That's all I could gather, I haven't had a doctor actually explain it to me . . . (pause) . . . in detail what's been wrong. All I know is that I've been real sick, and (pause) for a long, long time, and I couldn't stand up.

D: You walked in here today, I noticed!

P: Yeah.

D: A little bit shaky, but not too bad.

P: Well, (clears throat) the last time I was in the hospital, when they were finished with me, I couldn't get up. I was real dizzy when I would stand up. And I went home even though I was dizzy, and I stayed in bed at home. I could barely make it into the bathroom. Then I was in bed for a month and a half.

D: And then you were able to get up and walk around?

P: Then after a while I could, and I was allright, and I would do a little bit of work around the house. But then, a couple of weeks ago, well ah, this cold weather has really gotten me.

D: That's hard for you?

P: I started having trouble breathing.

D: I noticed. You know, you don't have to talk real fast. I see that you are breathing a little bit rapidly, and I don't know if this is your regular breathing rate or you're a little bit anxious?

P: No! It's usually worse than this, really. I'm breathing kind of easy right now.

D: Is that right? You feel pretty comfortable right now, or? (pause) a little bit on edge?

P: Yeah. (giggle)

D: I was on edge too, the first time I was on television.

P: (giggle)

D: I couldn't recognize myself. (both laugh)

D: But to come back to this problem you have with your heart; you say that the doctors have been giving you treatment for the angiosarcoma.

P: Radiation therapy for about five weeks.

D: Uh-hum.

P: And they stopped that on November the third.

D: November third?

P: And, ah, they've been talking, my doctor (pause 15 seconds) has been talking to me about taking a drug, but he isn't at this hospital anymore. He's at Veterans Administration Hospital now. And he was going to call another doctor, Dr. Smith, but I didn't talk to Dr. Smith before I came in. (pause) I talked to him on Wednesday, and I told him that I didn't want to come in the hospital (nervous giggle) because, ah, (nervous laugh) I really didn't.

D: Why was that, you didn't want to come in the hospital?

P: I just don't like hospitals. I'm just prejudiced, I guess. (nervous laugh)

D: You're entitled to a little bit of prejudice after a whole year of it, aren't you?

P: Oh, needles, and—well, here I am again. I just couldn't do anything at home at all. And my breathing just kept getting worse and worse and the cough (pause).

D: So it sounds like things have been a little bit up and down in the last year since you first got sick, and in the last few months it's been a pretty handicapping disease for you.

P: Yeah, I haven't been able to get around hardly at all.

D: Hardly at all? And you say that although the doctors told you what this was, this angiosarcoma?

P: They didn't tell me. I read it on the hospital admission slip.

D: Oh, you did?

P: (laughs)

D: You're one of those kind?

P: (nervous laugh) . . . I was curious.

D: That's right. Then nobody told you or you didn't ask anybody, or (pause) I was kidding, you know, about being sneaky, because sometimes that's the only way you find out things.

P: I don't know. I was a little bit afraid to ask. All I knew I was sick—ah—very sick, and . . .

D: What were you afraid of?

P: Lots! Somebody asks what's wrong with you and tells you you're going to drop dead, you know. (pause) All they will tell you is there's always hope, (nervous laugh) I guess.

D: That is a question. How do you have hope when you have a very serious disease.

P: Faith.

D: Faith?

P: Faith in God.

D: Has that played a role in your thinking about your disease and your future?

P: (pause 10 seconds) Well, it plays a role in all my life.

D: It does. How does it work? Can you tell me about it?

P: It's just ah (nervous laugh) you do what you have to do, that's all. Ah— I mean, (pause) if I'm sick, you know, if the doctors can't do anything for me (pause) . . . if they can they will.

D: So, you're coming to the hospital now again to get more treatment?

P: Well, I was thinking of taking this drug.

D: And you're hoping that taking the drug will help?

P: Yes.

D: So, when you say that you have some hope that drugs and the treatment will help, I guess you are thinking about how am I going to have faith in possible treatment, but, yet, how do I also deal with the fact that I've got a pretty serious disease—I've got to make some plans for my life.

P: Yeah, I guess so. (very low voice)

D: Have the doctors talked with you at all about plans for yourself and for your children, your husband, your family, in terms of your disease?

P: No, they just come and go real (low quivery voice) fast. (nervous giggle)

D: They do?

P: They don't ever sit down and discuss anything with me. How my life is.

D: I wonder. You know you have a very serious issue to deal with in your own life. I've been impressed that often-times, just as you were talking about the chart, sometimes it's more difficult for us to deal with our feelings if we don't know what it is we're dealing with. In other words, it's like in the dark, if you don't know what's in the dark then you may be very scared of it. If you know what's out there in the dark, then you can do something about dealing with it.

P: Yes.

D: And I wonder about your husband and your children. I understand you have three children?

P: My husband and I are separated.

D: You're separated? I see. So he's not involved in your life now at all?

P: No. He comes to get our baby. I was married twice, and we have one child by my second husband, and he comes to see the baby on weekends.

D: And who are the children living with?

P: My brother's taking care of my kids. He's 34, he used to teach, and he had a lot of psychology—child psychology. He's real good with the kids.

D: So he's helping take care of your kids while you're sick now. Does he know about your illness and what is wrong with your heart?

P: (nervous cough) I think so.

D: You haven't talked with him about it?

P: No (nervous laugh) He isn't a very talkative person.

D: Who is it that you talk with?

P: I don't talk to anybody.

D: Don't talk to anybody?

P: No, (pause 15 seconds) not at all about my problems (pause 10 seconds).

D: Yet you are able to sustain some faith and hope and courage while some people might be very depressed or very discouraged!

P: I think you just do what you have to do, that's all. (nervous laugh) There isn't anything else I can do! (clears throat, pause 15 seconds)

D: With this courage, then, you do what you have to do, which is a pretty good day-by-day way of tackling things. Now, have you talked with your brother about the management of your children, or plans to take care of them while you're so sick like this?

P: I don't have to talk to him, I just watch him. He's good with them, and they like him a lot. He's great with them. (pause 10 seconds)

D: One of the things about serious illness is the need for appropriate plans, with your family, with your kids. With a serious illness like this, you were sort of half kidding, and I assume maybe half serious, in saying, "gee, with trouble with my heart like this, I might possibly drop dead"—you might have a sudden heart attack. So, how will your kids be taken care of?

P: I don't know, I just figure that God will take care of them, that's all I can think. That's the only thing I can believe, anything else would frighten me.

D: Would frighten you?

P: Well, wouldn't it frighten you? (pause—ah) Well, sure it would.

D: I'm not sure what you're frightened of, that's why I'm not responding.

P: (clears throat) Well, (clears throat, pause 15 seconds) I can't worry about what will happen to the kids, you know. If I can take care of them, I'll take care of them; if I can't, I just can't. (coughs several times, clears throat)

D: Do you want a drink of water?

P: O.K. (40-second pause)

D: You're a pretty tough gal to try and handle a lot of this by yourself, (pause 10 seconds) someways courageous! What about your brother and your parents, what is their willingness to support or share with you the situation you're in today?

P: I don't know.

D: Have they tried to talk with you at all?

P: (pause) No. Just take the kids a lot.

D: They do!

P: Yep. (pause 10 seconds)

D: But they never openly share with you, talk openly with you about your illness? Do you think it would be helpful to them if they could talk openly with you?

P: I don't know.

D: Do they live around here?

P: Yes.

D: And they know that you're sick?

P: Yes.

D: You know sometimes we play the game of "you know that I know that we both know but we can't let each other know"—you know that sort of game?

P: I imagine. (pause 15 seconds)

D: So I would imagine they might have a lot of questions about your illness! How serious it is and what's going to be the outcome. Have they talked with any of your doctors about it?

P: A couple of times.

D: What's their understanding of your sickness?

P: I don't know. (clears throat) They seem annoyed.

D: Really!

P: Yeah.

D: Well, what happened?

P: Well, they have to take the kids a lot cause I can't take care of them. And, it just seems like you know, well, not that they don't want to be bothered, cause they always, you know, are good with the kids, and come to see them a lot and everything, but they've had to be bothered more than they used to, and ah, I don't think they like it.

D: Do they say so?

P: No, but (pause 10 seconds) it just seems to me, I don't know, maybe I'm being a bother, maybe they don't feel that way at all. I can't really say, you'll have to ask them.

D: That raises a possibility! I wonder how you feel about it. Sometimes when people have a serious illness like you have, we find it useful to get the family together, the brothers, the sisters, mom, dad. Sit down and talk together as a family about how we can handle things together, how we can be honest and open with each other, and how we can agree together to do the things that need to be done. How do you think they'd respond to something like that?

P: I don't know.

D: Do you think it might be helpful to them?

P: Helpful to them? I doubt it.

D: How about to you?

P: (pause 10 seconds) I doubt it. (pause 10 seconds) I don't know.

D: I'm not saying that should be done, but just a possibility for you to think about these things.

P: (clears throat)

D: The doctors apparently talked with your relatives, but you don't quite know what they've told them, and you haven't talked with them all that much yet?

P: No.

D: Any questions you'd like to have answered? That we could have your doctors tell you about your disease?

P: Oh! I don't know, I guess so when it comes right down to it.

D: What sort of things are the big hanging questions?

P: Whether or not I'm going to live, and if I am for how long, and if I'm going to die, how long do I have to live.

D: I don't know the answer to those questions myself. I do know that you have this cancer of your heart and I do know from my reading about this sort of cancer condition that it's unpredictable. Like you said half-joking, sometimes it does cause sudden death. You may have a heart attack suddenly, but we can't predict that. I'm no heart specialist—*human heart,* but not the anatomical heart. These heart tumors grow at different rates, so it's difficult to predict exactly how long a person may live until they die. (pause) But the issue is not whether a person dies or not, since we all die at some point or other in life. But the question is what we have to deal with, *human heart speaking,* while we look forward to the possibility of our own death—what are the emotional human heart problems we've got to deal with ourselves?

P: (pause 25 seconds, clears throat) I don't understand what you mean.

D: I'll try to explain—you were asking, when do I die and how long before I die? I don't know those answers specifically. But there are other things that we can deal with other than just death. How do we deal with our kids, our family, how do we deal with our own feelings about being sick, about having this serious disease? We've got these sorts of things to deal with, our own feelings, our feelings about the people we love, people we have some responsibility for, our kids.

P: Yeah.

D: How we can deal with these things. How we can be of help. We can't change the disease. I can't really help that.

P: No. (pause 10 seconds) I feel pretty secure that my brother has my kids, I think, cause he's good with them. (clears throat) I was frantic once because my mother couldn't keep them, but then he showed up on the scene and I guess that's why I feel confident that he's got them and will stay with them if something does happen to me, if I die. And I, I, feel relieved and I feel confident that he will, and he's real good to them, and they just love him.

D: Has he made that commitment to you that he will take care of the kids if you die?

P: Just, he hasn't actually said that he would, but he's been there, he's been there. He was gone in the daytime for awhile, but, ah, he's coming every night, he's keeping watch, cause he knew I was sick.

D: Yes! And he knew that this was a fatal disease that you have?

P: A-huh.

D: Does he know that you have the cancer?

P: (clears throat) I think so.

D: You think so? You're just not quite sure?

P: (pause) Well, he knows as well as anybody knows, as well as I know.

D: Yeah?

P: That's what they tell me.

D: Do you find that doctors find it hard to talk about fatal diseases and dying? To bring it out in the open so we can deal with it?

P: Doctors don't talk much about anything. (giggle) They make their own language.

D: Yeah.

P: They just come in and they start talking about stitches and your injuries, and all this business of well, I don't know what they're talking about. They don't say much to you, you know, just what you need in the line of medicine, how you feel and check your pulse and everything.

D: The reason I bring this up is because we doctors are just beginning to learn to deal with our own feelings about dying and death. Doctors have had as much trouble in dealing with our personal feelings and reactions to it as anybody else; and doctors have a great deal of difficulty in talking with patients who are dying, unless patients happen to be very old people, who are sort of wearing out at the end of the line. With young people that are dying, I think we often have a great deal of difficulty being very honest and straightforward or frank. It is almost as though we were afraid to talk about it, for fear that something bad is going to happen if we talk about it.

P: Well, ah, I know I would feel that way if I had to tell someone about death.

D: Uh-huh.

P: They're just human beings, you know.

D: Yeah.

P: They aren't superpeople, or anything, so it either frightens them or it doesn't, I guess.

D: Have you felt frightened about your own dying at all?

P: Yeah—have you?

D: Sure.

P: Do you feel frightened about your dying?

D: Yes.

P: O.K. then, you know. (giggle)

D: Yes.

P: (giggles again) Then you don't have to ask me. (nervous laugh, clears throat)

D: I guess what I was asking was really not how does it feel, because I know that you're right! But how are you dealing with it right now? Is it tolerable not to know just where you are going?

P: Just, I don't want to be alone, that's all, and do what I have to do.

D: In other words, you were more frightened about the idea of dying a while back than you are now?

P: Yeah.

D: Any other feelings that are bothersome now, besides the frightening feelings?

P: No, when you've been as sick as I've been and for as long as I've been, you just have to, to accept it, because there is a very strong possibility.

D: Yeah. That's right! But you've made some adjustments to the illness, in the sense that when you were first frightened you learned to deal with that and accept that frightened feeling, am I right in that? (pause) Or is it still bothering you?

P: It doesn't bother me now. (clears throat)

D: And you've gotten used to being sick and not being able to care for yourself and the kids the way you used to. And you have made some plans about the care of your children and your brother's going to take care of them.

P: I feel he's helped.

D: And these other things that need to be planned out or taken care of while you're still sick, before you have to face really getting very sick and dying?

P: (pause 10 seconds)

D: Do you think they are pretty well handled?

P: (pause 15 seconds)

D: So you're going to live it day-by-day?

P: Yeah.

D: Well, that's a pretty healthy way of doing things.

P: (nervous giggle) Yeah, that's the way I've always done it (clears throat) just what I've had to do.

D: The reason I mention this is that the nurses and other personnel at the hospital have been very on edge. They don't know whether to come to somebody and say "How are you feeling today", or say "Do you know that Mrs. so-and-so has a bad heart disease that is ultimately going to be fatal?" Then we start building up half-truths, where everybody gets on edge and tense instead of being able to be straightforward, honest, and respect each other.

P: They've all been great.

D: They're been very concerned about you.

P: Well, I certainly have been getting a lot of attention to me, today anyway. (light laugh)

D: Yeah. You get to be superstar today!

P: Yeah. (laughs) They told me a long time ago that I would obtain star billing from my illness, and it looks like I have. (both laugh)

D: Well, if not a huge star billing, at least a small one.

P: (laughs) A gold one. (laughs)

D: Well, we've been talking today about the whole process of dying and being able to talk about it and plan for it. But perhaps you have some questions you'd like to ask about things we haven't talked about.

P: No. (pause 10 seconds) I can't think of anything.

D: I very much appreciate your talking with us today. Your openness, honesty, frankness, and willingness is a real help to us.

The patient died suddenly the next morning.

COMMENT

Several major issues, common to many dying persons, are raised and illustrated in this interview I offer my comments and interpretations, while inviting readers to reflect on their own possible interpretations.

The Function of Denial

At the beginning, the patient alleges that she knows little if anything about her illness and her prognosis. As our discussion continues, it becomes obvious that she has much greater awareness of her condition than she intimates. Why is this?

One reason might be the social constraints on conversation. This is the familiar theme of "closed awareness." All parties possess personal awareness of what is going on, but there is constraint on sharing such mutual knowledge. For example, the patient refers to peeking at her chart, looking up her disease in the dictionary, and never obtaining any information from the doctors on their daily rounds. Thus, the subtle message may be that one is not supposed to discuss dying and death, even if you know about it. There seem to be elements of social constraint encouraging denial here.

A second reason, however, may lie with the patient herself. As she gradually talks more openly about her dying and death, she does not pursue her thoughts and feelings even after acknowledging and accepting them. Rather, after each bit of open acknowledgement she pauses, coughs, and withdraws back into her immediate self. To describe the process in a metaphor: We openly write her feelings and thoughts in the moist sand, which are then washed away in the next wave of denial. We write again in the sand, and it is washed away again by the recurrent wave of denial.

But should she somehow be forced into an ongoing open discussion of her thoughts and feelings? I certainly nudged and pushed along toward an open discussion. But then I moved back from a demand for open discussion—and supported her use of denial. What is to be gained from pushing and demanding some explicit open stance? I suggest that the need in this case was the doctor's need (my own need) to have the patient discuss issues in the same way that I wanted to discuss them; not her need. It is *not* her lack of awareness that is the major denial mechanism here. She *is* aware. She just wants to maintain herself without having to face that painful awareness all the time: "When you've been as sick as long as I've been, you just have to accept it." So she closes over, she suppresses, she denies. And it helps her to manage her daily hour-by-hour existence. Do we want to deny her the freedom and modest tranquility of her style of coping, by demanding that she continually endure the pain of her conscious full-in-the-face looking at her existence? Rarely do any of us look at ourselves in our daily life with such ruthless honesty. In this case, as perhaps throughout life, mechanisms of denial are useful and necessary.

The extent of this patient's use of denial was remarkable. *In fact,* her brother had formally adopted her children. *In fact,* her brother and parents had a precise knowledge of her diagnosis and prognosis. *In fact,* her personal physician had discussed her medical condition in exact detail with her. *In fact,* her relatives had been visiting regularly with her. *In fact,* she talked often and closely with many of the nursing staff.

This posthoc data indicates a substantial degree of denial of the major interest, involvement, and concern on the part of others. However, I do *not* consider this degree of denial necessarily dysfunctional nor pathological. Rather, it enabled her to maintain some degree of emotional composure. *she* set the level of awareness. I think that the interview demonstrates her need to maintain a high level of denial—but *not* total denial. And she can then continue to function so long as she can maintain denial along several fronts.

To summarize: I could push this young mother to discuss her thoughts and feelings about dying and death. I could engage her conscious awareness. I would momentarily broach her defenses of denial. However, she indicated that she needed those denial mechanisms. I would be inappropriate, inhumane, and irrelevant to suggest that she not use her denial mechanisms to maintain herself.

The Function of Withdrawal

Throughout the interview, the doctor (myself) continually came back to the patient's relationships with her family, and more specifically her children. In retrospect, my focus was out of place. I was influenced in my own thinking at that time about anticipatory grief and the problems of maintenance of relationships during the dying period. My concern was appropriate, but *out of phase.* Much earlier in her dying trajectory, this young mother no doubt was concerned about her children and family. But she is too sick now. Now she no longer has the energy or the ability to cathect others. She is withdrawing into herself. She can barely sustain herself. She has little available resource inside herself to invest in others. Time and again I tried to elicit her involvement with others. She appropriately resisted me: "I can't worry about what will happen to the kids, you know, if I can't take care of them." She is sicker than I realize. She is approaching death more quickly than I sense. I try to pull her into reality; while she is withdrawing from reality. I did not support her withdrawal, which was the only way she could now maintain herself.

The Function of Faith and Hope

This young mother says that her faith and hope sustain her. Does that mean she realistically believes she will be cured? I think not. She believes that her children will be taken care of. She believes that her doctors and nurses will give her the best possible care. She believes that it would be good to be cured, but that it is okay if she dies. Her faith and hope are not in the fantasy that things will change, but rather her assurance that her life is acceptable and her situation is tolerable as she is. She believes that it is all right to live just one day at a time. In my opinion, her faith and hope is that she is all right, she is affirming her sense of being at peace with herself.

Major Fears

It may well be that different issues provoke fear at different phases throughout the trajectory of dying. Some items suggest this in the interview.

Apparently, the fear of death did present itself early in the patient's illness. But she no longer is afraid of death. In fact, she is more comfortable than I. She challenges me when I inquire as to the fear of death. She knows—don't I know? Of course I do. But she is less afraid of death now than I am.

Early in her illness she feared for her children. But now she has attained separation from them and they are in good hands. She need no longer fear for the welfare or her relationship with them.

The fear of being a bother, a nuisance, and an imposition crops up in relation to her family. Apparently, she feared the possible anger of her family. But that has been resolved.

The fear of being alone, however, still remains. When I asked if it was tolerable to not know exactly what was going to happen, she responds: "Just—I don't want to be alone."

Finally, she repeatedly expresses her need to be able to manage—to cope, to deal with her own day-to-day existence. At the end of the interview we briefly kid about rewards for performance—star billing—or just the child's stickum star. She expresses what she needs: "A gold one." She, in my opinion, wants recognition and affirmation that she is doing a good job of doing what she can do. Recognition that she is a person doing the best she can do. She wants and needs our affirmation that she remains a person of integrity in her dying.

CONCLUSIONS

The lessons I have learned from this one patient include the following: First, that despite my years of talking with dying persons, my own anxieties about death and dying still remain close and undeniably real in my own sense of existence, ready to be stirred in every personal encounter, for this dying woman challenges my own denial of mortality. Two, that *awareness* may be confused with *denial.* I believe that this young mother demonstrated how a person can have awareness and still appropriately use denial mechanisms. I conclude that denial mechanisms are important and useful. Three, I learned that *withdrawal* rather than *engagement* becomes more important as one approaches death. Four, I observed that different fears and anxieties emerge at different phases of the dying process. In this case, I was *out of phase* with the patient, and failed to address fears of the present in the best way possible, because I was intent on fears that were no longer relevant to the patient. Five, I learned that a person needs *affirmation* of who they are. The dying person can cope with death but not loss of the sense of self-integrity.

CONCLUSIONS

II

EARLY CHILDHOOD

The first two chapters, by Carlin and by Wood, present the problem of dying in the young infant stage of life. The focus is on the family of the infant. Notice the feelings of guilt, disappointment, anger, and frustration that the parents express. In both chapters similar feelings are strongly expressed by the professional staff. In this social system there is a shared belief that the death of an infant is a tragedy. What is the meaning of bringing a malformed child into the world who will never attain normal adulthood? The struggle to make sense of this event appears to be a central issue. Ambivalence toward the infant is obvious: Shall we let the child die, or shall we struggle to keep it alive against insurmountable odds? Both authors suggest that the staff must resolve their own ambivalence and sense of helplessness before they can turn to appropriately assist the family.

The chapter by Seligman on the burned child gives an accurate picture of the primitive coping mechanisms used by the very sick child: hallucinations, delusions, manifest phantasies, and various obvious distortions of reality. These are not psychotic children but rather very sick youngsters experiencing severe stress. Thus, they rapidly fluctuate in using the primitive coping mechanisms available to the young child. Seligman illustrates the devastating emotional impact on staff and on families when the dying trajectory takes an unanticipated shift. The interaction between child, family, and staff is clearly demonstrated here.

The chapter by Towne and Wold is a contrast, with its focus on the home and family life of a chronic dying trajectory. Here they highlight the impact of dying upon the other children of the family as well as on the parents. They stress the importance of clear and accurate communication of information. They note how vulnerable the family members are to unexplored phantasies, hopes, fears, and expectations. They rightly point out that the care of the dying child involves care of the entire family system.

8

The Life of the Malformed Child

Jean E. Carlin

Unlike other chapters, which deal with conditions leading to the death of a previously normal and healthy person, this chapter deals with the dying of children, most of whom have never been normal and healthy. Many of the problems of developmental anomalies have their origins before birth and can be recognized at birth; others became apparent shortly after bith.

Thus, the primary concern will be with the unique problems faced by parents and medical personnel dealing with developmental anomalies severe enough to lead to a probable termination of life in days or months or a few years. These abnormalities are the results of genetic abnormalities; prenatal infections of the developing fetus; damage to the developing fetus as a result of toxins and drugs; damage to the developing fetus from oxygen deprivation; or interference with normal development from as yet unknown causes.

Although the etiologies (causes) are diverse, the abnormal children present many similarities with which parents and medical personnel must cope. Of primary importance is the problem of totally shattered expectations for a normal child after many months of pregnancy. Parents of normal babies are often seriously disappointed if their new baby is not the sex for which they had hoped. How much more profound is their disappointment when the baby is not "normal" as they had expected? No one can really know, unless he or she has experienced this overwhelming shock and disappointment. Much has been written on this (Gardner 1968; Menolascino 1968; Solnit, Stark 1961). *But*, little has been written about how these parents and the medical personnel cope with watching these abnormal babies live and slowly die. Also, many parents cease to have contact with these dying children, and so the medical personnel are surrogate parents.

Observations of new personnel, medical students, and resident physicians unaccustomed to facing the malformed and malfunctioning child give some clues as to how they come to terms with these realities. Parents go through similar sequences *if* they remain in contact with their children; but some parents and some employees flee the situation, and escape the denial. Denial is a frequently used method of coping, but since escape-avoidance tells little about the acceptance and integration necessary actually to care for these infants and children until their death, the option of massive and total denial will not be discussed here.

STAGES OF ADAPTATION

I have observed new staff unaccustomed to developmental anomalies progress through various stages in their adjustment. As in early childhood development, one may remain fixated at an earlier level, so, too, personnel may remain fixated at any of the following levels, thus hampering their effectiveness: Stage 1—Most medical students and uninitiated resident physicians do *not* want to see nor hear about people with severe physical and mental developmental problems. *They seek ways to avoid knowing,* trying not to come to hospitals or wards with this kind of patient, or by being late or ill. It is as if "out of sight is out of mind" will solve the problems—or *denial and escape-avoidance.*

Stage 2—When they do come and see, the next stage is one of *displaced anger*—anger displaced from they know not what, onto the hospital or ward caring for these patients, onto the doctors and nurses working with these patients, and onto the person or persons whom they perceive as responsible for sending them to work and learn in such a terrible place.

Stage 3—They enter a period of *depression* often clinically apparent and even picked up on psychological tests. Sometimes the depression immobilizes the doctor or medical student for a time to the point of being unable to get from his or her office onto the wards and he or she may even develop symptoms of physical illnesses allowing him or her to say home "sick." During this stage of depression, the whole problem of the meaning and purpose of life—everyone's life, the abnormal patient, other patients, one's family, and even one's own life—comes into focus and re-evaluation. The question of the ultimate meaning of life, which had been wrestled with in adolescence and thought to be well solved and permanently settled, again rears its threatening head and demands re-evaluation. If these maldeveloped patients are alive, why are they alive? And why am I alive? And what is life? and death? And if these anomalies exist, they *could happen to my children*! These kinds of existential meaning problems are what immobilize one's energy during this stage of depression.

Stage 4—This stage is again one of *directed anger*—but now anger directed at God or the Powers That Be, or at society for allowing such anomalies to occur and live. The problem of how can a God permit innocent babies (and families) to suffer so much haunts those who believe in God. Others become angry with a society the "allows" these children to live. And suddenly the unacceptable thought—they would be better off dead!—occurs to otherwise kind medical personnel, who are trained and committed to respecting and preserving life. This is often a frightening and unacceptable thought. Immobilization may occur because of ambivalence, that is, the strong desire to end the life of the severely maldeveloped plus the long training and commitment to saving life—all life. Anger is intensified by the ambivalence as a result of being forced to make such a choice, and one experiences a strong need for someone else to make that choice instead (a desire to be dependent).

Stage 5—*A period of resignation and helplessness*, which could be stated: These patients are people who are alive and are going to live for a time, but there are too many with too many needs; there is *nothing I can do*! This feels more comfortable than the preceding stages, but it also may immobilize for a time.

Stage 6—this stage is one of *acceptance and involvement*, which might be stated: All right, I *can't prevent* these problems yet and I *can't cure* them now and I *can't help all* of the people, but I *can begin with a few* patients and a few problems and see what I can learn and teach and accomplish. This stage is the beginning of the end of immobilization, anger, and depression. The task at hand is scaled down to bite-sized pieces and begun.

In much the same way, parents who remain involved with their retarded and/or handicapped children proceed through stages complicated by guilt and fears and misunderstandings, in addition to the above six stages.

CASE ILLUSTRATIONS

Conversations with ward personnel, medical students, resident physicians, staff doctors, and families of patients, all of whom are somewhere along the way proceeding through or beyond these six stages, have been valuable to observe. One psychiatric technician, a middle-aged woman, said "I never had any children and I have much love to give to babies, and these babies need much love. When I look at them I think it would be better if they would die because I know what is ahead for them if they live with their problems. But I learn to know each one as an individual and love him or her. And yet, when they die, I am glad."

When asked if that didn't create a conflict of interest—giving good care but hoping the patient would die—she answered, "Oh, no. I take good care of each one, and when God is ready He takes each child, and I didn't cause the child to die—we always try to keep it alive, but sometimes it is out of our hands."

An educated and sophisticated father of a profoundly retarded malformed child said, "I hope she will die soon. I want to know she is being well cared for, but I hope she will die." He claimed to be an atheist. He engaged in much discussion in his attempt to find *meaning* for this, his *third* child with the same defects. Finally, he began to ask if the hospital "experimented" on these babies. He clarified that he did not mean anything harmful to them, but rather if we attempted to learn anything from them that might eventually be of use to others. I assured him that we do study many things about our patients in an attempt to understand normal development; to study what happens when normal development has been interfered with at various stages, when enzymes are missing, or when unusual gene combinations occur. He then smiled, seemed relieved, and said, "You mean, like the sacrificial lamb—my baby's life and death might help someone else someday!" He had found a meaning to his existential problem.

One physician wrote the initial evaluation of a baby with multiple congenital anomalies, who was transferred from another hospital for care. The initial statement regarding the general appearance of the patient read, "Cute chubby little chappie, who looks perfectly normal with his clothes on." And, thus, the physician attempted to deny reality by focusing on what looked normal. This is a common phenomenon. One nurse, in discussing a baby with multiple facial and central nervous system anomalies, kept commenting on what a beautifully formed body the infant had. She had learned to attend to the few signs of normalcy to help her to keep her perspective.

One psychiatric resident insisted that he could not work with retarded patients because he himself was intellectually gifted and very verbal, and hence he has "nothing in common" with his retarded patient. After two months of almost daily contact between the patient and the resident doctor, both had changed. The resident doctor decided that the patient wasn't retarded! Because the two of them had related well and enjoyed each other, they were genuinely sad on parting. Since the doctor had not become less bright, he had to perceive that the patient was really bright to be of interest to him! The patient himself perceived that he could have friends who were not other patients, and he requested discharge to a foster home (after 13 years in the hospital for the retarded). The psychiatric resident was able to become involved with the patient's problems and only persisted in a verbal denial of his own uselessness in working with the retarded.

CONCLUSIONS

The multihandicapped infant or child with developmental anomalies, who is at or near death at all times, presents a very real threat to the inner security made up of beliefs and defense mechanisms of all who encounter him or her. Parents and medical personnel alike are forced into frequent re-evaluations of their beliefs and values and actions. It is painful and exhausting, for with each child's death, the personnel, parents, and family die a little. But, it can be challenging and rewarding. Some babies—few, but each one important—make it past the time of imminent death. An occasional comatose child awakens or a cardiac problem can be corrected. Then the child can start from there to proceed through the stages of development to the limit of his or her physical and mental potential. Others die, and their suffering has ended. And others linger on between life and death. Every tiny sign of development is noted and encouraged, and every new medical discovery is greeted with guarded optimism that some day prevention and cures might be reality. But in the meantime, what is one tiny step for mankind may be a giant step for a tiny needy patient.

It seems essential for parents and professional staff to pass through the above stages first before they can get on with the business at hand. Second, staff and families must be able to identify and appreciate those positive and normal aspects of appearance, personality, and behavior that are part of the child. Third, staff and families must be able to set short-term immediate goals that can be achieved and produce some short-term rewards. Fourth, staff and families must attain some resolution of the existential issues of ultimate meaning for their own existence and the meaning of the existence of the retarded and handicapped child—even though the life of that child may be short and unpredictable.

Once a sense of meaning has been established, even though at times that sense may be shaken, the life and death of the child with developmental anomalies become similar to the life and death of any other person.

REFERENCES

GARDNER, G., Psychogenic problems of brain-injured children and their parents. *Journal of the American Academy of Child Psychiatry* 9: 471-491, 1968.

MENOLASCINO, F., Parents of the mentally retarded. *Journal of the American Academy of Child Psychiatry* 9: 589-602, 1968.

SOLNIT, A., and F. STARK, Mourning and the birth of a defective child. *Psychoanalytic Study of the Child* 16: 523-537, 1961.

9

Meningomyelocele Infants

Paul E. Wood

The birth, life, and death of a deformed child in a family is always painful and traumatic, and such a child presents a complex emotional, social, and medical challenge. The problems encountered are not those of simple death, grief, and mourning, but they are the problems of how family, friends, and professional staff adapt and cope with the labyrinthine complexities of an oftentimes life-threatening, multifaceted, deforming handicap. In the deformity of meningomyelocele, the meninges (membranes that envelop the brain and spinal cord) and the spinal cord nerves protrude through a defect in the spine, resulting in hydrocephalus, loss of bladder and sphincter control, and varying degrees of decreased motor activity and sensation of the lower extremities. Secondary complications often include infections of the blood and/or meninges, blocked ventriculoatrial (involving the heart) shunts, eye muscle imbalance, urinary tract infections, deformities and fractures of the lower extremities, trophic ulcers, and obesity. In addition, mental retardation may also occur. The reported incidence of death in the first five years of life in these children ranges from 80 to 90 percent if untreated, down to approximately 20 percent with comprehensive medical and surgical treatment. The majority of deaths occur in the hospital in the first year of life, either in the neonatal period before the infant goes home or after repeated lengthy and costly hospitalizations.

The impact of the deformed child on the family begins at birth when the mother senses the anxiety and concern of the doctors and nurses in the delivery room. The newborn often will be whisked away to an isolation room, frequently without the mother ever seeing him or her. Later, after she asks many attendants, nurses, and doctors, someone will begin to explain honestly how her baby is different. Her shock, grief, confusion, and physical exhaustion will make it difficult for her to comprehend all that is said, but she will know that she has given birth to a deformed child. This fact will weigh heavily on her as she attempts to deal with her feelings of guilt and responsibility, which are mixed with confusion and a sense of personal inadequacy. No amount of professional reassurance or medical knowledge will assuage the guilt she feels. As one mother put it, "That baby came from my body. I made him that way. It's my fault." Another examined her period of gestation looking for clues as to what she had done wrong that caused her baby to be deformed. Many others view the deformed child as God's way of punishing them for sins they have committed.

In the midst of all this emotional turmoil, parents are confronted with the need for a decision regarding surgery on their newborn. Most commonly, physicians will advise in favor of surgery (especially in teaching hospitals), and the majority of parents will consent, feeling the doctor knows best and that the decision is really a medical one. This way, essentially allowing the physician to make the decision, reduces further guilt and responsibility of the parents, at the same time giving them a feeling that they are doing everything they can for the child. Unfortunately, most parents are so confused and ambivalent at this time that they do not adequately deal with whether or not they really want to do everything possible to save their deformed child.

The parents who refuse treatment and choose a likely death for their child are frequently of a higher socieconomic status. They may have experienced an earlier deformed child and wish not to repeat the process. In one dramatic example, a young middle class woman became pregnant out of wedlock and attempted to abort herself with an overdose of medication. She gave birth to an infant with meningomyelocele and has since devoted her entire life to the treatment and rehabilitation of her child. She shuns any adult social contacts for herself unless they are related to the treatment of her child, and in essence she has sacrificed her own life out of guilt over her deformed child. This kind of behavior does not become problematic until the child attempts to separate from the overprotecting mother, and then they both encounter serious problems. In three other similar cases, two became juvenile delinquents in adolescence and one developed psychosomatic symptoms, which forced him to stay at home with his mother.

Another example of "save the baby at all costs" behavior was a grandmother and grandfather who adopted their daughter's meningomyelocele infant and made a complete turnabout in their life-style to accommodate the child. The grandmother gave up a very good job, the family moved to the inner city to be near the hospital, and the 24-hour care of the child became their reason for living. They denied many of the child's limitations and would concentrate exclusively on her achievements. They isolated themselves from their old friends, and their only social contacts became parents of deformed children. In our group therapy, it became clear that both of these people felt very guilty about the way their own three children had turned out. Their daughter ran away at age 17, became pregnant, and was not sure who was the father of her child. Of their two sons, one had been shot to death in a drug raid and the other was in federal prison for murder. It is little wonder that they wished to devote themselves to exclusively to their daughter's grossly deformed baby in an effort to absolve themselves of some of their guilt feelings.

Less dramatic are the families who appear to accept the deformity quite routinely. These are most commonly the lower class minority families, who have known of deformity in their local community and who may, indeed, have had a sibling or relative with the deformity. They tend to appear very accepting, yet there are many evidences of denial in their behavior. They often isolate themselves and avoid talking about or revealing that their baby is deformed. An interesting example of this is the way these mothers wrap the head of their hydrocephalic baby so that only the face shows, thus concealing any evidence of deformity. In addi-tion, they are excessively overprotective and frequently allow little or no self-sufficiency or independence in the child. They also tend to overfeed the deformed child in an attempt to make him or her look fat and healthy. Behaviors such as temper tantrums, demanding one's own way, and retention of infantile habits are viewed as cute and appropriate, and therefore, do not require any intervention or confrontation from the parents. These parents tend to view their deformed children as incapable of any kind of normal, age-appropriate behavior, and they infantilize them. They do not allow them the opportunities for growth experiences that other children receive. This becomes a problem as the child reaches school age and the parental views of the child's incapability conflict with the views of his or her doctors and school officials.

A good example of this type of behavior is a 30-year-old Mexican-American mother of five, whose husband had told her not to have any more babies after the third. Her sixth infant was born with a midthora-columbar (chest and abdominal regions) meningomyelocele with hydrocephalus, incontinence, and no motor ability in the lower extremities. Her guilt over having a deformed child was expressed in thoughts when she repeatedly stated that it never would have happened if she had just done what her husband had told her.

Her behavior toward the deformed child was remarkable in her over-protectiveness and isolation of herself and her infant. She grossly overfed the baby so that at 14 months the child weighed 45 pounds and could do nothing but remain in the position in which she was placed. As the child grew older, she became the center of the family's attention, demanding and receiving anything she wanted. At age six she was still taking all her milk from a bottle, sleeping in her parent's bed, and refusing to go to school. When the school officials demanded that the child attend school, the mother came to our group for help. She quickly perceived how she was allowing her daughter to manipulate and control her, but it was with great reluctance that she was able to take a firm parenting stand and demand that the child go to school. Interestingly, after a few months in school, the child gave up many of her infantile ways and behaved quite appropriately. Her mother became depressed over the loss of her baby, and again the group helped her to understand and be a part of the growth and progress that the child was making.

On the other end of the spectrum is a middle-aged mother of three, who gave birth to a meningomyelocele baby and refused to acknowledge the infant's existence after one look at his deformed body. She referred to her infant as not yet born and denied that the deformed infant was hers. She refused to consent to any treatment for the infant, and he died shortly thereafter. In this example, the husband was interviewed and was in agreement with his wife's position. He stated that if the baby upset his normally easygoing wife to that extent, then he felt that what she was doing was best for herself and her family, and he supported her.

In another somewhat similar case, an upper-middle class mother of a normal two-year-old gave birth to a badly deformed infant and stated that she wanted nothing to do with the infant, that it would seriously intrude into her life, and she would not accept it. After this woman left the hospital, the baby was treated and some minor improvements in his condition were made. His mother later visited him at the urgings of her own mother and broke down in tears when her baby made eye contact with her. She then visited regularly and became involved with her child. However, after much thought and consultation with her husband, the woman maintained her original feelings and asked for placement of her child, with a fund to be established to pay for his care so that she would not need to know whether he was alive or dead.

The problem of ultimate death for the families of deformed children is a continuation of their problems in life. For many families, death comes as a relief from the painful, trying, daily existence they have suffered. For others, who have invested so deeply in the child, death is felt as a great loss and is mourned and grieved extensively. For still others, whose personal guilt over the deformed child is so great, the death only compounds the guilt, and these people frequently try to make up to their lost child, in death, what they feel they did not do in life. There is no set pattern of behavior exhibited when a deformed child dies, but the following case examples will serve to illustrate some typical reactions.

CASE STUDIES

CASE 1.   A young, black, professional woman gave birth to a meningomyelocele infant as her first child. Her husband left her when she refused to give up the child for placement. The child had repeated shunt infections, brain abscesses, pulmonary and urinary tract infections, and his mother stayed by his side all the time making plans to take him to the best specialists in the world. When she was told that he had a very poor prognosis with his final infection, she renewed her intensive involvement with him, spending long hours at his bedside caring for him. However, as the weeks drew on and he changed little, she decreased her visits and became less and less involved with him. At that time his condition worsened, he weakened and died. His mother accepted his death as best for both of them and resumed her professional life. It appears that her tapering off of contacts with her son demonstrated a reality-based recognition of his true status, and this helped her to deal with his death.

CASE 2.   A multiple deformed meningomyelocele baby was born to a middle class family as their first child. Because of the many deformities, he had to be hospitalized many times in the first year of his life, and he finally died at age 14 months. His family was deeply grieved at his loss because they had tried very hard to accept him and love him, and to overcome their own guilt over conceiving him. In spite of genetic counseling, this woman became pregnant again soon after the death of her son and later gave birth to an even more deformed baby. She originally tried to deny the baby and did not visit him in the hospital, but as his condition became critical, and she was notified, she visited regularly taking pictures and involving herself with her infant. He lived only six weeks, and the family appeared relieved at his death. This family did not give up, however, in their desire to have a child. They further underwent genetic counseling, established a major contributing factor in the husband's heredity, and sought artificial insemination, which proved successful and gave them a normal healthy child. Not all cases have such a happy ending, however, as demonstrated in the following two examples.

CASE 3.   An 18-year-old girl gave birth to a meningomyelocele baby with many deformities and a very poor prognosis. She demanded that every attempt be made to save her baby, claiming that it was the only thing that could hold her and her boyfriend together. After she left the hospital, she visited the baby once and was not able to be reached at the time of the baby's death. It appears that she had very little investment in her baby because most of her energy was tied up in trying to meet her own infantile needs.

CASE 4.   In another tragic case, a woman gave birth to her fourth child, a badly deformed meningomyelocele baby. Her husband rejected the baby as not being his and refused to live in the same house with the baby. When she brought the baby home, her husband fled, taking the three other children and leaving her with nothing. She tried desperately to love and accept the baby, but her grief over the loss of her husband and three children made it very difficult and she began neglecting the infant. The baby died a few weeks later, and this guilt-ridden distraught woman borrowed a large sum of money for an elaborate funeral for her dead baby in an apparent attempt to relieve her guilt.

The families of deformed children are not the only persons who become deeply involved. Hospital staffs, because of their multiple and often lengthy, intensive contacts, also face many problems in dealing with their feelings and behaviors related to deformed, dying children. No one can remain neutral and objective dealing with these children. Because the doctors, nurses, social workers, and attendants are all very human, their responses tend to be individualized and personal. They do, however, tend to fall into two major groups, which are the "every life must be saved at all costs group" and the "some babies are better off dead group." A few examples will help to clarify these feelings and behaviors.

A nursing student became intensely involved with a poor prognosis, badly deformed child who was hospitalized for a shunt revision. In her vigorous efforts to help, she regularly propped him up in an infant seat, which, unknown to her, applied pressure to his back which led the meningomyelocele to breakdown, infection, and eventual death. She was very upset when she discovered that she had contributed to his death because she had such a strong conviction that she could really help him, although others had given up.

A similar feeling was expressed by a junior resident during his stay on the ward. He expressed the view that to him death meant a medical or surgical failure, and since he viewed himself as a very fine physician and surgeon, he expected no deaths on his service. He ran into major conflict with the head nurse, a very compassionate and sensitive person who viewed death as a legitimate function of life. When a new multiple deformed infant was admitted to the service, the resident and nurse talked to the parents, who asked that no heroic measures be performed to save their baby. The resident informed them that he was the doctor in charge and would make those decisions. The infant was then placed on electronic monitoring of his vital functions with instructions to the nursing staff to notify the resident at the first sign of any abnormality. The infant underwent numerous medical and surgical procedures and treatments, and finally died three weeks later when the resident was out of town. The nursing staff and parents were relieved at the infant's death, but the resident maintained that he could have saved the life if he had been there. What he did not know was that the child had stopped eating nearly two weeks before and the nurses were not force feeding him or reporting his poor intake.

A very different view was held by the thoughtful, humble woman resident who succeeded the above resident on the ward. She did an extensive work-up on each new child and then held an in-depth interview with the parents to try to determine their honest feelings about their deformed child. She always accepted their decision to allow their child to die, and in those cases where the issues were confusing she held further conferences to clarify their feelings. This physician was loved and respected by the parents, the patients, the staff, and the other residents. The determination to turn off a respirator or not to perform heroic measures when a child dies in a hospital is always difficult, but when it is made in concert with the parents and physician it appears to be more acceptable.

A technique that has been extremely helpful and successful in dealing with the families and involved staff is regular group meetings. It is always impressive to see the interactions between families, and it is eye opening and sensitizing to the staff. The most popular themes of the groups are the successes and achievements the children have made. They share ideas and information, which is helpful to all, and frequently bring up problems and concerns, which the group handles. The issues of overprotection, isolation, sibling rivalry, discipline, marital stress, and guilt are also common concerns. The issue of death is usually avoided in favor of talk about how well the children are doing in life. When a death occurs, the group supports the bereaved parents but does not want to talk about the possibilities of it happening to them. It appears that this denial may be very important in sustaining the motivation, high energy, and sacrifice required to live day-to-day with a seriously deformed child.

REFERENCES

AMES, M. D., and L. SCHUT, Results of treatment of 171 consecutive myelomeningoceles, 1963-1968. *Pediatrics* 50:466-470, 1972.

FORD, F. R., *Diseases of the Nervous System in Infancy, Childhood and Adolescence (5th ed.). Springfield, Ill.: C. C. Thomas, 1966.*

HEWETT, S., *The Family and the Handicapped Child.* London: George Allen and Unwin, 1970.

MATSON, D. D., Surgical treatment of meningomyelocele. *Pediatrics* 42:225, 1968.

WALKER, J. H., M. THOMAS, and I. T. RUSSELL. Spina bifida—and the parents. *Developmental Medicine and Child Neurology.* 13:462-476. 1971.

10

The Burned Child

Roslyn Seligman

No sooner had I entered the Intensive Care Unit than I caught myself leaving and stopped.* I realized that my behavior was in response to the atmosphere of tension and apprehension! I remained for one hour and observed.

Carl, 10, is dying. He is on dialysis and does not respond to verbal stimuli. He appears in a great deal of distress. There is much activity and medical care around him, yet the sensed prognosis is dim and frustrating.

Bob, 11, is confused and disoriented as to his age, the time, and his father's visit two days ago. As I question him, he gets upset and then suspects that his dad is around but won't come in to see him. Bob seems to be dealing with Carl, the dying patient, by identifying with the dying and then projecting his own behavior onto his dad in expecting that his dad will ignore him. Bob looks at a dried spot of blood on his leg and becomes concerned that it will start bleeding. At the same time he compulsively covers and uncovers his genitals. This same apprehension has kept him from sleeping last night. His apparent brain syndrome, which may be organic in burned patients, seems more likely an adaptive withdrawal mechanism to this painful situation. Sam, 10, is sleeping more

*Acknowledgments: These data were collected from the Cincinnati Unit, Shriners Burns Institute; however, opinions expressed are solely those of the author. I am indebted to the Unit nursing staff for their cooperation and observations; to Bruce G. MacMillan, M. D., who dedicated so much of his life to the care of burned children and is largely responsible for the existence of the Unit; to Shirley S. Carroll, M. S. W. for gathering social history and giving moral support; to Joseph Rauh, M. D., and Barbara Allen, B. A., for critical review of the paper; and to Pat Lewis for manuscript preparation.

and Art, 15, is complaining. Librium has assisted in keeping his anxiety within manageable limits.

After observing, I talk with the nurses about this tense atmosphere. One nurse, recognizing my supportive and empathic position, acknowledged that the situation was so tense that she too had had to leave the Intensive Care Unit (ICU) for awhile this evening. In quarters as close as our ICU, apprehension is contagious. Therefore, I talk with the captain of the evening shift, hoping that a focus on the apprehension of the nursing team might lessen their anxieties and hence those of the patients.

Over the next three days, Carl improves—he can follow verbal commands. At the same time the tense atmosphere diminishes and Bob's confusion clears. Something new develops. Bob notes the condition of one of his hands, the less severely injured one. He speaks of how terrible it looks and complains of bugs crawling around it. His concern three days ago about his leg must have been a downward displacement of the apprehension he felt when he learned that parts of his fingers from both hands were missing. In addition, his concern about bleeding, likely related to anxiety about dying, is greater than his concern about his real mutilation.

The next day Carl dies. A nursing note states: "There is comparatively little confusion surrounding this event. External cardiac massage and artificial respiration are administered. The other patients appear to be sleeping. Carl's family arrives to see the body. His mother weeps loudly. The visit lasts five minutes. The curtains are pulled around his bed. Art is awake. Since the dying event, he has not asked for attention in any form and seems overly cheerful. His father visits this morning."

The morning after, another recently admitted 10-year-old, Brad, dies. The same procedure is followed. Art is on his abdomen and appears to be sleeping. His eyes are closed and he doesn't answer when his name is called. An hour after the removal of Brad's body from the ICU, Art asks his father, "Where's Brad?" The nurse, being unsure of the policy for telling patients of a death, replies, "Brad isn't here now."

Art drinks his provomalt and says no more. An hour later he asks if he too is going to die. He wants to know how many kids get out of the ICU. The nurse reassures him that Carl and Brad had been much sicker than he and that sometimes children with very large burns cannot get well. She also tells him that he is getting better and will soon move out of the ICU just as Bob and Sam have. His father is present and seems nervous but reinforces what she says. Art reveals his continued anxiety about dying in his curiosity about when he will go to the operating room, and he asks repeatedly, "How many kids get out of here?" He seems more relaxed and less demanding after his talk with the nurse.

STUDY OF A BURN UNIT

The material upon which this chapter is based comes from my observations as the child psychiatrist for children admitted to the Cincinnati Unit of the Shrine Burns Institute. In February 1968 the 30-bed Shrine Hospital opened, and my observations were made from that time until July 1972. There I saw patients on rounds, for consultations, and chaired two weekly meetings with the nursing, social service and physical therapy staffs, the dietician, and the teacher contributing. Some families were interviewed either by me or the psychiatric social worker. Much of the material is taken verbatim from nursing observations, which were recorded in a log. We used the log to get a better picture of the children's reactions and interactions within the group, a vivid and rich picture not fully appreciated by observations isolated in each individual patient's chart.

Plan of Procedure

From the initial ICU scene of responses to a dying patient, I will now describe our unit and discuss some technical aspects of burns, such as mortality rate, total body surface (TBS), total body burn (TBB), full thickness burn (FTB), and postburn day (PBD). These technical aspects are important for the understanding of the expectations and anxieties of all those involved with burned children. Hereafter, the abbreviations TBS, TBB, FTB, and PBD will be used to represent the burn terminology. Also, the fraction TBB/FTB will follow the patient's name and will represent the percentage of total body burn as the numerator and full thickness burn as the denominator.

After briefly discussing the technical aspects, I will present my case material dealing with the *potentially* dying patient. Some of these will have lived, some died. They will be divided further into those who were themselves grieving for the loss of a parent or sibling killed in the same fire. Others will be patients who responded to a death of another patient. Burns, like cancer, span all age and sex groups so that these cases will not be confined to any one age or sex. In one of our studies (Seligman, Carroll, MacMillan 1971), no survival trends related to age or sex were found.

Description of the Unit

Children, 1-day-old to 16-years-old, are admitted to the unit for acute and reconstructive treatment of burns. The unit occupies one floor of the 4-floor hospital and consists of two mirror-image wards of 15 beds each. At certain times all patients in reconstructive treatment have been housed in one ward and all acute patients in the other; at other times patients have been intermixed.

Each ward has a central nursing station that is surrounded by a semi-circle of glassed-in rooms: two 4-bed rooms, one 4-bed intensive care unit (ICU), and three 1-bed rooms. The ICU has its own nursing personnel, separate from those of the rest of the ward. The outer sides of the patients' rooms face a surrounding glass-enclosed, walkway visiting area (Seligman, Carroll, MacMillan 1972).

Mortality Rate

MacMillan states: "The mortality rate associated with flame burns in children is 25 percent, as opposed to 5 percent for hot liquids. In the absence of other associated injuries, thermal injury by itself has a predictable mortality. A child with a burn of 25 percent of the body surface will almost invariably survive in spite of inadequate therapy, whereas a burn of over 70 percent of the total body surface is associated with a mortality rate that is formidable under even the most optimal circumstances. In the 25 to 50 percent group, proper medico-surgical management will result in the survival of the majority of these patients" (MacMillan 1972).

In a recent report (National Commission on Fire Prevention and Control, 1970) to Congress and the President, the Commission stated that of all the two-year-olds treated in general hospitals for second- and third-degree burns over 45 percent of the body, only 1 in 10 survives. Of the small proportion of these children who are treated in burn centers (such as ours), more than 6 out of 10 survive. Among eight-year olds suffering second- and third-degree burns over 60 percent of the body, the national survival rate if only 2 out of 10. In burn centers among patients in this category, half survive.

In our unit, the mortality rate over two identical time periods, February 1968 through December 1969 and February 1970 through December 1971, as correlated with TBB is illustrated in Figure 1.

In 14 of the 17 children who died in the 1968-69 period, the deaths occurred between postburn day 16 and 48 (Seligman in press). Hence, my case material will include postburn day. The mortality rate of those

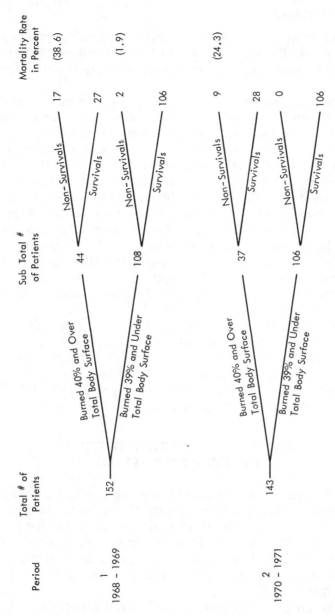

Figure 4

123

burned 40 percent and over TBS is further divided into a group burned 40 to 59 percent TBS and those burned 60 percent and over TBS (Figure 2). As can be seen from this figure, mortality rate is not a constant figure.

Percentages of total body burn and full thickness burn in children over 15 years are determined by a simplified method of estimating the amount of body surface that is burned—"the rule of nines" of Pulaski and Tennison. Each arm represents 9 percent; each leg, 18 percent; the anterior trunk, 18 percent; the posterior trunk, 18 percent; the head and neck, 9 percent; and the perineal region, 1 percent. The method of Lund and Browder (Manteuffel, Berkich 1969) is used in children under 15 years to account for their growth and, hence, their changing body proportions. Full thickness burn, according to Manteuffel and Berkich (1969, p. 4), "involves the destruction of all epithelial elements and is characterized by a dry, pearly white, or charred anesthetic surface" They further state, "Diagnosis of the depth of the burn injury can be extremely difficult, since the thickness of the skin varies according to both its location and the age of the patient."

In consideration of the factors relevant to mortality rate and the difficulty in assessing percent of full thickness burn, we acknowledge that all large burns 40 percent and over TBS are *potentially* dying patients. This fact is known among all staff, and quickly comes to be known by the patients and their families. These patients are admitted to the ICU where tensions are high until patients become well enough to move out.

RESPONSES TO DEATH AND DYING
BY PATIENTS WHO LIVED

Earlier I described the responses of Bob and Sam to Carl, the dying patient. Bob and Sam had been together 23 days in the ICU prior to Carl's admission, on their 38th PBD. Both boys had had losses; Bob lost his mother, brother, and a friend in the car accident in which he was burned, and Sam lost a friend in an accident just prior to his own injury. The conversations of these patients were filled with themes related to death and dying.

Following are two of the conversations Sam had with the nurse, one on PBD 24 and the other on PBD 38. I found it interesting that Sam took 14 days after talking of Bob's losses before he could speak of his own. His own death anxiety is revealed as he identifies partially with his friend who died. This is seen in his concern about the doctor not being available.

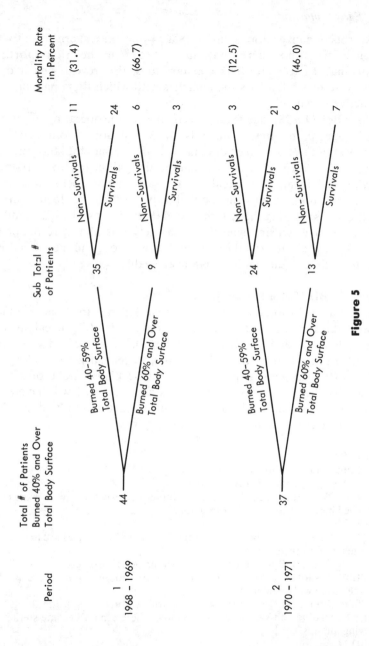

Figure 5

125

Excerpts of conversations during that 14-day interval are given to help us sense the atmosphere that Sam 61/61 (in the high mortality group)—had to tolerate. The conversations also reveal why a dying patient who dies intensifies the anxieties with which these patients have been actively dealing.

When Bob (40/28), age 11, has been taken to the operating room, Sam (61/61), age 10, inquires, "Nurse, is it true that Bob's mom died? Does he know about it?" Fourteen days later, PBD 38, Sam told the nurse that the day before he was burned, he had been a pall bearer for a friend of his who died in an auto accident. He said that a doctor was at the accident and took care of this boy's brother. When the doctor finished with the boy's dressing, he left. Sam said that this was why his friend had died. The nurse, sensing what Sam's anxiety was about, responded by saying, "We are going to take real good care of you, and there is a doctor here all the time." Sam replied that he knew this.

Excerpts: PBD 25 (for both boys)

Bob: Nurse, do you know my mother was killed in the accident? Guess she went through the windshield. She was so good. Will you call my dad? I must talk to my dad. Cover my peep (penis). I wish I could get up (said to another patient who was getting up in a wheelchair). I would not cry. Will you (to that patient) pray for my mom? (Then spoke of Jim, his younger brother, who was killed.) Jim's my brother. I will have to ask him to move my hand. It is falling down (had been complaining of pain in his badly burned hands).

PBD 26:

Bob: Get the doctors in here.
Nurse: They have already been here.
Bob: Well, they should be in here doing their work on us. I want out of this bed because this one is burning up.
PBD 27:
Bob: Get me out of here. I am tangled up in wires. My legs are in a vacuum cleaner and it squeezes them.
Sam: Shut up, Bob. You are crazy. Get me some earplugs.
Bob: I want to get out of here because this room is going to explode in flames and I will go up in flames.
Sam: (to nurse) Do you think these burns will make my urine sterile? (We later learned he had seen a television show where a man became sterile after having mumps.)
PBD 32:
Bob: When can I go home? Can I go today?
Nurse: No.

Bob: Tell my dad to come and see me. Daddy, daddy. (later) I am sorry for screaming so loud. I have to do this once in awhile at home to let off steam.
PBD: 33:
Bob: (talking of accident) Luckily, I am going to be all right. (later) Why can't I have a drink of water?
Nurse: You are going to surgery.
Bob: But, I am not Bob, I am Jim, Bob's brother. I am eight years old and the baby of the family.
Nurse: Where is Bob?
Bob: I do not know. Bob, Bob.
Nurse: What grade are you in?
Bob: He is in the second, he is little.
Nurse: Who are you?
Bob: I am Bob.

RESPONSES OF A BURNED GIRL, HER FATHER, AND THE UNIT STAFF

Martha (53/49), an 11-year-old who seemed more like 13, was burned when she got too close to her mother's Christmas gift, a commercial fireplace. Her mother, who had been ill for 18 months following the discovery of a lump in her breast (carcinoma), was admitted to the hospital four days prior to the patient's burn. Since the mother was known also to have a growing brain tumor, our patient, the oldest of five children, was being groomed to take over her mother's role. The patient's father believed that Martha did not know of her mother's tumor or of her mother's death during our patient's hospitalization. From her responses, I thought she did know.

Martha's father had described his wife as inadequate as a woman and not demonstrative. He described Martha as a tomboy and expressed concern that she would feel negative about being a woman.

Responses to a Structured Interview

Following are Martha's responses during an interview:

Dr. S.: Pretend you can have three wishes and state them.
Martha: One—to get well. Two—For mom to get well. I miss her, need her at home, and love her. And three—for all of the family to stay well and together. It is lonely without everybody together.
Dr. S.: When you grow up, what would you like to become?
Martha: An airline stewardess (her father is a travel agent who travels a lot by plane).

Dr. S.: What one person would you take to a desert island?

Martha: Nobody. I do not want to take anybody else from the family.

Dr. S.: Pretend you had a dream in which you felt ashamed.

Martha: I ran away from home because I was mad at my mother for making me do the dishes.

One day after admission (18th PBD), the following nursing note was recorded:

During her dressing change, Martha told me she had come downstairs in her nightgown to get warm by a gas logs fireplace. Her gown caught fire; the babysitter failed to put the fire out with water and ran to the neighbor's for help. Martha thought of rolling in a blanket but was afraid, and besides she did not know where a blanket was. The sitter and neighbors returned and put out the fire by putting her in water in the bathtub. I thought that was a long time to be burning, but she said it was not because the neighbor lived only a few doors away. Her brothers' and sister's screaming and crying upset her more. I inquired where her parents were. She said her mother was a patient in the hospital and her father was visiting her mother. As to why her mother was in the hospital, she stated she did not know because she did not think her father wanted her to know. Later a friend of the family visited. I told the visitor of my conversation with Martha. The visitor seemed surprised because she knew Martha's father had told two of her brothers that the mother would not be returning home because she had a brain tumor and was not expected to live. The visitor added that she had never heard Martha speak of her mother returning home, either before her burn injury or since.

Excerpts From Martha's Clinical Course

On her 24th PBD, Martha's father surprised her by visiting a day earlier than expected. She cried, then asked about her mother. Her father said her mother was the same. (Actually, her mother had died a few days before.) Later that day during dressing change, the conversation was as follows:

Martha: Daddy, I am sorry. I am a bad girl.

Nurse: You are not a bad girl.

Martha: Yes, I am bad and I am stupid.

Nurse: Are you mad at yourself?

Martha: Yes.

PBD 28: During whirlpool and dressing change:

> Nurse: Martha, cry instead of screaming.
> Martha: I cannot cry. I do not know how to cry.
> Nurse: Could you cry before you were burned?
> Martha: Yes, but I have not cried since.
> Nurse: Crying would be easier on you than screaming.
> Martha: I cannot. I just do not know how to make tears.

NURSE'S NOTE. Martha is very uncomplaining. She grits her teeth and hyperventilates and then screams when the pain gets too severe. As soon as the episode is over, she immediately stops screaming. While being buttered, she screams only when touched. Last week patient stated, "It isn't fair; it isn't fair." She was referring to the pain she was going through. She further stated, "It feels like everybody is so mean and that they want to hurt me, but I know that they don't. They all work so hard for me."

One patient in the ICU was moaning and groaning loudly, another was crying as blood was being drawn, and then Martha cried out, "I'm going to die." She continued, "Daddy come save me. I'm sorry." Two days later when Martha was being moved out of the ICU to a room where she could be weighed on a special kind of bed, the patient who earlier had been crying asked, "Why are they moving Martha out?" After the nurse explained, this patient replied, "Okay." I think he was anxious that she had died and, if she had, that his crying had been the cause.

ANOTHER NURSING NOTE. Martha's course is slowly downhill. She has been alert but talking as though her tongue was very thick. She cries for her father and continues saying that she is sorry for everything, like putting us to so much trouble. I explain that this is our job and we are glad to help to get her better. Her father called last night and arrived at two A.M. He visited for an hour. An uncle visited for five minutes and left saying, "I can stay no longer. It is too much for me." Her father returned and visited for a brief period. Later, Martha was apologetic for having fallen asleep during her father's visit. She cried and asked for him to come back.

A LATER NURSING NOTE. I met Martha's father in the gowning room. He asked me how Martha was, and *he* said, "It is only a matter of time, isn't it?" I told him that we were doing our best and that the best we could do right now was to pray. He agreed. He was very emotionally upset, shaking, and near tears. He visited alone briefly with Martha. I noticed he was sitting there crying silently, and so I joined him for awhile. I told him it was not necessary for him to stay, and he said he just wanted Martha to know he was there. I told him she knew. He replied yes and said he would be leaving. He lingered a few more minutes while crying and kissed her saying, "Goodbye Martha, I love you." He left crying heavily. Fifteen minutes later she passed away.

Reactions the Next Day

The day following Martha's death, the following note appears:

Walter (51/49), an almost seven-year-old, continually starts screaming and sitting up in bed for no apparent reason. This time he was screaming for dad. When I asked him why, he said, "I am going to die. I am going to bleed to death and I want my daddy." Even though this patient had not been in the ICU with Martha, he must have sensed the gloom that surrounded the unit in response to her death.

Sixteen days later he celebrated his seventh birthday and was noted to be feeding himself and pleased with his birthday. On PBD 41, three days later, he was noted to be in good physical condition. His parents visited and he ate a large meal. He then became nauseated, vomited, sat up in bed, turned blue, and once again cried out, "I'm going to die," and expired. The response to this unexpected tragedy is not noted in the log. I do not recall this patient. I do wonder if the unexpected and sudden death of a patient who was thought to be doing well was too much for the group to note our response, especially since Walter's death followed so soon after Martha's.

RESPONSES OVER A 10-DAY-PERIOD TO TWO UNUSUAL DEATHS

The responses to the deaths of Bessie and Scot are separated into those of the staff, the other patients, families of the two children, and families of other burned children still living.

This separation is for clarity, but the reader should remember that all of these actions and interactions were going on simultaneously, one response feeding into another, yielding a complex picture.

The Sudden and Unexpected Death:
Responses of the Staff

One Saturday evening Bessie (35/25), a six-year-old, died on her 90th PBD. She was the Unit's first death in a patient who had gotten better, moved out of the ICU, and was beginning to walk. The next morning the charge nurse called to tell me of Bessie's death and to ask how to respond to the other patients who were beginning to ask questions. I indicated I would come in. I did so to learn more about the Unit responses to the death as well as to learn more about the issues that were inhibiting the nurses in handling the situation.

As I talked with three nurses together, I realized they were identifying with the nurse who had been caring for Bessie last evening. They had some conflict around the issue of whether or not this nurse had been negligent, and they feared that other staff, patients, and their families might share this concern. One nurse kept saying, "Im afraid of what the children might ask." When I asked what could be so terrible in the children's questions, she answered by an association. She recalled that while she was caring for Bessie in the ICU, Bessie threw a temper tantrum, quit breathing, and turned blue for a moment. In other words, Bessie could easily have died under her care at an earlier time. During still another temper outburst in the ICU, Bessie had had to have her closed tracheostomy reopened.

After looking at the other nurses' identification with this nurse and their feelings that she might have played a role in Bessie's death, we were able to move on to more of the reality factors involved. Twenty minutes had elapsed between the time Bessie had been given her capsule and the time she had vomited and aspirated. Recognizing this somewhat relieved the nurses, who then were able to respond to the questions of some of the children, and the apprehension of others, who could not yet acknowledge what they had either observed, heard, or sensed.

That evening I phoned the nurse who had been caring for the now deceased patient. She did not sound responsible for the death either in the description of her own feelings or of the event. She described having given the patient her capsule, which she swallowed, and then 20 minutes late complained that she was having trouble getting it down. Then she gave Bessie some bread; Bessie began to request water, which she received. She demanded more water and then threw a temper tantrum, stopped breathing, and turned cyanotic. The doctor arrived quickly and pressed on Bessie's chest, only to have fluid ooze from her mouth and nose. With the failure of these resuscitation efforts, she was pronounced dead. Bessie had complained earlier of having trouble breathing but at that time was not cyanotic.

Five days later in my regular staff meeting, Bessie's death and its surrounding events were still disturbing to the Unit staff; clearly they wanted to talk more about it. They asked what had happened and I indicated that their version of the story was as good as anyone else's. With encouragement they were able to volunteer their ideas. Many thought the nurse caring for the deceased patient had been at fault. Only one of the nurses had been able to approach this nurse to ask directly about the event; the others felt that asking would put the nurse on the spot. I saw this as a reflection of their own feelings that this nurse was responsible in some way.

Excerpts from Bessie's Life: Understanding Death Through Life

Since Bessie should not have died when she did (she had lived through 90 days since being burned), the nursing staff and I explored the meaning of living (versus dying) for Bessie. We did this through looking at Bessie's previous role and her anticipated role in her family. In the history was marital rift. At the time of the fire the evening Bessie was burned, her father was out. Her two-year-old brother, Shep, died in the fire. Prior to Bessie's mother being able to visit her (the mother was being treated elsewhere for burned hands), one nurse wrote, "There appears to be sincere love in this father for Bessie." On an early PBD, Bessie's father heard by phone from her mother that a television news item reported Bessie as having died. (She had not.) When her mother was able to join the father with Bessie, joy and sorrow prevailed. Together they cried over the loss of Shep and then sang, "Swing Low, Sweet Chariot." Thereafter, mother and father talked frequently of replacing Shep with another baby.

This tragic story appeared in newspapers across the country. Gifts poured in. When her mother would visit, even before asking how Bessie felt, she would say, "Oh, we got so many packages, Bessie." Throughout, the message I heard the mother giving was that illness and death have more value than life.

Responses to Bessie's Death by Her Parents and Parents of the Other Burned Children

Many of the families of our burned children live far away. To accommodate their visiting over a prolonged period, the Shrine Unit has found a boarding house within walking distance of the hospital. In this close living situation, these families share each other's suffering, anxieties, and even some joyous moments. Each person's response to the other is not only predicated by the daily events, including death and dying, but also on individual personalities and how they rub each other.

Bessie's mother had moved into the boarding house the evening before Bessie's death. Following Bessie's death, her mother came to the glass-enclosed walkway visiting area and banged on the window, while screaming "My God, my God." Those mothers in the boarding house whose children were getting better became apprehensive. They had had the feeling that after their child had gotten beyond the acutely ill stage, they could give a sigh of relief.

This unexpected death on a 90th PBD reawakened all previous parental fears. Now the feeling was one of hopelessness. Each became concerned that her child might do the same as Bessie. One of the mothers, closely attached to her seven-year old son, fainted in our lobby prior to visiting her son. We had been trying to loosen this attachment, but this event only cemented it. Her son's response was to have abdominal pains.

Responses by the Other Patients

Having presented Bessie's death, the responses of the nurses, the behavior of her mother, and the intensified apprehension of the other parents, we can now view the responses of the other children within the context of this social interaction. In general, two initial responses occurred. Either the other children acknowledged that they knew by asking questions or they acted as if they knew nothing and wished not to know. In the room next to Bessie were three boys. They had witnessed the behavior of Bessie's mother. Sam (61/61) asked questions; his two younger roommates could do so only a day later. A nine-year-old boy (41/18) in a recovery stage, who had observed the resuscitative efforts, could also ask questions; Bessie's roommate, a six-year-old, could not talk about her observations. Jean, a teen-ager in the ICU, asked questions; Scot (55/47), a 14-year-old, was much sicker and did not appear to know.

Two days later, Scot and a nurse conversed.

> Scot: I am glad that little girl died like she did. She died like my daddy, instantly.
> Nurse: What little girl, Scot?
> Scot: Bessie. May I have some water?

Nurse: Just one minute, please.
Scot: I wish every voice was as reassuring as yours.
Nurse: Thank you, Scot.

Scot was injured in an auto accident in which his father burned to death at the wheel. The man who pulled Scot from his jammed seat belt said, "You're lucky. That man at the wheel burned to death."

Scot would vacillate between grieving the loss of his father and denying that his father was dead. However, his unconscious never denied that death. He continually dreamed of his father bursting into flames as he was reaching out to him.

While having much pain on his 15th PBD, Scot conversed with the nurse.

Scot: I want to die and I will try all day tomorrow to kill myself. Is my father okay? Is he dead? My mother told me he was not, but I'm not sure. I believe her.
Nurse: You will have to ask your mother.
Scot: Please show me the pictures of my father.

NURSE'S NOTE.   Was unable to reassure Scot and calm him. After receiving Demerol, he slept.

During the month prior to Scot's death, his surgical resident and he became very attached. Scot told this doctor that he had replaced his father. The doctor rotated to another service shortly after Bessie's death. Scot responded by saying that he could not deal with losing two fathers in one month.

Several days later he told his mother that he was praying to die and hoped to join his father. He asked if she would forgive him. She prayed with him. He also learned that he would have two stubs for hands and might lose a leg. He told her that most of his life he had been ridiculed for being fat, and now he could not take the ridicule he anticipated for having two stubs and one leg. Two days later, while talking to the doctor, he suddenly stopped breathing. Resuscitation attempts failed.

Five days before Scot's death, his legs showed no evidence of Pseudomonas (a bacterial) infection. At autopsy he had Pseudomonas infection on his legs, but "surprisingly there is no Pseudomonas of the viscera (internal organs)," the prosector stated. Even though Scot's 57-year-old mother and I had excellent rapport, her communication that she wanted to see me the day before his death never reached me. No nursing notes were recorded in the log revealing Scot's desire to join his father.

Scot's mother looks at life in a very realistic fashion. She exuberates both warmth and hardness in that she feels that if you really love someone you cannot wish for them to live and be a cripple if that would bother them. She felt that his death was really the best answer to his prayers. She explained this by telling me about his family and their "sensitivities." These sensitivities referred to suicide attempts and successful suicides in members of the family. I sensed she had communicated to him what I was hearing; namely, that it might be better if Scot did not get well because she might not be able to tolerate having a crippled son. She feared that she did not have many years left and Scot left alone as a cripple would commit suicide as had other relatives. She much preferred the natural death that occurred.

Unit Responses the Next Day

Mike (41/18), whose mother had been close to Scot's, and Sam asked questions about who was in the ICU. Only gradually could they ask directly about Scot. Mike would ask his mother where Scot's mother was. Our approach was to answer these questions simply and truthfully. We did not tell the sick children who were not asking; we felt not asking meant "I am not ready to hear." Jean, the teen-ager, said how brave Scot was with all his burns. Now she seemed ashamed to complain. During dressing change she stated, "Scot, oh Scot. Where's Scot?" She was asked what she meant. She replied, "I know he is in heaven with his dad, but where are they keeping him? His mother is so brave. She is such a wonderful woman."

Two days later Sam and I had a discussion regarding the time the children should be told. He thought waiting until they asked would be better because telling them before they were ready might be too upsetting.

PERSONAL RESPONSES

Two other cases I wish to comment about briefly are a 14-year-old-boy, Tim (87/44), and a five-year-old girl, Beth (47/43). Tim was remarkable, as was the staff's response to him. In spite of extensive burns, operations, and amputations, he survived for 55 days. On the day he returned from the operating room with his scalp covered by a surgical dressing (his scalp had been the only site of his body previously without an injury), the nursing staff was shocked and angered. Their anger was directed at the surgeon. They felt that Tim had been through so much that injuring the only untouched spot was unfair. Shortly thereafter, Tim died. I believe he sensed the change in the nurses' attitudes and then gave up his hope and desire to live. In contrast to Tim's intense relationship with the staff, Beth never responded and never protested. She related only to her older sister, who traveled 300 miles to visit, but she was not part of Beth's current household; no other family member came. Her mother had no phone. Beth showed no desire to live; she lingered until her quiet death.

The deaths of all the children described affected me, but two were especially difficult. The one that was most painful and still has effects today, many years later, is Scot, who prayed to die. His qualities, to which I could make meaningful associations within my own life, made my response to his dying and death an intense one. My understanding then of the dynamics of my response did not lessen the pain. In his feelings about being painfully teased about his obesity, I could identify with a favored relative. In his desire to be an oceanographer and contribute to science, I saw that which I value. In his mother I saw the strength, warmth, and concern for her child that reminded me of my own parents. The day after Scot's death, when I talked with his mother, she did not weep; I did. Months later when she visited and called, we had dinner together. With no other family has that occurred. My failure to help Scot was troublesome to me as a doctor, whose role is to help people live, and especially to me as a psychiatrist, whose role was to help Scot deal with his grief about his father. In both of these, I had to accept my failure. My associations with this family intensified the loss. I received some comfort from his mother's position; I knew she understood Scot enough to judge what was best for him. Even so, when at dinner that evening she talked of her loneliness, I knew she was in the midst of her own grief work.

In contrast to Scot, I never knew Beth; she never gave me a chance. Again, I was a failure but in a different way. The frustration and disappointment of not being able to help a lonely and dying child is, indeed, painful.

Fortunately for us on the Unit, we meet some who through their will to live let us help. For example I was called to see a teen-age boy, Ralph, burned over 90 percent TBS, the result of an industrial accident. He had requested to see himself in the mirror, and the nurse wanted to know whether he should or not. After talking with Ralph, I said, "Let him do whatever he wishes." In my interview with him I was impressed with his strengths and ability to accept his position. Later I called to ask what his response had been. The nurse stated he said, "Gee, it's not as bad as I thought it was going to be." This boy came from a very warm, close family. His mother was caring for him each day. His girlfriend, as well, faithfully visited. Ralph emphasizes my impression that we can help those patients who through their families or through our staff find enough warmth and interest to wish to live. In contrast, Scot and Beth emphasize that those who do not have hope for whatever reason do not live no matter what our efforts are.

In summary, I have presented variations on the living, dying, and death theme in a burned child's life. I have seen, as I have tried to indicate by case material, many different ways of coping or not coping. In my own opinion, we have not adequately studied dying and death. Neither have we dealt adequately with the dying patients and their families. In the Shrine Unit, when the child dies, the family returns home. I have no follow-up data except in Scot's instance to say whether or not these families are able to grieve adequately. Money and professional time for and interest in dealing with the emotional understanding and needs of burned children and their families have lagged far behind the medico-surgical advances. Three of my previous studies (Seligman, Carroll, MacMillan 1972; Seligman in press; Seligman, MacMillan, Carroll 1971) report on this neglected area and present some ideas to help remedy the situation.

REFERENCES

MACMILLAN, B.G., Management of burns in children, in *Pediatric Therapy*, ed. H.C. Shirkey. St. Louis: Mosby, 1972.

MANTEUFFEL, S.V., E.J. BERKICH, *The Burn Patient: Management and Operating Room Support.* New York, Ethicon Corp., 1969.

National Commission on Fire Prevention and Control, 1970.

SELIGMAN, R., A psychiatric classification system for burned children. *American Journal of Psychiatry,* 131: 41–46, 1974.

SELIGMAN, R., S. CARROLL, B. G. MACMILLAN, The burned child: emotional factors and survival, in *Proceedings of the Third International Congress for Research in Burns,* ed. P. Matter. Bern, Switzerland: Huber Publishers, 1971.

———, Emotional responses of burned children in a pediatric intensive care unit. *Psychiatry in Medicine* 3:59-65, 1972.

SELIGMAN, R., B.G. MACMILLAN, S. CARROLL, The burned child: a neglected area of psychiatry. *American Journal of Psychiatry* 128:84-89, 1971.

11

Childhood Leukemia*

Brenda D. Townes / David A. Wold

In the past two decades, there has been about a 50 percent increase in the incidence of cancer in childhood. Accompanying this increased frequency, the life-span in childhood leukemia has been increased from an average of three months to a current median of over 21 months. Thus, replacing the past expectation of imminent death, parents of a youngster with leukemia are now exposed to the prolonged anxiety of a critically ill child for whom painful medical procedures, hospitalizations, remissions, and ultimate death are predicted.

In a seminar in 1965, the director of the hematology program at Children's Orthopedic Hospital and Medical Center in Seattle asked, "Why do some families and some individuals within families disintegrate in the presence of prolonged illness and death of a child with leukemia? Why do other families appear to draw closer together? Can mental health professionals help by identifying factors that facilitate and interfere with adjustment to the death of a family member?"

Participants in the seminar responded, "How can you evaluate death; it is not a researchable question?"

ADAPTATION OF FAMILIES TO LEUKEMIA STUDY

A few months later, in the summer of 1965, a three-year investigation was initiated to study the adaptation of families to a child with leukemia. Parental interviews and multiple tests and questionaires were completed

*This work was supported in part by grants MH 12548 and CA 04937 from the USPHS, and grant 5 107A66 from NIH.

by eight families at yearly intervals. Findings have been reported elsewhere concerning parental (Townes, Wold, Holmes in press; Wold, Townes 1969) and medical staff (Wallace, Townes 1969) responses to the dying child. This chapter discusses the impact of the degree of parental communication about the diagnosis and prognosis of childhood leukemia upon siblings' adaptation to the dying process.

Subjects

Sixteen families, each with a child under treatment for leukemia at the Hematology (blood study) and Oncology (tumor study) Division located at Children's Orthopedic Hospital and Medical Center, were approached to participate in a study of sibling adjustment to the prolonged illness and death of a child. Of the 16 families, 4 had no healthy siblings, 2 did not wish to participate in the study, and 2 had only one sibling less than two years of age. The remaining 8 families, with a total of 22 healthy siblings, were followed at yearly intervals.

At the onset of the study, 6 out of 8 of the children with leukemia were of preschool age, two were of school age. Five were males, 2 females, and the data on the last child was incomplete. Of the 22 healthy siblings, 3 were 4 years of age or less, 11 were between the ages of 5 and 8 years, and 8 children were 9 years of age or over. There were 10 males and 12 females among the siblings.

Methods

The healthy siblings of the children who had leukemia were tested individually during the summers of 1965, 1966, and 1967; this was on the average approximately 10, 20, and 32 months, respectively, following the diagnosis of leukemia. The parents rated on the Communication Questionnaire each sibling's knowledge that the child with leukemia was ill, had leukemia, and might die; parents indicated how much the sibling had been told, how much the sibling had asked questions, and how much the parents thought the sibling knew about his or her brother's or sister's disease. Both parents completed for each sibling the Symptom Checklist (Wimberger, Gregory 1968), a quantitative measurement of each sibling's academic and interpersonal adjustment. The sibling then estimated on the Silhouette Test (Colvin 1964) the adequacy of his or her own and the ill child's health and his or her expectation concerning the longevity of him- or herself and the child with leukemia.

The Child with Leukemia

All parents were concerned about the handling of their child with leukemia. Many questions arose from the parents' uncertainty of the ill child's understanding of his or her condition and the amount of information he or she should be given. Parents almost always told the preschool child only that he or she was sick and did not explain either the diagnosis or prognosis. For the older child with leukemia, the question was how to provide information relevant to leukemia while still maintaining hope:

> Gary H., 13 years old, was so inquisitive about the true nature of his disease (he was told he had anemia) that nurses had to make sure the whole clinic area was devoid of any materials mentioning leukemia. After two years of treatment, he walked in front of a car. Although he was not injured seriously, suicide, based upon knowledge of the seriousness of his condition, was considered as the motive. Susan S., age 15, was never told about leukemia by anyone right up to her death, but she wrote a paper for school on leukemia and death and talked freely to an adult friend of the family about it. Noel L., age 13, finally was told about his illness a few weeks before his death and was noted by the staff to be calm and serene at his moment of death. Mrs. S., mother of Alan S., related to an interviewer that her son asked her what he would be "next time" while receiving a transfusion only three weeks after diagnosis of leukemia. He was very pleased and relieved that he could be anyone he wanted to be, including himself, once again (Wold, Townes, 1969, p. 5).

The clinical impression was that avoiding a child's question about the nature of his or her illness may increase the child's distress and anxiety. Relevant information in response to specific questions from the dying child provided relief and reassurance to that child.

The Healthy Sibling

At the period closest to the time at which the diagnosis of leukemia had been established (approximately 10 months from diagnosis), the greatest amount of parental communication concerning the disease was directed toward the sibling over 9 years of age. Communication decreased with age, with little parental communication to the sibling of less than 5 years of age. By the second evaluation period (approximately 20 months from diagnosis), there was no difference in the amount of parental communication relevant to the disease between the 5- to 9-year-olds and the oldest siblings. By the final evaluation period (approximately 32 months from diagnosis), 5 out of 8 of the children with leukemia had died; the siblings were aware of the diagnosis and prognosis regardless of age.

The healthy sibling's understanding of the seriousness of leukemia also was related to the age of the sibling. The sibling older than 9, early in the progression of the disease, understood that the child with leukemia was in poor health and would live a short time. In contrast, the younger sibling at the time of diagnosis thought that the child with leukemia would live a long time and that he or she was not very sick. A year later, however, both the younger and older siblings saw the child with leukemia as being very sick and as having a short amount of time to live. As parental communication about the implications of leukemia increased, and the sibling experienced the illness of his or her brother or sister, the sibling realistically evaluated the illness as life threatening.

The shift toward a realistic understanding of leukemia was not the same for boys as for girls. Between the 10-month and 20-month period following the diagnosis, boys as a group saw the child with leukemia as becoming healthier; girls expressed a realistic understanding of the ill child's deterioration. Simultaneously, a greater amount of parental communication was directed to boys, while parental communication remained constant toward girls. Parents' communication to their sons may have conveyed misinformation with a resulting distortion in boys' understanding of the disease. More likely, however, parents may have increased communication to their sons to correct misperceptions and to avoid maladaptive denial of the stress upon the family.

Although the direction of the relationship between parental communication and boys' development of a realistic understanding of leukemia is not clear, our results showed a relationship between parental communication and adjustment as measured by the Symptom Checklist. Early in the course of the disease, poor adjustment was associated with little communication from mother concerning the nature of the disease; more adjusted siblings regardless of age or sex had greater communication from mother. Poor adjustment also was associated with an unrealistic concept of the seriousness of the illness. Thus, those siblings who adjusted best, immediately following the diagnosis of leukemia, were those who obtained information about leukemia and who achieved a realistic understanding of the nature of the disease.

Following the death of the child with leukemia, poor adjustment among the siblings was related to age and sex. Boys and older children had more academic and interpersonal problems than girls and younger siblings. Thus, family communication concerning the nature of the disease interacted with sex and age in determining the adequacy of siblings' understanding of illness and their adjustment to the dying process.

Following the death of the child with leukemia, poor adjustment among the siblings was related to age and sex. Boys and older children had more academic and interpersonal problems than girls and younger siblings. Thus, family communication concerning the nature of the disease interacted with sex and age in determining the adequacy of siblings' understanding of illness and their adjustment to the dying process.

One goal of the study was to begin to identify factors facilitating and inhibiting adjustment of the healthy siblings to the prolonged illness and death of a child with leukemia. In doing so, the expectation was that this information would assist medical personnel in counseling parents and siblings faced with a prolonged terminal illness. Several factors were identified that were associated with relatively poor adjustment following the death of a child with leukemia. In the following composite picture, no one factor or no combination of factors are meant to imply that a sibling will or will not have difficulty; it represents a beginning attempt to identify a group of siblings with a high probability of having a difficult adjustment to the stress of a dying child.

The sibling who had most difficulty adjusting to the illness and death of a brother or sister was a first born male who was over 6 years of age at the time the diagnosis was established. His mother tended to be extremely anxious, particularly during the initial phases of the disease. If he was over 10 years old, he also received little information from his parents about the nature and seriousness of the disease during the first year of his brother or sister's illness. Over the two- to three-year period, this sibling's concept of the disease shifted away from a realistic understanding of it. He viewed the child with leukemia as becoming less healthy; he saw the dying child's longevity increasing or his own decreasing. His parents noted behavioral disturbances at school and at home or they were afraid such disturbances might occur at some time in the future. Following the death of the child with leukemia, this sibling was most likely to have academic and interpersonal difficulties as a response to the prolonged anxiety and family disruption resulting from a critically ill child who experienced painful medical procedures, hospitalizations, remissions, and ultimate death.

Summary

Eight families of children with leukemia were studied over a three-year period to begin to identify factors that determine the adequacy of healthy siblings' adjustment to the dying process. *The amount of parental communication was found to be one central factor determining the adequacy of adjustment.* The type of information imparted to the siblings relative to the disease was not studied; this remains a critical problem for parents, physicians, and mental health personnel to explore. Our experience implied, furthermore, that children's responses to the dying process is a researchable phenomenon. *Parents, staff, and children can and need to communicate with one another so as to cope with and understand the dying process.*

REFERENCES

COLVIN, R. W., A study in family diagnosis and treatment for preschool retarded children and their parents. *International Copenhagen Congress on the Scientific Study of Mental Retardation.* Denmark, August 1964.

TOWNES, B. D., D. A. WOLD, and T.H. HOLMES, Parental adjustment to childhood leukemia. *Journal of Psychosomatic Research,* in press.

WALLACE, E., and B.D. TOWNES, The dual role of comforter and bereaved. *Mental Hygiene.* 53(3):327-332, 1969.

WIMBERGER, H. D., and R. J. GREGORY, A behavior check list for use in child psychiatry clinics. *Journal of the American Academy of Child Psychiatry* 7: 677-688, 1968.

WOLD, D.A., and B.D. TOWNES, The adjustment of siblings to childhood leukemia. *The Family Coordinator.* 18(2):155-160, 1969.

MIDDLE CHILDHOOD

The three chapters in this part raise a number of similar points in the care of the school age child. First, the child at this age has acquired considerable skills in reading, rational understanding, and environmental sensitivity. Thus, the child at this time is most likely to respond to many of the cues about him, although he does not necessarily tell other people how much he really knows. Therefore, the authors repeatedly stress the need for clear and accurate sharing of information with the child, his family, and with staff in the hospital as well as in the community.

Second, the authors stress that the child does acquire a sense of his or her own death. Yet the focus of the child's concern is much more on everyday activities, his own personal friendships with siblings and friends, and concern with his own body. All the authors stress the importance of maintaining valued everyday activities, the importance of avoiding too much attention to the disease process, and the maintenance of peer relationships.

Third, these chapters highlight the importance of the family relationships. The chapter by Mattson carefully documents the family dynamics that exist before a fatal illness, which may then disable family function when stressed by a dying child. Similarly, in the chapter on accidents, Easson points out how guilt, blame, anger, and confusion can be generated between parent and child. Finally, Toch describes how successfully the dying child can cope with his or her illness when there is a carefully orchestrated effort among all those involved with the child.

Fourth, in terms of dying trajectories, it would appear that the acutely ill child needs support and reassurance, whereas the chronically ill child needs more specific information and carefully guided daily living. Furthermore, the chronic living-dying interval should be geared as much as possible toward life as usual, rather than as a preparation for death.

12

A Death in a Family
of Hemophiliacs

Ake Mattson

This chapter describes the impact of death and of fears of dying in a family with two hemophilic boys. Hemophilia is a life-long serious illness, almost exclusively of males, and characterized primarily by bleeding into the soft tissues and joints. The bleeding tendencies are due to clotting defects transmitted as sex-linked recessive traits by carrier mother to recipient son. Consequently, half of a carrier's sons are hemophiliacs and half of her daughters are carriers.

There are two types of hemophilia—classic hemophilia and Christmas disease. Clinically, the two types are practically indistinguishable. Most patients with hemophilia show an onset of symptoms in early childhood. They are subjected to repeated bleeding episodes, often causing severe pain, requiring immobilization, hospital admissions, and various treatment procedures. Despite recent improvements in the treatment of acute hemorrhages with concentrated plasma-fractions and greatly increased chances for a normal life-span, the constant threat of a bleeding episode that might prove fatal looms over the young hemophiliac and his family.

Working as a liaison child psychiatrist to pediatrics, I was introduced to the family when their two hemophilic sons, Andy and Bill, were 8 and 10 years old. Both boys showed a high clinical severity of hemophilia; that is, their antihemophilic blood level was less than 1 percent of normal. A sister, 11 years of age, complemented the family, who were devout Catholics. The father worked long hours as a security guard, while the mother augmented the family income by a weekend job as a supermarket clerk. Both parents were in their late thirties. Bill was found to be a hemophiliac at 8 months of age, and his family history showed that his maternal grandfather and two maternal cousins were known hemophiliacs. During Bill's first 10 years of life, he required about 30 hospital admissions, mainly due to hemorrhages into his large joints. Some of these admissions had lasted for several months due to protracted orthopedic treatment. Bill's bleeding episodes were more serious than those of his brother. Both Bill and Andy showed cycles of increased bleeding tendency several times a year. From the time that Bill was 8 years old and Andy 6, they would assist each other in taking care of minor bleeding and bruises. Bill was described as calmer, less daring, and less active than Andy. When the boys began to play outside by themselves, the mother ceased to watch them constantly, as she had done earlier, worrying about hurts and hemorrhages.

Andy, the younger brother, had experienced 20 hospital admissions by the time he reached 8 years of age. Most of his bleeding episodes involved the soft tissues and muscles, and infrequently the joints, in contrast to his brother Bill. The mother stressed that Andy seemed more happy, more alert and spirited than Bill, even at times of painful bleeding episodes.

The developmental milestones of both boys were described as normal. The parents had tried to raise them as normally as possible and had allowed them a fair amount of physical activities with their peers after age 3 to 4. The boys had always related well to other children, and often joined in neighborhood baseball games, using plastic bats and balls to minimize the risk of injuries.

The mother was the main disciplinarian in the family, although both boys often expressed fears of causing their father to get angry at them during his brief periods of time with the family. No behavior problems were reported in either son. With certain pride, the mother mentioned that Bill and Andy often took care of small injuries themselves by applying ice packs to bleeding sites and assisting each other. Indeed, from about age 6, both boys showed much evidence of a good psychosocial adjustment to their chronic illness.

Before her marriage, the mother knew she was a carrier of hemophilia, for her father was a hemophiliac and her two sisters had hemophilic boys. In the presence of his sister, she had told her future husband of the possibility for bearing hemophilic sons, "so that all would be out in the open and honest before we got married." In retrospect, both parents felt that they had counted "a little too heavily" on the odds of having boys who were not hemophiliacs. Occasionally, the father would mention his wish for healthy boys with whom he could roughhouse.

Clearly the mother has assumed most of the child rearing responsibilities and allowed the father to work long hours away from home. She also excused the father for his infrequent visits to their sons during their hospital admissions for hemorrhagic episodes.

The mother often spoke in glowing terms about her hemophilic father's stoic attitudes toward his serious illness. She recalled his telling her how he, as a teen-ager and unaware of what was ailing him, often would go to the slaughterhouse to drink fresh blood from killed animals in the belief that this would cure his bleeding disorder. Her father seemed to have minimized physical discomfort and fears associated with his hemorrhages all through his life, and managed his life situation quite well until he died of cancer of the stomach at age 63. The mother's admiration for her father and his seemingly adaptive denial of his chronic disease probably were reflected in her own tendency to minimize her sons' disorder and remain hopeful even at times of critical bleeding episodes.

When observed in the hospital, visiting one of her ill sons, the mother always seemed calm, cheerful, and efficient in attending to her child. In addition, she had been remarkably successful in soliciting blood donors to replace the large amounts of plasma that often were required to treat her sons.

At 9 years of age, Andy had enjoyed a good year with no serious bleeding. He was proficient in many age-appropriate sports and games. Following a strep throat infection, he was admitted to the hospital for the care of bleeding into the soft tissues of his pharynx, which caused breathing difficulties and soon required a tracheotomy. After a few days, exchange transfusions became necessary, as Andy developed circulating anticoagulants. He remained alert and cooperative, despite the tracheotomy and strict bed rest, and appreciated any opportunity to engage with various ward staff members in playing games, reading, and watching television. Andy's good cooperation seemed to be sustained by the parents' assurance that both they and Andy should leave "things in God's hands," which included assisting the doctors and nurses in carrying out their duties. During this serious bleeding crisis, which lasted for 10 days, Andy remained in a cheerful mood most of the time, to the point of being prankish on occasion. On the 10th day of his admission, an attempt was made to remove the tracheotomy tube because of considerable bleeding around it. Profuse bleeding ensued, and, after a few hours, Andy died from aspiration of blood and subsequent asphyxia.

At the time of Andy's death, Bill was 11 years of age. The parents declined our offer to provide some psychological assistance to the family in their mourning process, and for the next year and a half we only had contacts with them at times of Bill's bleeding episodes.

Then, to our surprise, the mother called me and reported that Bill was showing problems in the parochial school that he attended. His male teacher had become concerned about Bill's declining grades. Bill had impressed the teacher as "miserable if not depressed." His reply to the teacher's admonitions was, "Why should I bother to study? I'm going to die anyway." The teacher's immediate reponse had been, "God will take you when he wants to," whereupon the teacher had tried to elicit more information about Bill's misconception concerning hemophiliacs dying at a young age, as had been the fate of his brother.

The parents and the teacher were shocked by Bill's repeated references to his brother's death "such a long time later." The mother had tried to reassure Bill about his future by telling him about the steady medical progress in the treatment of hemophiliacs. She admitted, however, that she as well as her husband had tried to avoid any discussion about Andy's death and never openly recognized the possibility that Bill might worry about his own condition and safety.

During my interview with the mother, which preceded the brief psychiatric intervention with Bill, she recalled how Bill had cried upon learning about Andy's death almost two years ago. At the funeral, Bill went up to the casket, looked at his brother, and remarked, "He seems to be sleeping." Following the funeral, Bill had asked few questions about his brother. Occasionally, the mother would show Bill a picture of Andy taken a few days before his death, portraying Andy in bed with a smile on his face, and displaying his tracheotomy tube to the surgeons. The mother had continued to carry this picture in her purse at all times, and she also showed it to me during the interview.

Whenever friends of the parents brought up the subject of hemophilia or referred to Andy, Bill would listen with interest, make no remarks, and often leave the gathering with his eyes filled with tears.

Before Andy's last hospital admission, he and Bill had shared a bedroom. Upon learning of Andy's death, Bill moved into his sister's room and for several weeks he shared her bed. Three months later, Bill told his mother that he was ready to sleep by himself in his old room.

During the years following Andy's death, Bill became more open, more daring, and more involved in play activities with friends in the neighborhood. He enjoyed roller skating, bicycling, playing baseball, and even practicing football with caution. When needed, he would apply ice packs to his bleeding sites, and he seldom complained about pain and immobilizations. Obviously, at age 13 he showed a healthy independence in terms of self-care.

Commenting on her and her husband's reluctance to allow any family talks about all the memories surrounding Andy's last bleeding crisis, the mother recalled that only once during the intervening two years had the father broken down and cried about the demise of his son. At this time the father had been under the influence of alcohol. Religion had continued to play an important role in the family's life. The parents frequently told their children and their friends that "We have two children here and one angel in heaven." The parents had felt that Bill accepted these parental views, and he often prayed to Andy to intervene "because Andy is now closer to God, and he can help me when I am bleeding." Bill also seemed to share the notion that all of them would sooner or later join Andy after death.

At this point in my interview with the mother, she spontaneously wondered if she should have spoken more directly to Bill about Andy's death in the intervening years. She added that she had continued to rely on her cheerful, matter-of-fact approach in regard to hemophilia, the approach she seemed to have learned from her own father. At the same time, she was definitely in tune with Bill and his upset feelings, and she had acted immediately on the alerting signals from the school teacher.

When I saw Bill a few days later, he seemed well prepared by his mother for his visit with me. Bill was a cooperative, verbal 13-year-old boy, and he readily told me about his present school situation, minimizing his academic difficulties, particularly in science, referring to the fact that "I don't like to read so much about the human body." This provided me with an early opening into the area of hemophilia, and Bill complained that, "I haven't been told much about hemophilia by anybody." Bill thought that he had been about six years old when his mother first tried to explain it to him, relating his frequent black-and-blue marks and joint swellings to a blood disorder. He then asked me many questions about the healing of cuts, of oozing tooth sockets, and of sprained joints. Bill knew that hemophilia was hereditary and mentioned the long life of his hemophilic grandfather. He then remarked that his two older cousins suffered from hemophilia and seemed to do fairly well.

In my second meeting with Bill, we approached the death of his younger brother, a topic that Bill introduced by telling me that he missed Andy a lot, that they had been very close, and that "God wanted it to happen." Bill recalled his sad and frightened feelings immediately following the death of his brother and his refusal to sleep in the same room that he and his brother had shared. For a long time Bill had held on to a big teddy bear that used to belong to Andy, and he had imagined that the teddy bear was his deceased brother. Especially at night, before going to sleep, these thoughts had helped Bill "to make it easier missing Andy." Everybody at home seemed to have missed Andy very much, according to Bill, so "It was too hard for us to talk about Andy's death and his and my illness."

Bill then recalled situation after situation in which he and Andy had played together, had helped each other out when one of them was bleeding, had stood up for each other toward other children, and also allied themselves against their parents and their sister.

Bill felt uncertain about his chances to have a normal life-span due to the fact that his brother had died at a young age. He remembered visiting Andy once in the hospital, seeing the tracheotomy tube, and he also mentioned the mother's photograph of Andy. Bill knew that this fatal bleeding episode had not been related to physical injury but was caused by a throat infection. No wonder, Bill said, that he had been very scared several times in the intervening years when he had suffered from colds and sore throats. He had imagined the worst outcome, that is, a complication of pharyngeal bleeding that might lead to his death just as had happened to Andy.

In the subsequent four interviews, Bill repeatedly asked many questions about his clotting defect and the effects of plasma transfusions, about progress of research dealing with improved treatment of bleeding disorders, and the possibility of a "once and for all cure" of hemophilia. In addition, he wanted to learn more about hereditary illnesses and the specific genetic explanation of hemophilia. He went over his family background in great detail and recalled many early memories of his hemophilic grandfather and two hemophilic cousins, and, of course, his deceased brother. Bill remembered his mother telling him about her role as a carrier, which was followed by a reflection on his part about the likelihood that his mother had "sad feelings" about this fact. Toward the end of these sessions, and also repeated a few years later when I again met Bill, he stressed that his mother had three healthy brothers who did not have hemophilia. This important fact convinced him that his possible future sons would not have the same disease as he had.

Toward the end of the short period of psychiatric intervention, Bill began to speak about his interest in a trade school after high school graduation, and more specifically about learning to become a baker, a job in which "you can both make good money and don't have to be afraid of getting hurt." It should be noted, too, that any attempt on my part to bring up the likelihood that, on occasion, Bill and Andy had had their scuffles and that Bill might have resented his brother, resulted in incredulous and irritated responses, such as "So what? It doesn't matter now; he is dead . . . Andy was my best friend, we had the same illness . . . and I think he is alive in heaven and knows what's happening to me . . . and I can pray to him, too, and he can hear me, I think. . . ."

When I arranged for a follow-up two years later, Bill was a healthy looking 15-year-old, doing satisfactory work in school, participating in biking, baseball, and softball, and enjoying many friendships. With a certain pride, he told me that he seemed to be in much better shape than most of the other hemophilic teen-age boys he knew in our area. At this time, he had an excellent recall and understanding of the clinical and hereditary characteristics of hemophilia. He admitted that he worried at times about "bleeding around my throat" as a complication to throat infections, similar to the fate of his brother six years earlier. Otherwise, memories of Andy seldom occupied Bill's mind. Bill, his sister, and his mother seemed to be able to speak about the years when Andy completed the family without experiencing undue distress or a wish to avoid the topic. The father, however, continued to resent any mention of Andy except for the perfunctory ones included in the family's religious practices. Consequently, the father's psychological isolation had deepened, which the other family members were keenly aware of but felt unable to change. As Bill remarked, "Dad can never accept Andy's death . . . Sure, it was a bad blow to me and Mom, but I think we have licked it; Dad still can't talk about it."

DISCUSSION

The effects of Andy's death on his family and on his brother Bill in particular are similar to those reported in several studies of children's reactions to a death in the family. Binger's recent reports contain a summary of these studies in addition to accounts of his own observations of emotional disturbances in children who have suffered the loss of a sibling due to leukemia (Binger et al. 1969; Binger 1973). Following his brother's death, the 11-year-old Bill showed an incapacity to sustain a mourning process, just like his parents, strong attempts at denying and suppressing his sad and frightened feelings, inability and unwillingness to accept the reality of Andy's death—the latter continued to "live on" in a highly personalized way, being able to communicate with Bill in accordance with the family's religious beliefs. The slowly developing learning problems of Bill were directly related to his feelings of futility regarding school work as he saw himself doomed to repeat Andy's fate.

Bill's scholastic problems and despairing self-attitudes finally conveyed to his environment his long-standing sadness, worries, and confusing conceptions of hemophilia and their relationship to Andy's fatal bleeding crisis. Its impact on Bill had overtaxed his ability to cope mentally with his "own" chronic disorder and attendant psychologic stress. Particularly noticeable were his inefficient—maladaptive—use of the essential coping techniques offered by various cognitive functions (for example, memory, speech, judgment, reality testing) and his crippling reliance on certain psychological defenses, such as denial, avoidance, and identification with his deceased brother rather than with living and well-functioning hemophilic and healthy peers (Mattsson 1972). Bill's failure to mourn Andy's death and to maintain a hopeful, positive outlook on his own future could be related to his family's conscious efforts to avoid any relevant, interpersonal sharing of memories and emotions related to Andy and his hemophilic condition. It was striking to observe how Bill's release of a host of pent-up feelings and bewilderment in regard to his brother and his death promptly enabled him to remobilize his good cognitive resources to cope successfully with the past and the present stressful situations. Simultaneously, with a lessening of his denial and avoidance of distressing feelings and his overidentification with Andy, he demanded and could retain many facts about his familial disorder in all its ramifications. Subsequently, he began to look to his future academic and vocational goals, clearly viewing himself as a potentially independent and productive young adult.

Bill was confused by Andy's death on many levels. His strong dread of his bleeding episodes was partly related to the failure to provide him with factual and sensible explanations about the illness, its complications, and medical management. On a deeper level, Bill wondered why he had been spared while Andy had succumbed. To attribute this solely to guilt feelings seems an inadequate answer in view of the unique closeness that had existed between him and Andy. The early and deep feelings of solidarity between hemophilic brothers are remarkable to watch in their behavioral expressions: from age 6 to 7, most brothers watch out for each other in play and games, assist each other in home treatment of hemorrhages, discuss their symptoms and treatment, and as they get older increasingly share views on dangerous, reasonably risky, and safe activities, including vocational choices and family planning (Mattsson, Gross 1966). In other words, the boys seem to gain substantial emotional support from each other, which is especially impressive at times of bleeding crises. Competitive, resentful, and hostile attitudes toward each other, as seen among healthy siblings, usually appear only in subdued and sublimated fashions in hemophilic brothers who are over 6 to 7 years of age. These observations suggest that the mourning process of a surviving brother with hemophilia will differ from our expected "norms" in terms of its observed and subjectively felt manifestations of guilt and ambivalent attitudes toward the deceased brother.

During the two years following Andy's death, the mother had been well aware of the family's deficiencies in not heeding Bill's many references to his frightened and sad state. Her reluctance to listen and respond to him, as she normally had done to both her sons before, was related to her great concerns about the father's emotional fragility, increasing drinking habits, and his steadfast refusal to allow himself or others to vent any expressions of grief about Andy and his fate. For years, the mother had accepted her husband's frequent absence from the family, his minimal assistance in raising their two boys, and his view of a lingering blow to his self-esteem caused by begetting two "not normal" boys. The mother wanted to protect the father, as she was openly afraid that family discussion about hemophilia and Andy's death would make him seriously upset. Her many attempts to get him interested in psychiatric counseling had been futile.

As soon as Bill signaled his distress through his teacher, the mother was able to assume an active role in opening up some communication among the family members in regard to hemophilia and its effects on the two boys. An additional helpful factor behind Bill's rapid psychologic improvement seemed to have been his mother's early acceptance of herself as a carrier of hemophilia. She had not hidden from her family her fearful, at times self-accusatory, feelings about her genetic responsibility for her sons's serious illness. Finally, her experience in growing up with a hemophilic father, who stoically had coped with his serious physical condition, made her prone to minimize the emotional impact of Andy's death on Bill and the other family members. She expected Bill to continue his satisfactory psychosocial adaptation to his disorder, just like her father had in the past. Despite these complex earlier experieces with hemophilia, the mother became an important ally in the brief psychiatric work with Bill, and she gained much satisfaction from watching him change to a better adjusted, more content, and hopeful teen-ager who wanted to strive toward achieving social and scholastic goals for himself; that is, Bill again could cope with his chronic illness in a realistic, adaptive way.

REFERENCES

BINGER, C. M., A. R. ALBIN, R. C. FEUERSTEIN, J. H. KUSHNER, S. ZOGER, and C. MIKKELSEN, Childhood leukemia: emotional impact on patient and family. *New England Journal of Medicine* 280: 414-418, 1969.

BINGER, C. M., Childhood leukemia—emotional impact on siblings, in *The Child in His Family: The Impact of Disease and Death,* eds. E. J. Anthony and C. Koupernik. New York: Wiley, 1973.

MATTSSON, A., Long-term physical illness in childhood: a challenge to psycho-social adaptations. *Pediatrics* 50:801-811, 1972.

MATTSSON, A., and S. GROSS, Adaptational and defensive behavior in young hemophiliacs and their parents. *American Journal of Psychiatry* 122:1349-1356, 1966.

13

Accidents and Trauma

William M. Easson

"Mommy, I didn't mean it."

She was only seven years old. The bandages almost covered her face, but her lips were visible, swollen, and cracked. She had just two more days to live, yet all she could say, over and over again, was "Mommy, I didn't mean it." By the little girl's bedside, her mother waited for the agony to end. She could only whisper numbly in reply, "Of course, you didn't. Mommy knows. You are Mommy's good girl."

It had all started so happily. The little girl had been camping with her friends in the backyard of her home. The children lit a fire to cook weiners for their supper. As the evening grew darker, they danced and sang around the fire and their laughter echoed into the night. Suddenly the little girl's dress caught fire and she was enveloped in flames. A happy, joyful child—a shrieking terror—a whimpering mass of bandages that cannot be held because it is too painful—"Mommy, I didn't mean it"—and death.

What happened to those playmates who also danced around the fire? Three little girls ran screaming home for help and for protection, one little boy fled down the street to hide somewhere, anywhere, and the other little boy tried vainly to catch his flaming, shrieking playmate. When it was all over, five young children had lost a friend; they had to continue living and growing.

In most American cultural and ethnic groups, the grade school period is a time when the growing child begins to move away from the security of home and out into the relative uncertainty of society. The youngster starts to go to school and begins to spend more and more time with peer friends. Although the child is becoming more independent, the youngster is still very closely involved with the family. The life of the child at this age level is family, school, and play. Even though friends are very important, to the child it is still more significant what mommy or daddy

157

want. It is only with this assuredness of continued family support and protection that the elementary school child can experiment and test, experience new pleasure and pain, grow and develop—and take risks.

When the grade school child is hurt, he or she knows it is possible to return home for comfort and support. After all the fights and the squabbles, the latency age (a period from about five years to puberty) child comes home for dinner. The eight-year-old girl enjoys balancing on the top of the wall, but, if she falls, she knows that mommy will hold her tight. The seven-year-old boy may fight and win or lose, but he is not too proud to run home for a cookie and a cuddle. The grade school years are the time of "dares" and "I bet you can't," but this is also the period when the child lives with the security of parental protection.

THE VICTIM'S GUILT

Sometimes all the protection of family and society is not enough to keep the growing child from serious injury or death. The adventurous little boy who wants to climb to the highest branch may fall to his death. The little girl who is so proud of her swimming ability may swim just a little too far and drown. The youngster who really enjoys her new skill at twisting and turning her bicycle might unexpectedly veer into the path of a car. Matches bring fun and excitement to little boys, but matches can also lead to fire, pain, disfigurement, and death.

Death in the latency age period very often is a result of accidents, and these accidents tend to occur when the youngster has been disobedient or has not heeded parental warnings. So often the child has been told repeatedly, "You keep off the busy street," "Don't climb that tree again," "Don't go swimming in that river," but still the youngster wanted to try. They disobey. They get hurt. They die. When the grade school child has been fatally injured, the dying child often realizes that he or she is largely to blame for what has happened. The young boy who has fallen knows that he took a forbidden risk; the burned little girl remembers that mommy told her not to touch the oven. Often the fatally injured child pleads with the parents, "I did not mean to do it."

THE ACCIDENT—A PUNISHMENT

The elementary school years are a time when the growing youngster is developing and stabilizing his or her conscience. Initially this conscience is relatively rigid and inflexible, and tends to dictate "an eye for an eye and a tooth for a tooth." In the conscience of the grade school child, bad behavior still merits and often brings bad punishment; to such a child, bad punishment usually means that bad behavior must have occurred somewhere. What punishment could be worse than a life-threatening accident or a potentially fatal injury? The seriously injured elementary school child is liable to believe that only the worst behvior on his or her part could have brought on this accident, this form of punishment. Any child realizes that, of course, he or she has been bad—and we have all been bad in some way. With the natural striving for knowledge and for independence, every grade school youngster has experimented rashly, acted secretly, and sometimes done what parents or teachers forbade. In the minds of injured youngsters, *somebody* must have known and *somebody* must have punished them. "Mommy, I didn't mean it." "Please forgive me." "Do not hurt me." "Do not punish me even more than I have been punished."

When a youngster has been fatally injured, the last few hours of the child's life may be haunted by these feelings of guilt and responsibility. This inner emotional pain may be shown outwardly by restlessness, by unrelieved physical pain, or by unresolved misery. The child may be withdrawn and hopeless. If the child is to die as comfortably as possible, the youngster must know that his or her injuries and death are not an awful punishment from some punitive parent or authority. Dying children should believe firmly that they are loved and always have been loved, no matter what they have done or been. Parents will say some of this needed love in words but never can really express all the youngster has to know and feel. The dying youngster is better reassured by the parents' presence, by the feel of their touch, and by the intensity of their caring. By being strong, loving, comforting parents even in their child's final hours, the parents of a fatally injured child will help their youngster to die in peace (Easson 1970).

THE PARENTS WHO FAILED

In the eyes of society, the grade school child is still very much a part of his or her family. He or she may be doing things more and more away from home, but everyone knows—the child, the parents, and the community—that the parents are still responsible for him or her. If an elementary school child is fatally injured, one of the first responses of the parents is to feel that they have failed in their most basic parental responsibility. They are to blame in their own eyes, and this blame is inescapable and intolerable. They have not been strong enough, motherly enough, or fatherly enough. They feel that they have not known enough or done enough. Because they have failed, their child is dying. Such feelings of self-blame are almost unbearable for most parents, so, in a very understandable fashion, they often try to make life tolerable by blaming someone else. If they can displace this blame, they will be able to live easier with themselves. Father can still feel that he is a competent man, mother can still cling to her self-confidence if someone else can be blamed—the teacher, the driver, those peer friends, and sometimes even the child him- or herself. "Who was responsible?" is often the cry of the child's parents, parents who desperately need to believe that someone else was responsible for this accident that is taking their child from them (Martin, Lawrie, Wilkinson 1968).

Because the parents need to shift blame to others, they may show seemingly illogical anger toward any person associated with the child. In the most unreasonable fashion, these parents may go to great lengths to make someone else responsible for their child's injury or death. Even though the injured youngster was beyond hope when brought to the emergency room, the parents may claim that it was bad care that caused the death. When these parents are stating that they wish to make someone "pay" for the accident, they are really saying that they want someone else to take this burden of responsibility for the child's death from their shoulders. They need someone to relieve them of some of their intense guilt. When they lash out in their guilty anger, the people around must restrain themselves from attacking back. Such retaliative anger from caring professionals or from the community is liable to make the parents feel even more anxious and guilty. People dealing with these parents do not have to tolerate destructive anger, but they must recognize that these deeply hurt parents need support and understanding. The injured child is dying or is dead, and these parents will have to live with the constant thought "I was to blame."

One way that many parents have of handling their anguish is to ruminate "If only." "If only I had been there." "If only we had taught him or her." "If only—" And in this way they can feel that they really were strong, sensitive, and caring, but circumstances somehow were against them and their child. "If only" fate had dealt differently with them, they could have shown to everyone (and to themselves) that they really were good capable parents.

Since these parents enjoyed, in a normal healthy parental fashion, the increasing independence and ability of their grade school child, they often gave the youngster the very opportunity that led to the fatal accident: this reality may be a profound reason for parental anxiety and guilt. Because the father was so proud of his son's fishing skills, he gave him that nice new fishing rod—and then his joyful son went off to the lake and drowned. For months now, the little girl had been fussing to get a bicycle, so her parents saved and eventually bought her that bicycle. They were so proud and she was so happy. It made them feel so good to be parents—and then she rode off to her death. He was such a confident young man, so father let him sit on the tractor—and the tractor overturned. All growth-oriented parents want to see their child develop and mature, but sometimes they learn, to their bitter grief, that their expectations and hopes unavoidably have led to the youngster's death. "She was so sure of herself." "He had a mind of his own"—and now he is dead.

THE PARENTAL ANGER

"If I told you once, I have told you a thousand times."

Yet with all the tellings, many young school children will try just that one last time, and that one final time may be the fatal time. When parents face the shock and the anguish that their child has been fatally injured, often they recognize bitterly that the youngster has brought this accident on him- or herself by disobeying what he or she had been told. They see that their son is dying and they know that their son really is to blame. The parents look at their dead daughter and remember that she had been told so very many times not to do those things. When parents and family members face the sorrow of a fatally injured child, they must also struggle with their realistic anger at the child's disobedience or willfulness that has now led to this fatal accident.

> One deeply distressed father of a six-year-old drowning victim spoke for many parents when he said, "I am so mad at him for disobeying, I could kill him—but he is dead anyhow and I didn't want that to happen."
> The mother of a fatally injured eight-year-old boy could not allow herself to go into his hospital room. Eventually she confessed to a sympathetic nurse that she desperately wanted to see the dying youngster, but she could not stand by his bedside without the overwhelming urge to "beat the hell out of him." She had told her son repeatedly to keep away from the farm machinery. He had disobeyed her orders and had been fatally injured in the moving mechanism. How could he do this to himself and to her?

This parental theme of "How could he (or she) do it to me?" is often unspoken but is always present. These children carry the hopes of the parents. As parents grow older, they gain much of their joy and gratification through the achievements of their children. How could this child hurt the parent so badly—by getting injured and by dying. How could the youngster be so disobedient and bad? How could he or she be so stupid?

THE SURVIVING CHILDREN

When they deal with the tragedy of the fatally injured child, caring personnel, relatives, and neighbors are usually very aware of the emotional needs of the dying youngster and of the grieving family. However, there are other people involved who are often ignored and who may be even more important—the surviving children. When a school child is fatally injured, often this accident has occurred during play with other children; these playmates are markedly affected by this accident.

The elementary school age period is the time of emotional maturation, when the growing youngster is developing a sense of group responsibility. During these early school years, these children become more aware that they have an obligation to support, care for, and protect each other. They become part of an accepted code of mutually dependent and socially responsible behavior. When a playmate is fatally injured, these surviving children are left with their own emotional burdens from the accident. The fatally injured child and his or her playmates have planned together, experimented together, disobeyed together, and fought together, sometimes in fantasy and sometimes in act. The surviving children often feel a profound personal responsibility for the fatal accident that has occurred. Even though the survivors may not have been directly involved, they may assume all the blame and all the guilt, and few people may be aware of their emotional burdens.

Sometimes, in an apparently illogical fashion, a surviving child will appear to be anxiously blaming everyone else for the tragedy. "Paul pushed him," "I told him not to climb the tree," or "I had gone home." Other children usually understand and so can adults if they are sensitive and listen. It becomes apparent that the youngster is frantically trying to unload or displace the blame he or she feels. Because of this feeling of responsibility, the surviving child may become deeply depressed. Since their experimentation has lead to the friend's death, a surviving youngster may stop exploring, trying, or even growing intellectually and emotionally. When disobedience has resulted in this fatality, the surviving child may become a numbed paragon of virtue, rigidly compulsive, and emotionally stunted.

A grade school child will say openly about his or her friends, "We think the same." This close identification between school age playmates also means that they can feel the same identification in death and in vulnerability. The surviving child knows now that he or she too can be killed and that no one can protect him or her completely. The world has become much more frightening, and the child is now more obviously fragile. The surviving child may show many outward signs of this increased vulnerability. Since the world is not really safe, he or she may develop phobias or undue fears. Nights are no longer tranquil and may be broken by nightmares or restless sleep. Because the child knows that he or she needs protection, he or she may be less eager to move away from the protection of parents, family, or teachers. The surviving child often becomes much more clinging and dependent and frequently more obviously childlike. The youngster who was toilet trained may wet the bed again. The eight-year-old may suck his or her thumb once more.

Wise parents and sensitive teachers know that this identification with the fatally injured child has wide-ranging effects among the schoolmates of the dying youngster. Classmates will wonder and worry and show many of the symptoms of the survivor child. Some of these school children become depressed and withdrawn. Other surviving children who carry this emotional burden of self-blame or anxiety become irritable or "bad" and often bring punishment on themselves.

Often parents or neighbors are so concerned with the fatally injured youngster and the mourning family that they tend to be insensitive to the surviving friends and peers of the dying child. These other children, who have a life yet to live, need added support, reassurance, and caring to help them deal with their anxiety, their sadness, and their fears. These surviving grade school children have just learned what can happen to a child their age, once very much alive like them but now dead or dying. To grow emotionally and intellectually, these surviving youngsters need to be doubly sure that they are protected and that they do have security. They must be certain that it is permissible to experiment, to try, and sometimes even to take risks.

SUMMARY

When a child is fatally injured, no one is prepared emotionally. Grade school children are not expected to die. They are healthy, active, and energetic; when an accident leaves them maimed, ugly, and dying, the reactions of everyone to this tragedy are acute, intense, and unmodified.

Frequently the intensity of these emotional responses heightens the anxiety of those involved.

In this chapter, we have dealt briefly with the emotional reactions of the fatally injured child, the grieving parents, and the surviving peers. These reactions are all remarkably similar, and each person affects the other and all with whom they come in contact.

Human beings are bound by a common bond of humanity and by a shared vulnerability.

REFERENCES

EASSON, W. M., The dying grade school child, in *The Dying Child.* Springfield, Ill.: C. C. Thomas, 1970.

MARTIN, H. L., J. H. LAWRIE, and A. W. WILKINSON, The family of the fatally burned child. *Lancet* II:628-629, 14 September 1968.

14

Cancer in the School-Age Child

Rudolph Toch

In drawing the profile of preadolescent children who have some form of cancer from which they are likely to die, the first difficulty encountered is the lack of uniformity. Except for the diagnosis they share, children with cancer are as varied as their peer groups, and the following generalizations become automatic oversimplifications. While striving for more independence, they also become more social and peer-oriented. Segregation by sex becomes more pronounced and intellectual interests expand: a lengthening attention-span permits more reading. Better self-control emerges and more realistic short-range planning becomes evident in daily activities: long-range goals may still be unrealistic and influenced by "hero worship" and what used to be called "crushes" for selected adults. Nevertheless, reliability and responsibility grow even while disdain for authority increases. Throughout these years the concept of individuality both for him- or herself and those around him or her develops apace, and some attitudes and character traits evident toward the end of the preadolescent phase will carry over into adult life.

Preadolescents are aware of their own mortality, although a great deal of fantasy is mingled with factual information. For many, illness is equated with punishment, usually as the product of ill-advised parental attempts at discipline or coercion. The most memorable example for me was a 10-year-old girl who had a neuroblastoma (a malignant tumor) removed in early childhood and whose parents ever since attempted to improve her eating habits by warning her that if she did not eat well she would get leukemia. Why they used this particular threat they could not explain, but the girl did develop acute leukemia and nothing could persuade her that it was not a punishment for eating too little. Her therapy was generally unsuccessful, and the year she lived after the diagnosis was one of unhappiness, depression, regression, and ultimately complete withdrawal. We must remember that children are likely to accept adult statements as factual and literal and that only extreme exaggerations will be recognized as such. Their particular sense of humor will often baffle adults while being readily understood by their peers. They are very sensitive to ridicule and criticism, which they can read into the most innocuous statements, and they begin to display the swings of mood that will become more characteristic during the adolescent phase.

Their concern with their own bodies becomes more pronounced. The boys like to display their muscles and like to have them admired, while the girls are embarrassed by their budding breasts and want to hide them by a slouching posture and loose clothing. Both sexes are concerned with threats to their bodies and indulge in fantasizing about their changes.

CHILDREN'S THOUGHTS ON DEATH

McIntire, Angel, and Struempler (1972) have made an outstanding contribution to our understanding of what children know and think about death. The role of fantasy, religion, and experience in the conceptualizaiton of death by the child are documented. The authors emphasize that in their study the significance of life was "enjoyment of life's pleasures and interpersonal relationships. This might reflect a denial of anxiety, persistence of immature demands for instant pleasures, or simple acceptance of the satisfactions of life." They also observe that by the age of eight, death was no longer considered to mean total oblivion, but a large percentage of their sample (up to 80 percent) displayed an increasing belief in spiritual immortality. The study also bears out the truism that the great cultural, religious, regional, and socioeconomic diversity of American children prohibits simple generalizations. It is imperative that the personnel dealing with a specific child make every effort to assess his or her specific beliefs and comprehension and total background to the end that his or her management may be tailor-made to his or her needs.

THE CHILD'S REACTION TO HIS OR HER ILLNESS

There are common denominators in the reaction of children to their own illness that they may perceive as life-threatening. Guilt, fear, anger, and anxiety are displayed to some extent by each child, although not always in the same order. An analysis of the child's self-image may help in anticipating some of the reactions and thereby lessen their impact. The child who has set high goals for him- or herself, usually in sports at this age, will resent the disability that cancer may produce and will react with anger and resentment. By talking honestly with him or her and by describing as fairly as possible the prospects of continued participation in the activity, the impact may be lessened. But most importantly he or she must be permitted to resume conditioning exercises and activities as soon as conditions permit, to restore hope. This may be in clear conflict with parental attitudes, to whom rest and avoidance of exercise so often are synonymous with sound medical care. They must be persuaded to see that any real or imaginary danger that may result from physical activity is less important than the psychologic harm that results from enforced inactivity. The sad memory of the crippling effect produced by radical curtailment of all natural physical activities in children suspected of having rheumatic fever should serve as a reminder not to repeat past mistakes. Fear, particularly of the unknown, is an inherent component of the human's emotions. The preadolescent will usually have outgrown the unreasonable fears of earlier childhood, but being struck down by an inexplicable illness may revive some of them—for example, that of darkness—and add new ones. They may relate closely to the nature of the illness and express themselves in objections to hospitalization, necessary procedures, limitations of activity, exaggerated concern over minor physical symptoms, and occasionally even by imaginary complaints sometimes used to assess the degree of concern they may evoke in parents or physicians. A 12-year-old girl who know that she had acute leukemia used to complain of aches and pains, particularly sore throats, even while in complete hematologic remission, which were usually attended to in the appropriate manner by her physicians. Once she was seen by a physician who had not seen here before and who rather brusquely told her that anybody with leukemia had to expect these minor problems as part of the disease. This was a crushing blow to the child, who understood the broad implications of her diagnosis but had rightly understood that while in remission her problems were not related to the leukemia. She then assumed that she had relapsed and that this fact had been kept from her. It took some time to convince her that nothing had changed in her status and that the physician's comment was more general than specific. This episode highlights the need for awareness of the limits of a child's understanding and the great care that must be taken in the choice of explanations and, indeed, of words used to avoid creating an unintentional misunderstanding.

It is my practice and advice to minimize the complaints of the children rather than to launch full-scale investigations into each minor symptom: even the child with cancer will suffer the minor illnesses of children in their age group. Nothing is lost by deferring exhaustive studies to prove that a bout of fever or an ache or pain are not due to the spread of the basic disease but to an intercurrent and transient infection and by doing only those tests one would do if the child did not have cancer.

Anxiety

The question of increased anxiety in children with cancer who do not know the nature of their illness has been raised often, and it appears likely that children perceive that something serious is wrong with them by a nonverbal transfer of anxiety from all people who deal with them. It is often the most emphasized wish of the parents that their child remain ignorant of his or her fatal diagnosis. I may say categorically that this cannot be achieved and no promise should be made that it will be done. With their natural curiosity, children will investigate things that interest and affect them, and it is impossible to structure their activities in a manner that would keep information out of their reach.

A hospital in particular is the last place where any secret can be kept. The ways by which children learn what is going on are many. They can read and will do so. One 10-year-old boy was left with his chart in his lap while waiting for some tests. Of course he leafed through the record and read some of the notes, and the carefully withheld diagnosis was there for him to read. Other children will listen to the discussions by the staff making rounds and pick up enough information about themselves and other patients to make any secrecy a farce. The effect of presumably nonverbal transmittal of anxiety was studied by Spinetta, Rigler, and Karon (1973) in 6 to 10-year-olds whose parents asserted that their children did not know the fatal nature of their illness. They concluded that:

. . . even though the concern of the 6- to 10-year-old leukemic child may not take the form of overt expression about death, the more subtle fears and anxieties are nonetheless real, painful, and very much related to the seriousness of the illness. . . . To equate awareness of death with the ability to conceptualize it and express the concept in an adult manner denies the possibility of an awareness of death at a less cognitive level. If it is true that the perception of death can be engraved at some level that precedes a child's ability to talk about it, then a child might well understand that he (or she) is going to die long before he can say so.

This expression may take pictorial form. Figure 1 shows the drawing of an 11-year-old boy in his third year with leukemia. He was not symptomatic at the time he drew the picture, and his parents reported that he had drawn it as he had drawn many other pictures of the kind all children draw—houses, animals, people—without emotional reaction or comment. When asked about the drawing, he just shrugged his shoulders and said it had seemed like a nice scene to draw. He died within three weeks of making the drawing, never expressing fear or even apprehension.

Death Concepts

There have been several studies on children's concepts of death, some of which I have listed (Alexander, Alderstein 1958; Gartley, Bernasconi 1967; Jackson 1968; Maurer 1966; Schilder, Wechsler 1934; Von Hug-Hellmuth 1965; Waechter 1971). Although death is the most dramatic aspect of a fatal illness, the process of living with it is infinitely more trying. Being ill is unnatural, and children resent or even deny it. Physicians caring for children with diabetes experience this more often, but as

Figure 6

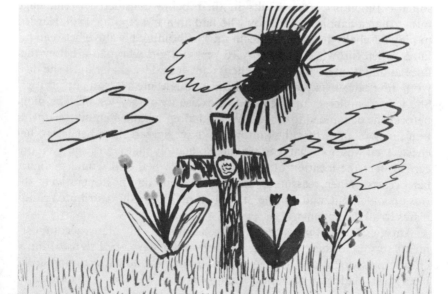

cancer treatments become more complex and demanding, our young patients are becoming more resentful, and the problem of medication not taken and appointments not kept grows. The problem of disfigurement looms large; children learn to cope with the loss of a limb or an eye, but the persistent loss of hair that attends most tumor chemotherapy (treatment with chemical agents) causes difficulties for both boys and girls. The latter take more easily to wigs, while boys often prefer hats or caps to hide their bald heads. Some tumors do produce unsightly masses and lesions, and the patient must be helped to disguise or hide them. One nine-year-old boy developed large projecting scalp lesions from his type of cancer, which the wearing of a baseball cap 24 hours a day made bearable. He worried more about these visible masses than about being confined to a wheelchair when long bone lesions made walking impossible. Fortunately, pain is not a constant feature of childhood cancer, but when it does occur it should be controlled promptly with all palliative measures available. In many tumors local radiation will bring relief, and analgesics should not be spared. Schlesinger's Solution is a singularly effective oral medication that has made it possible for many children to stay at home even when pain becomes a significant problem.

Many other complications that accompany cancer present still more concerns to the child. Interference with locomotion, vision, or other somatic functions often results in their being considered a challenge rather than a handicap. One boy who had an arm amputated still learned to play baseball, developing a technique of holding his glove between his knees when throwing the ball. A 10-year-old girl who had a below-the-knee amputation became an excellent dancer and ice skater until she died from lung cancer six years later. She also taught me a lesson in priorities. She was to undergo an operation to excise a solitary lesion. The night before, she demanded to see me. We had already talked about the operation and she knew that the tumor may have spread from her leg to her chest. That was not what troubled her so acutely that night; she was concerned over the location of the incision and whether it would disfigure her breasts. When reassured, she relaxed. One day postoperatively she was up and about, and it being St. Valentine's Day, she distributed candy kisses to all the patients.

Another boy's story is remarkable because of his many accomplishments in spite of overwhelming handicaps. He developed signs of intracranial pressure at age nine. A diagnosis of pinealoma, a tumor in the head, was made and radiation therapy given. Within a few months he developed many complications, including tumors elsewhere. He responded remarkably to chemotherapy and radiation but was left bound to a wheelchair. Nevertheless he participated in most activities of his peers including playing ball and swimming. He attended school by two-way telephone; but when he had to attend classes in a building with stairs he developed a technique of going up and down by sitting on a step and hoisting himself up with his arms. Although no hope for regaining the use of his legs seemed justified, he insisted on trying to walk with crutches and mastered the technique. Fortunately, at about age 16 he stopped developing more metastases. Eventually, he discarded the crutches, attended college, and is now in theological school. He was quite aware of his life-threatening disease, but his faith in God and in his ultimate recovery was unshakable.

COMMUNICATION PROBLEMS

Communication with preadolescent children is often difficult. Not only are their powers of verbal expression limited, but their thoughts often do not follow adult rational patterns. We must also recognize that children use other than verbal communications. These are the years when they are intrigued by codes and cyphers and secret messages. They use all manners of signs and symbols and will often approach a subject obliquely. Their desire for information is intense but rather specific. When they want to know something, their interest is usually limited to the specific item and it is a mistake to try imparting information for which they have no use at the moment. The proper choice of words is important because they have already learned some emotionally charged words, as for instance "cancer" or "leukemia," and it is important to know what each one means to them.

A discussion (condensed to essential elements) may be structured in the following manner:

Physician: "Well, Johnny, what do you think is wrong with you?"
Johnny: "I don't know."
P: "You must have thought something about it. A bright boy like you does not stay in the hospital and have all those tests and X rays without thinking that something is wrong with him."
J: "I guess so. I saw a picture on T. V. where a guy had all those tests and the doctors said he had cancer."
P: "What does that make you think of?"
J: "Well, maybe I have cancer. Do I?"
P: "Just what does cancer mean?"
J: "I guess it is some sort of bad disease from which people die."
P: "Do you know anything else about it?"

J: "Well, maybe a person with cancer has to have an operation to cut it out."

P: "Do you think that all patients with cancer have to have an operation?"

J: "I don't know. David (another boy on the ward) has cancer and he had an operation and now he has no hair and has to get needles."

P: "Well, Johnny, cancer is a very big word that can mean many things. Not all people with cancer have operations and not all people die from it. Do you know what an operation is?"

J: "Yes, that's when they cut you open. Do I have to have an operation?"

P: "After all the tests have been done, you may have to have one so that we know definitely what is wrong with you. See, David had an operation and look how happy he is!"

J: "Do you think I have cancer? Do I have to have my leg cut off?"

P: "No, you will not have your leg cut off, but we have to take some of the lumps off your neck. After we find out what they are made of, we'll know whether you have a form of cancer."

J: "Will you tell me if I do?"

P: "Yes, Johnny."

After the biopsy proves he has Hodgkin's disease, Johnny will be prepared to accept the diagnosis and will reluctantly agree to a course of treatment presented to him a step at a time. He is not asked whether he wants to be treated because his refusal could not be respected. It is amazing how often people ask children to do something by the ploy of couching the order in the form of a question—"Do you want to see the doctor?" when they really mean "Let's go see the doctor"—and never intend the child to have a choice. The child, however, in his or her literal interpretation of an adult's question and having firmly said "No," resents his or her refusal being ignored, and this cannot help but diminish his or her self-respect to some degree. But the most important result of a discussion as sketched above is the establishment of rapport and mutual respect between physician and child and the implicit assurance that the doctor is willing to listen, to answer questions, and that he or she speaks honestly.

One of the most elemental fears of children is that of separation and isolation. The preadolescent usually has learned that his or her being separated from parents is temporary and reversible, but under the stress of illness old fears may be rekindled and there is constant need to reassure him or her and above all to be honest.

The mother who leaves the child's bedside with an "I'll be right back," and then goes home instead can hardly expect the child to trust her the next time she leaves. Often in the initial phase of a child's fight against cancer, there is a surge of interest by family and friends, and if the child is unfortunate enough to become the object of journalistic attention, a great many strangers will also respond with letters and gifts.

As the illness continues and the first outburst of sympathy wanes, the child, now used to having a great deal of attention paid him or her, feels deprived and neglected. The harm that sensational newspaper reporting can do to such a child when he or she reads the lurid and usually inaccurate reports about him- or herself is considerable. Physicians also contribute to this sense of isolation when they become closely involved in the child's care and then, their job done, rarely if ever see him or her again. The plaintive "Why doesn't Doctor A. see me again?" "Doesn't he like me anymore?" may be forestalled by the care of the child being managed by a team of physicians, all taking continuous interest in the patient. Another form of isolation that is being used increasingly in the care of some children is the life-island isolation unit, which is employed for protection against infection. Important as this may be, the isolating effect must be kept in mind and a conscious effort made by all personnel to overcome this effect. The withdrawal and unhappiness of children in such situations, who learn very quickly that whenever a physician, nurse, or technician comes near them, it means a painful procedure and not just a friendly visit, often persist long after their return to a less germfree but more companionable environment.

THE ROLE OF SCHOOL

Next to family, school occupies the major time and attention of the child. With the concept of "leading as normal a life for as long as possible" as our goal, the question of what to do about schooling comes to the fore soon after a cancer diagnosis has been established. I advocate that schoolwork be resumed as soon as feasible and be pursued by teachers in the hospital, tutors at home, and by return to regular classes, albeit modified to meet the child's needs, at the earliest moment.

The fact that schoolwork continues to be important imparts a sense of assurance to the child, to whom ignoring what was so central to his or her preillness life cannot help but be disturbing. The execution of such plans requires coordination, but I have found most school systems willing to cooperate. If at all possible, only a few key persons—the principal, the teacher, and the nurse—should know the diagnosis to avoid problems of overreaction, which may range from excess attention to outright shunning.

Going to school may present some problems that can be anticipated. A very bright 12-year-old girl returned to her classroom after the diagnosis of acute leukemia had been made. She had not asked any questions concerning her illness and only knew that she needed ongoing medical care for a blood disease. Unfortunately, her plight had been the topic of conversation in her small hometown, and one day a classmate, piqued by something the girl had said, blurted out at her, "You have leukemia and you're going to die." The patient was obviously upset but did not speak of the incident until her next clinic visit, when she asked whether the girl had been right. When she was told that she did have a blood disease called leukemia and that nobody could tell her what of or when anybody would die, although people did die of leukemia, she made the extraordinary remark that if her parents had wanted her to know that she was going to die they would have told her so. Since they did not, she was not going to let them know what she knew. For several years while she was in remission, the topic was not again discussed. Only during her terminal relapse did she tell her parents what had happened and how she did not want them to worry about her.

The increasing publicity given to the possible infectious quality of leukemia has had the unfortunate side effect of considering children with leukemia a potential hazard, and they may be shunned by schoolmates and former friends. The need for better awareness by the public of the lack of any evidence for a simple transmission of leukemia or any other form of cancer from person to person is obvious.

THE ROLE OF RELIGION

The role religion plays in the life of the preadolescent varies with the denomination in which he or she has been reared. McIntire (1972) found significant differences between Protestants, Roman Catholics, and Jews in their beliefs in personal or universal spiritual continuation after death, with most Roman Catholics and very few Jewish children expressing such beliefs. Conversely, Jewish children had the highest percentage of belief in death as total cessation, Roman Catholics the lowest.

Religion does affect children in many ways, some of them less obvious or unexpected. When a seven-year-old rushed into my office to ask what was wrong with him, he did not give me a chance to reply before saying: "Everybody tells me that they are praying for me but nobody prays for my sister."

Although I firmly believe in the power of prayer, I do advise parents to tell their friends not to share their prayers with the patients. Some religious tenets do profoundly influence the child's life during illness. One child from a family where the mother practiced Christian Science but the father did not was treated medically for leukemia, but at home his illness was never spoken of. He led a normal life, unencumbered by frequent references to his illness or queries about his state of health. He died very suddenly, having taken care of his paper route a few days before while in profound relapse. Although I saw no evidence that his physical state was influenced by any extramedical forces, his spiritual well-being certainly was enhanced by his healthy assertive home environment.

If we succeed in teaching parents to adopt a positive, hopeful outlook early in the child's illness, we will improve the quality of his or her life considerably. When we fail in this, we may well encounter the extreme situation that I have seen only once: upon being told the nature of their child's disease, the parents and a numerous family of grandparents, aunts, and uncles donned mourning clothing and literally sat at the child's bedside as if at a wake, crying and chanting and acting as if the bewildered and frightened seven-year-old were already dead. Although the child lived several months, the aura of death continued to prevail. The child was confined to her bed in a darkened room, and nothing that physicians, social workers, or nurses said could shake the family's conviction that their course of action was proper.

CONCLUSION

The composite portrait of the preadolescent child dying of cancer is then really not so very different from that of his or her healthy peers. If we provide the child with love and respect, a sense of belonging, an assurance of being honest and fair with him or her, a mode of life as close to the norm as physical problems permit, and a cheerful, hopeful, and confident home life, we will make the child's, be it measured in weeks or years, a happy and satisfying one.

With the great progress that has been made in the treatment of childhood cancer, we must remember to structure each child's life in such a way that he or she will be able to grow up emotionally undamaged if he or she should be the one who has been cured.

REFERENCES

ALEXANDER, I. E., and A. M. ALDERSTEIN, Affective responses to the concept of death in a population of children and early adolescents. *Journal of Genetic Psychology* 93: 167-177, 1958.

GARTLEY, W., and M. BERNASCONI, The concept of death in children. *Journal of Genetic Psychology* 110: 71-85, 1967.

JACKSON, N. A., A child's preoccupation with death. *American Nursing Association Clinical Sessions* 172-179, 1968.

MCINTIRE, M. S., C. R., ANGEL, and L. J. STRUEMPLER, The concept of death in midwestern children and youth. *American Journal of Diseases of Children* 123: 527-532, 1972.

MAURER, A., Maturational concepts of death. *British Journal of Medical Psychology* 39:35-55, 1966.

SCHILDER, P., and D. WECHSLER, The attitudes of children toward death. *Journal of Genetic Psychology* 45: 406-451, 1934.

SPINETTA, J. J., D. RIGLER, and M. KARON, Anxiety in the dying child. *Pediatrics* 52: 841-845, 1973.

VON HUG-HELLMUTH, H., The child's concept of death. *Psychoanalytic Quarterly* 34:499-514, 1965.

WAECHTER, E. H., Children's awareness of fatal illness. *American Journal of Nursing* 71:1168-1171, 1971.

IV

ADOLESCENCE

In each of these three chapters on adolescence it is apparent that the adolescent faces death in the contradictory and perplexing ways adolescents seem to face life. There is heightened philosophical and religious concern and often intense interest in the meaning of life and death. The adolescent makes frequent use of strong denial and repressive mechanisms to cope with dying. Humor appears as a useful device. Both Coppolillo and Schowalter clearly point out how the adolescent uses denial mechanisms in appropriate ways to maintain his emotional equilibrium. In fact, frank depression and suicidal ideation, often seen in adulthood, are relatively lacking in the dying adolescent.

The chapter by Galdston gives a remarkable picture of how medical technology has changed the dying trajectory for adolescents with heart disease. Here the total uncertainty is changed to a partial uncertainty, which results in renewed hope and vitality in living, even though the possibility of death remains.

Coppolillo presents a careful description of the process of partial grief, *which has been ignored in management of organ transplant does not eliminate the possibility of death, but it does provide a partial certainty, which allows the adolescent to proceed in living life.*

On the other hand, Schowalter points out that for the adolescent with cancer who has a certain death prognosis, the focus must shift to the maintenance of daily life and personal concerns and interests.

All three chapters highlight the importance of body image to the adolescent. Furthermore, the dynamic interplay between the adolescent, his family, and the professional staff is repeatedly demonstrated. It is clear that one cannot only care for the dying adolescent; rather, care must be provided for all the people in the social system of the dying.

15

The Effects of the Cardiac Pacemaker in Adolescence

Richard Galdston

INTRODUCTION

The observations upon which this chapter is based were made during a study of 17 children and two adults who received internal cardiac pacemakers during the years 1960-67.* The study has been supplemented by subsequent anecdotal follow-up and was made against a background of clinical experience gained in the provision of psychiatric consultation to the ward services of The Children's Hospital Medical Center, Boston, Massachusetts, from 1960 to 1972 (Galdston, Gamble 1969).

The data gathered by a psychiatrist working in a medical facility cannot be freed from the constraints that serious illness places upon patients in their representation of their experiences. The psychiatrist is a member of a medical-surgical team and, although patients and their families may allow themselves a greater measure of candor and spontaneity in their expressions to him or her, the anxiety inherent in the position of dependence due to physical illness influences the patient's perceptions and statements. The intimidating effect of serious illness upon the patient's relationship to his or her physicians will inevitably cause the patient to alter his or her portrayal of personal experiences to them.

*I wish to express my appreciation to Walter Gamble, M. D., whose help and counsel made this study possible.

179

CONCLUSIONS

The hypothesis with which this clinical study was undertaken was that the threat to life that necessitated the implantation of a cardiac pacemaker would be a source of anxiety sufficient to cause a high incidence of the signs and symptoms of dysfunction and regression in the ego. *The data derived from the study not only failed to support this hypothesis but indicated that the contrary was the case.* The experience of an implanted cardiac pacemaker, with all of its attendant care, appeared to protect against regression in the ego functions compared to children with congenital heart disease without pacemakers and children with other forms of chronic disease such as a type of diabetes. This contrast in the adaptation of children to life-threatening stress has indicated some conclusions about the power of relationships to protect against the ravages of uncertainty upon the adolescent ego (Galdston 1973).

DISCUSSION

Consideration of the factors that might account for the unexpected absence of regression in ego function should start with the basis for anxiety in the danger of heart block. The reason for implanting a cardiac pacemaker is the failure of the heart's capacity to conduct its electrical impulses to achieve proper contraction. Whether the cause is unknown, congenital, or acquired through disease or as a complication of cardiac surgery, the threat is the same—that the heart will stop suddenly.

The regular beat of the human heart affords a biologic basis for a sense of security. Constancy in rate and rhythm of the heartbeat allows the individual to pursue daily life free from awareness of his or her heart and its functioning. This state of ignorance, of unawareness of what goes on inside, facilitates the maintenance of attention to what goes on outside. It enables a person to assume a predictable experience of cardiac function that does not require his or her recognition. Only when that state of predictability is interrupted by a missed beat is the patient confronted with the conscious acknowledgement of uncertainty in the functioning of his or her heart. This form of uncertainty is the biologic counterpart of the mental state of anxiety, "My heart stood still with fear." A patient who receives a pacemaker has known the experience of feeling his or her heart stand still, an experience that may or may not have been obscured by resultant loss of consciousness.

The implanting of a pacemaker restores some measure of certainty.

The source of power in batteries gives promise of a predictable rhythm and rate of discharge with a potential decay that can be anticipated with replacement in time. Thus, the authority for cardiac function is shifted from an internal biological origin to an external, technological source. With that transfer of authority, the physician who cares for the patient, the surgeon who implants the device, and the cardiologist who services it become heirs to attitudes and expectations that had hitherto been reserved for the forces of nature or the divine.

The doctor-patient relationship for the patient with an implanted cardiac pacemaker has certain unique features. The medical and surgical skills needed to implant and maintain a pacemaker are highly specialized. Most any physician can adjust the insulin schedule of a juvenile diabetic or regulate the medication of a patient in cardiac failure, but the training necessary to determine the responsiveness of a pacemaker to its requirements is usually available to but one or two physicians in any center for cardiac care. Thus, the patients, the doctors, and their relationship become very special.

This specialness in relationship affords an important element in the patient's adaptation to his or her stress. Although the threat of sudden death from untreated heart block is very real, as we said earlier, a pacemaker affords very significant protection, albeit at the cost of frequent operative procedures to correct the recurrent problems of battery failure, disruption of contacts, broken wires, and the many other possible complications. The physician provides the patient with a *future of limited certainty against an alternative of total uncertainty.* His or her physician becomes the patient's guarantor of a life with a limited future. The outer edge of the limits are not only approximate but there is every reason to expect that the limits can and will be extended with the improvement in technology. Since 1960, when the first pacemaker was implanted at The Children's Hospital Medical Center, 42 patients have received pacemakers, with only 7 deaths. The expectation of a longer life and an improvement in the quality of that life affords a realistic basis for hope, which further intensifies the patient's attachment to the physician.

The maintenance of hope for the uncertain future is supported by a relationship with a physician that has three distinguishing factors functioning in concert to afford the patient relief. These are: (1) identification with a medical attitude, (2) intellectualization, and (3) denial of emotion.

The very prominence of the technology involved in cardiac surgery affords eloquent example of the enthusiasm of the medical profession for its treatment of heart block. The optimism and the expenditure of prodigious amounts of time, money, and energy demonstrate a posture with which the patient can readily identify. Such identification is facilitated by the alternative choice of abandonment to a future marked by a sense of hopelessness.

Cardiac patients in general and pacemaker patients in particular quickly come to emulate their physician's behavior in speech and in attitude. The stance of active affirmation, of "doing something," affords the patient an example with which to identify not only as regards his or her heart disease but the conduct of life in general. The very idea of corrective cardiac surgery taps into the deeply seated fantasy of rebirth, of the rising of the Phoenix out of the ashes. A number of parents of children for whom corrective cardiac surgery was being considered promoted the operation, advancing the expectation that surgery also might improve conditions ranging from faulty school performance to an ornery disposition in their children.

Not only is the attending physician a source of identification in his or her presence, but even in absence the patient and family refer to the physician as a source of guidance. "Now what would the doctor think about this or that?" is a question often posed about matters that have little direct bearing upon the cardiac condition. The whole topic of electrical conduction by the heart, of electricity in the environment in forms ranging from lightning bolts to walkie talkies, allows for a richness in speculation about medical opinions on questions that defy anticipation by the physician.

Intellectualization, the exercise of the mind to master anxiety through the process of thought, is a prominent feature in the relationship of the patient with a pacemaker and his or her physician. Patients and their parents, who gave no sign of particular interest in thinking about other questions, displayed a deep interest in cardiac structure and function and electricity. They posed frequent and sophisticated questions about the autonomy of the pacemaker and its vulnerability to interference from external sources of electrical power. Implicit in these questions appeared to be a deeper concern about the ultimate sources of life.

The aspects of time, not only as rate and rhythm of the heart beat, but as watches and clocks ticking, seasons passing, and the intervals between clinic appointments appeared to have acquired a special importance in their thinking. Much of this intellectual activity had a repetitive, compulsive quality, circular and limited in its scope. The thoughts about the questions posed appeared to function as a means of keeping the mind busy in a fashion that resembled the example the doctor shows in concerns for his or her patient.

Denial of emotion, both in manifest behavior and by parents' report, was another attribute that distinguished the realtionship of these patients with their physicians. In view of the rigors of their illness and its treatment, the frustrations and disappointments of their lives, there is adequate reason to anticipate intense emotional reactions. Such was not the case. One can only assume, since the children and their parents did not appear to be a particularly isolated or schizoid group, that they denied those emotions associated with their cardiac status. This selective use of denial did not preclude the experience of intense emotion about other issues of concern. Indeed, displacement of affect allowed for the expression of intense feeling and strong opinion about items that appeared quite insignificant to others. One adolescent girl with a pacemaker and her parents were adamant in their desire for the surgical correction of her lop ears.

In some instances, the denial of emotion was supported by counterphobic activities. Three patients caused themselves electrical burns by short-circuiting the wires of electrical appliances shortly after they had received pacemakers. One woman gave herself a serious electrical shock by plugging in her washing machine while taking a bath during her convalescence.

Many of the children used humor, referring to themselves as "Ever-Ready," "Dry Cell," and "Hot Shot." One boy signed a Valentine's Day card to a girl "To my transistor sister!"

The quality of this denial of emotion was the more noteworthy for its coincidence with a generally informed and realistic appraisal of cardiac status. The dissociation of facts from feelings allowed for an effective mobilization of energies in compliance with a demanding treatment regimen. The patients, whether out of concern for their relationship with their parents or with their physician or for their own personal needs, found it necessary to deny the conscious knowledge of any strong emotion about their cardiac status.

Efforts by physicians to circumvent this denial of emotion appeared to have been misguided and counterproductive. When attempts were made to encourage the patients to share their "inner feelings," they became manifestly anxious and reacted to the questioner with anger. Only when the initiative came from the patient did the acknowledgement of emotion appear to be useful.

The relationship of the patient with his or her physician, supported by the practices of identification with the medical attitude, intellectualization, and the denial of emotion, appear to be the most important adaptive measure utilized by those children and adolescents confronted by the stresses of having to live with an internal cardiac pacemaker. The cost of maintaining this means of coping with adversity appears to be a constriction in imagination. It is difficult to estimate the potential range of curiosity, the possible limits of fantasy, the maximum freedom available to any group of children under ideal circumstances. Whatever those parameters might be, the requirements of contending with an acute and chronic threat to life expectancy appear to constrict the outermost limits of the mind's freedom to manipulate images. This self-imposed limitation may well be an advantage, for it spares the patient from frightening imagery as well as more creative speculation. The result is a certain literalness and an adherence to the immediate present of here and how. This does not preclude making plans for the future, but those plans appear to be dictated more by the need to have a plan rather than out of a free exercise of imagination about the possibilities for the future.

SUMMARY

Children and adolescents with heart disease requiring the implantation of a cardiac pacemaker do not appear to think much about death or dying. They think about leading their lives, and they rely heavily on the relationship they have with their doctors to sustain this habit of mind. They plan for the future as if it were guaranteed, even as they also realize the possibility of living a foreshortened life. It appears that the physician who can join his or her patient in this attitude can make the most useful contribution to sustaining hope and thereby promoting fulfillment in the face of uncertainty.

REFERENCES

GALDSTON, R., Growing up with cystic fibrosis, in *Fundamental Problems of Cystic Fibrosis and Related Diseases,* eds. J. A. Mangos and R. C. Talamo. New York: Intercontinental Medical Book Company, 1973.

GALDSTON, R., and W. J. GAMBLE, On borrowed time: observations on children with implanted cardiac pacemakers and their families. *American Journal of Psychiatry,* 126: 104-108, 1969.

16

Renal Transplantation

Henry P. Coppolillo

From shortly after birth until the time a person dies, grief is a companion of life. The intensity may vary or the issues about which one grieves may be different, but it would be difficult to imagine human life, as we know it, to exist without grief as a ubiquitous phenomenon. As awareness of the world grows, the infant grieves for the mother, however brief the separation. The lost or broken toy, the playmate who moves away, the frequently tearful goodbye to the beloved teacher when the child is promoted are other examples of the way the child comes to know grief. As maturity and understanding increase, the process becomes more complex, for now symbolic or abstract concepts must be grieved as well as concrete objects and possessions. A cherished friend is found to be wanting in loyalty or integrity, and the experience is that of a loss. A parent is found to be less than perfect, and that image of the perfect parent must be mourned and replaced by a more realistic one.

In adolescence and early adulthood, a process begins that is of specific interest here. The individual becomes considerably more self-evaluative and in so doing his or her physical attributes and integrity become more discrete as objects for his or her consideration. The "I" portion of the person scrutinizes and responds to the "me" portion in a more marked and conscious fashion. The task of creating an image of ourselves is completed with the completion of adolescence, and we carry that image of the self within us as we do that of every person to whom we relate. As life proceeds, we need to change that internal image of the self to keep pace with that which happens to our body in reality. The change in that self-image is sometimes accompanied by subtle grief and mourning. Gradually and slowly, the 50-year-old comes to realize that his or her body is not the same as that which was his or hers some 30 years before. Usually this process is gradual, and the ability to surrender sexual, physical, or intellectual prowess to time is achieved without undue disturbance and with compensations by investing in "more mature" interests and activities. Sometimes, however, there are disturbances in our ability to mourn our youth and its vigors and accept the wiser if more sedate mantle of age. One dramatic instance of disturbance is the situation in which an acute illness tumultuously accelerates the process and confronts the individual with the image of death before he or she is prepared to contemplate its existence. Naturally, this can happen not only when the self is threatened but also when there is a threat to someone so dear that the subject identifies in part or wholly with the victim.

It seems that we in the helping professions have not contemplated or dealt sufficiently with these aspects of the human condition. Often when there are disturbances in the person's ability to grieve for themselves or for a loved one, we find ourselves in perplexed discomfort. In fact, one could question the ability of the culture in general to manage the "normal" grief of everyday living. A clinical study may be instructive in raising some issues in this regard.

A CASE STUDY

Brian T. was 16 years old when an acute kidney illness left him in peril of death. Dialysis was begun and transplantation was planned. Work-up indicated that Brian's mother was the most suitable living donor. She immediately volunteered to be the donor, and it was decided that after the family was evaluated psychiatrically, Dr. Jack Metcoff, the pediatrician in charge and I would tell Brian of the plan.

The psychological evaluation revealed that Brian and his family were as free of conflict, stress, or psychopathology as any family or group of individuals can be expected to be. They loved each other and were capable of demonstrating affection. Irritation and quarrels occurred, as in any family, but reconciliation followed in short order and the predominant mood in the home was one of harmony.

Mother was the more actively communicative parent and she obviously set the tone for the family's comfort in effective communication. Father was somewhat less communicative and was not the first person to whom the children turned. In this sense, the mother could be considered to be the dominant person in the family, although the father could not be considered to be passive.

Brian was the oldest of three children, with a sister of 12 and a brother of 7. Brian was a tall, well-built, and communicative youngster, who showed no signs of the seriousness of his illness. In fact, his patient good spirits and the optimistic trust he communicated to his doctors heightened the poignancy of the situation. Life-threatening disease always seems cruel in one so young. It was outrageous in one so vital.

There were no signs of psychopathology in Brian. He had always been an intelligent, active young man, who had done well in school and with his peers. He was active in sports, played the guitar well, and had begun to date on a relatively regular basis. Adolescence was as pleasant as it ever is while one is living it, with the gratifications outweighing the problems he felt he had to master. From the point of view of temperament, Brian was an activist. If anything posed a barrier or a problem, his modus operandi was to meet it head on and actively master the difficulty. After he became ill, he read and collected all the information he could find on kidney disease. He then attempted to figure out all that he needed to do to help himself. If we were to put a label on his life-style vis-à-vis stress, we would call it counterphobic.

Mrs. T. was a tower of strength as we prepared for the transplantation. She participated actively in deciding who would present the plans to Brian, and after it was decided that Dr. Metcoff and I would speak to her son she made some excellent suggestions as to how she would follow up our communication with her availability.

Dr. Metcoff and I then met with Brian and told him our recommendations. The poignancy of his responses was matched only by Jack Metcoff's gentle sensitivity. Brian worried about whether this would hurt his mother and how much danger there was in it for her. Behind some of his questions there were distant rumblings of the questions he had about his own pain and future. These, however, could not be tackled until we were well into the interview, after we had talked at length about the possible consequences to his mother. During the preparatory phase, there were opportunities to reopen some of these personal fears and concerns. Again, however, there was nothing that suggested psychopathology in Brian or his mother.

The procedure went without a hitch. During the long recovery period in the sterile room, Brian was visited daily. Aside from some irritability at the isolation and appropriate concern about how his mother was doing, Brian complained only of the boredom. His return home was joyous and uncomplicated. There occurred only one moment of concern in the staff when it was discovered on one ambulatory visit that Brian had albumin in his urine and that his blood urea nitrogen was slightly elevated. Subsequent questioning revealed that the youngster, finding himself free from the shackles of a restricted diet, had gone on an eating binge. He had consumed an enormous number of eggs garnished with prodigious quantities of bacon. With only slight reassurance that the "freedom to eat" law would not be repealed, he became more moderate, and the alarm bells quieted.

Brian's progress was excellent for the next several years, but an incident occurred that startled us into the realization that there was an area of difficulty in the management of this family that we had not even begun to contemplate. After Brian's discharge from the hospital, there were several conversations between Mrs. T. and various members of the medical team. Inevitably the painful issue of Brian's life expectancy arose. Generally, Mrs. T. was told that this was impossible to predict and that each year the results were better. At sometime, however, someone mentioned "three years" as an expected survival time. As time passed she *seemed* less invested in the question.

After Brian completed high school, he elected to go to a college several hundred miles from our medical center. Arrangements were made between our medical center and the one attached to the university he planned to attend for his continuing care. A part of this planning was that both medical enters would keep a two-week supply of an antirejection drug (Azathioprine) that was at that time still considered experimental and sometimes difficult to obtain. It was felt in this way that if either center ran short they could procure the medication from the other institution. This arrangement, and the arrangements for blood counts and his chemical checks, were implemented without difficulty. Brian did well physically and socially, enjoying his college experience and gradual return to a self-concept of healthy vigor.

In the midst of this calm, Dr. Metcoff received a phone call from Mrs. T. one morning in which she anxiously stated that the University Medical Center had depleted their supply of Brian's medication and that she feared he would die. Dr. Metcoff called the attending physician at the university immediately and was told that while there had been some difficulty in obtaining the last batch of medicine, the shortage was in no way critical and that Brian would continue to be well cared for. Although slightly surprised, since Mrs. T. had never been an alarmist, Dr. Metcoff ascribed her concern to some kind of miscommunication. He confidently called Mrs. T. back to inform her that all was well, only to have his serenity shattered by an outburst of anguished and unreasoning bitterness from her. He was accused of insensitivity and lack of concern. The medical team was thought to be interested only in the procedure and the experiments, and certainly not in Brian. We were indicted for lack of interest in peoples' feelings and disinterest in Brian's life. Mrs. T. said many other things that day that were powered by the impetus of her explosive anguish rather than motivated by reasoned pain.

Being the competent clinician that he is, Dr. Metcoff did not become defensive or counteraggressive or attempt to hammer back with cool logic. He rode out the storm by listening with that part of the human apparatus that resonates to human suffering and sought only to keep communication flowing. By the time the conversation was finished, he had a good idea of what the problem was and the area about which we had more to learn. Even as he was talking to Mrs. T., he became aware that it was three years *to the day* that Brian had had his transplantation. Later as we reviewed the conversation and the course of our interventions, we were convinced that we could formulate what had happened, for Mrs. T. taught us a bit more about what occurs in human beings as they face death throughout life.

Mrs. T. was a mature woman. She was close to 40 when we first came to know her. Everything we saw indicated that she had faced and mastered those developmental steps that permit humans to groom and leaven their narcissism so that they can develop the wisdom, humor, and identifications needed to face their own impermanence. She had achieved that transformation of her sense of self that Kohut (1966) talks about in his article "Forms and Transformation of Narcissism" She had become a happy and productive woman, wife, and mother. She was invested in her husband and children as individuals separate from her and cherished their presence as well as their accomplishment. This serenity was shattered by the illness that assaulted the family through Brian. The situation was doubly cruel because it required not only that the family feel the threatened loss of Brian but also that it face the suffering and threat to Mrs. T. What we had not contemplated was that due to the need to mobilize her resources and because of the nature of the medical intervention, the ability to grieve two issues had been inhibited in Mrs. T.

After being initially stunned and aggrieved by her son's illness, Mrs. T. had to "pull herself together" and support herself and Brian emotionally. She had to react with hope and optimism to the notion of transplantation. This interfered with her ability to grieve the imminent loss of her son. Once the procedure was undertaken, the concern about Brian's recovery, his postsurgical management, and the business of his resuming a "normal life" interfered with the process of grieving the accelerated loss of her own physical integrity. It is on this latter form of grief that we should dwell, since medical practitioners have not contemplated it sufficiently, our culture does not foster its expression, and it is a nearly universal phenomenon in acute illness.

THE PHENOMENON OF GRIEF

To understand this phenomenon, we must recall that in 1920 Henry Head articulated the neurophysiologic concept of the "body image" (1952). He pointed out that sensations from the periphery of the body constantly reach the cortex to form a "schema" or mental representation of the body, which is used as a reference for interaction with the physical world. These stimuli from the periphery of our body have come to be so taken for granted that we no longer contemplate their presence but find interference with them most disruptive to everyday functioning. If we think of the disruption caused by lesions to these sensory pathways in illnesses such as multiple sclerosis or the discomfort caused by local anaesthesia in a mandibular (jaw) block, we get an idea of the importance of this neurological mechanism about which we are largely unaware.

In the course of the child's development, psychological qualities are added to this essentially neuroanatomical schema. Anna Freud (1952), Willie Hoffer, (1949, 1950), Paul Schilder (1935), and others have written on this integration of functions. Through the pleasure his or her body affords the child, the pain when it is abused, and the delight he or she shares with mother as she nurtures, grooms, fondles, and gazes adorningly on it, the child comes to experience his or her physical attributes as objects to be cherished. In the early years of life then, neuroanatomical, physiological, and psychological phenomena combine to produce a relatively stable, psychologically significant, internal image the person carries of his or her own body and its attributes.

For an example of the relatively stable nature of this body image, think of the surprise we experienced when we took a college tuxedo or ball gown or service uniform out of the trunk after about 10 years and discovered how much *it had shrunk!* More serious phenomena such as the "phantom limb" attest to the relative difficulty in changing body images. Thus, as mentioned above, this relatively stable, cherished, and mostly unconscious body sense participates throughout life in constituting the part of the self that is experienced subjectively as an object. I [subject] am a healthy person [object].

The second concept to be reviewed if we are to understand grief's role in life is that of bereavement or mourning. Both in clinical and personal experience we can observe that when a person loses an object, whether it be an object relationship in the external world or a body part of function that is experienced as a cherished object, he or she experiences grief in a process called mourning. Although painful and unhappy, this process is essential for reestablishing the person's capacity to relate comfortably to other objects in his or her world or qualities that he or she possesses. A bereaved person cannot and will not accept a substitute until he or she has successfully mourned the lost loved one. A traumatized person who has lost a function or a body part cannot successfully undertake the use of compensatory faculties (or a prosthesis) until he or she has successfully mourned the lost function.

This mourning process has certain characteristics that can be observed in almost every situation of loss: It must go on over a period of time and is not a constant or linear process; it manifests itself in a series of paroxysms that gradually become less intense and more widely spaced, and leave the mourner feeling somewhat exhausted and in a state of relative quiescence; there is a gradual reinvestment in objects if the process is successful.

For example, a beloved grandmother dies relatively suddenly, leaving a family shocked and bereft. Following an acute period of grief during the wake and funeral, the family returns to its home and attempts to restore emotional order. All goes well until bedtime when seven-year-old Johnny recalls that Grandma would always inspect his hands, ears, and neck for cleanliness before kissing him good night. His memory brings a wave of grief to the family members, and together they acknowledge how much they will miss her. This subsides and only Mother, next day while cooking, recalls Grandmother's comforting presence, and she weeps for loneliness. At dinner the family notes her absence from the table and some members find it impossible to eat. Then perhaps several days pass. While watching a T. V. program, someone recalls how much Granny enjoyed a certain show and mentions her comments. Again there are tears and sadness, but gradually each episode is more brief and they are further apart until warm tender memories rather than grief are evoked by recalling Grandma. Simultaneously, one can watch Johnny become more attached to an elderly teacher. Mother begins to show warmer and friendlier feelings to an older neighbor lady and Father not only tolerates but even occasionally enjoys the ministrations of his hovering maiden secretary.

Thus, the human psyche in dealing with the grief of a loss tends to fractionate the trauma and to master it with repetition. Simultaneously, the emotional investment focused on various qualities of the lost object are gradually withdrawn and reinvested in new objects.

Let us again recall that parts of the body and their functions are experienced as objects. Any loss of a part of a function then must be subjected to mourning. If mourning it not successful, the patient cannot regain emotional equanimity and commit him- or herself to developing compensatory skills or functions. Watson and Johnson (1958) vividly described this reaction in young children with acquired physical deformities.

Actually, except for time, this is not much different from what happens in the process of aging. As cherished functions, such as sexual and physical vigor, or perceptual acuity or tolerance for fatigue, are slowly eroded by time, the person changes his or her sense of self and desires and values. Almost imperceptibly, he or she mourns the passing of youth even as he or she replaces those lost joys with an appreciation for the wisdom, security, and serenity that should come with middle and advanced years. Freshmen swell with pride at the quantities of beer they can drink. We—in our middle years—must enjoy the sensitivity with which we sip vintage wines. In a loss occasioned by an acute insult, such as illness or trauma, the time interval is, of course, much shorter and the mourning process must be more intense.

Besides the fact that we have until recently been less than thorough in our medical institutions in exploring these issues of grief, we have an additional problem in our culture. Rather than explore human grief objectively, our culture has sought to protect itself from its impact (as indeed it has with all intense human effect). There has been relatively wide acceptance of the positive value of the "stiff upper lip" and that suffering in silence somehow ennobles people and connotes, if not actually develops, strength. Conversely, "feeling sorry for one's self" indicates that a person is weak and unproductively self-indulgent. Consequently, social pressures inhibit rather than facilitate expressions of grief.

In an acute illness then, this process of gradual, fractionated grieving that goes on throughout life and leaves a person competent to face death is either precipitously accelerated or massively inhibited. In the former instance, the person accelerates the process until the work of mourning the specific issue is accomplished and the pace of everyday living and mourning is reestablished. In the latter case, the task of reestablishing those patterns of living that will permit mourning throughout life is impeded, and until those inhibitions are removed optimal functioning and adaptation are virtually impossible.

In Mrs. T.'s case, we inadvertently participated in the inhibition of grief for her son and for her lost kidney. By focusing on Brian and his pain almost exclusively, we reenforced her conviction that her grief about herself should not be voiced. We left her alone to struggle with her reactions to her scarred body and we were not sensitive to what her reactions would be when she realized that the transplantation would not insure a total restitution to full life expectancy for Brian. Had we removed some of the road blocks in her path, she may well have been able gradually to mourn the loss of Brian's health, vigor, and physical integrity, and the loss of a part of her body. Then perhaps she could have accepted and cherished the additional years she had with Brian and the contributions she made to the continuation of his young life.

Mrs. T.'s reaction should be instructive to us for a number of reasons. Some have been mentioned, but I should like to add two more. I believe we have come to be so afraid and distrustful of subjectivity in our medical and scientific institutions that we have all but forgotten that it is an objective fact that human beings are in constantly fluctuating subjective states. Furthermore, these subjective states are an enormously important variable in determining the human's illness or health as well as the use he or she makes of the faculties he or she possesses. The evaluation of these subjective states often provides the answers to why one man with a leg amputation can adjust to a prosthesis with maximum benefit and be able to dance with his wife, play with his children, drive his car, and so on, while another with almost identical physical attributes becomes essentially an invalid. It also may help to explain why when the time comes, as it must to all, to gaze on that pale and fearsome spectre called death, one person can do so with composed competence, while another struggles with a heart-rending anguish that robs him of her even or her even of a single moments peace.

Finally, in transplantation's with human donors, the situation is generally more complex. Both donor and recipient are assailed by grief from two directions; they must grieve themselves and the person they love. The complexity of their relationship has been studied by Crammond (1967), Kemph (1969), and others (Abram 1967; Castel, Nuovo, Tedesco 1971; Cobb, Lindeman 1943), and our clinical postures should be influenced by these observations. We must acknowledge that to date transplantation cannot be considered a definitive cure for renal disease. It does, however, offer a period of vitality and life that would have otherwise been lost to the recipient. Life in general, and especially when it is so brief, is too precious to be marred by fear of grief.

REFERENCES

ABRAM, H. S., *Psychological Aspects of Surgery.* Boston: Little, Brown, 1967.

CASTEL, NUOVO, TEDESCO, P. *Psychiatric Aspects of Organ Transplantation.* New York: Grune and Stratton, 1971.

COBB, S., and E. LINDEMAN, Neuropsychiatric observations. *Annals of Surgery* 117: 814-824, 1943.

CRAMMOND, W. A., Renal homotransplantation—some observations on recipients and donors. *British Journal of Psychiatry* 113: 1223-1230, 1967.

FREUD, A., The role of bodily illness in the mental life of children. *Psychoanalytic Study of the Child* 7:69-81, 69-81, 1952.

HEAD, H., *Studies in Neurology.* London: Oxford University Press, 1952.

HOFFER, W., Development of body ego, *Psychoanalytic Study of the Child* 5: 18-23, 1950.

———, Mouth, hand and ego integration. *Psychoanalytic Study of the Child* 3-4, 49-56, 1949.

KEMPH, J., E. A. BERMAN, and H. P. COPPOLILLO, Kidney transplants and shifts in family dynamics. *American Journal of Psychiatry* 125: 1485-1490, 1969.

KOHUT, H., Forms and transformations of narcissism. *Journ. American Psychoanalytic Association* 14: 243-272, 1966.

SCHILDER, P., *The Image and Appearance of the Human Body: Studies in the Constructive Energies of the Psyche.* London: George Routledge, 1925.

WATSON, E., and A. JOHNSON, The emotional significance of acquired physical disfigurement in children. *American Journal of Orthopsychiatry* 28: 85-97, 1958.

17

The Adolescent with Cancer

John E. Schowalter

Fortunately, cancer is not common during adolescence, but when it does occur the patient is extremely difficult to manage emotionally.* Adolescence is the time of life for fulfillment, and the prospect of one's body killing one presents the patient with a most cruel paradox. It is this tragic quality that predominates or stifles the reactions of a majority of dying adolescent patients, their parents, and the caretaking staff. In our experience most dying adolescents deny their fate, while a more remarkable minority adjust best within the realistic context of their despair.

PATIENT BEHAVIOR

For the most part, patient questions about their diagnosis and prognosis are conspicuous by their absence. This is more true for younger than older adolescents. Adolescents are in general very inquisitive and demanding patients, and it can be assumed that the passivity characteristically exhibited by cancer victims stems from the fact that they know they have a fatal illness, or that they have picked up cues from others indicating they are not supposed to ask questions, or both.

Cindy was a 15-year-old girl who had a widespread cerebral tumor. Even after extensive brain surgery on two occasions and with moderately severe increased intracranial pressure and evidence of general deteriora-

*This work was supported by the Maternal and Child Health Division and the Mental Health Administration of the DHEW, the Connecticut Department of Health, and USPHS grant 5 T1 MH 5442-20.

tion, she kept a cheery disposition. Being a bright girl, there was no way she could not have realized her prognosis. However, keeping a smile and a stiff upper lip was an important feature of the character of her family, and loyalty to this expectation was more important (and perhaps more protecting) than facing her destiny and entering into mourning.

Besides this reluctance to inquire directly into their fate, few other characteristics seem to differentiate cancer victims from other severely ill adolescents. Some are docile "good" patients, some whine, and others are rebellious. Our experience suggests that the patient's premorbid disposition most influences his or her behavior. Other influences are the type, extent, and rapidity of involvement. Debilitation, like anything that keeps an adolescent from being active, is resented. More specifically, loss of strength or coordination for athletic boys and attractiveness for pretty girls cause great shame. We have found that to provide wigs, cosmetics, and appropriate clothes for patients who show the ravages of their malignancy can have great impact on behavior. Barbara, for example, lost most of her hair following radiation treatments. She became increasingly withdrawn. A psychiatric consultation revealed that her surface concerns focused more on the ridicule caused by a poor-fitting wig than on whether or not her tumor had been eradicated. A more natural wig led to a sudden and prolonged brightening of her behavior.

When discussing adolescent cancer patients' feelings and thoughts, a distinction must be made between those patients who acknowledge that they are dying and those who do not. In our experience the latter group keep their personal thoughts and feelings vague. They want to be closed in, and they defend equally against telling or being told about themselves. They cannot usually allow themselves extremes of behavior. One is less likely with them to witness either the rage or the calm seen in some patients who show disdain for denial and either grapple with or give in to the idea of their own death.

Once the adolescent patient acknowledges he or she is dying, the most universal thought expressed is "Why me?" There is a tremendous pressure emotionally to answer this usually unanswerable question, and much of the patient's subsequent behavior is based on the answer. We have heard some religious adolescents curse God, some curse the devil, and some find solace in identifying with Job. It is usually inconceivable to the patient that such an unspeakable horror as their cancer is not the fault of something or someone. Our clinical experience corroborates that of others in finding self-blame to be very common. Sexual fantasies or experiences, arguing with parents, getting bruised in fights, and poor physical hygiene have all been suspected by our patients as causing their malignancies.

Another common feeling expressed by the dying adolescent is "It isn't fair!" If blame is stripped from the disease, the patient must face the awful fact that his or her cause of death makes no sense. As a patient with Hodgkins disease said, "I can take everything except the damnable fact that there is no earthly reason why this should be happening to me instead of you or anybody else."

The realization that they are dying before fulfillment haunts the thoughts of many dying adolescents. Although most adults view childhood as a time of relative freedom, many children and adolescents see it as something akin to indentured servitude. If they follow the rules and put in their time, they will become adults and be able to do what they wish. One patient wept at the thought that he could not live to age 16 and fulfill his dream of owning a sports car and driving around the country picking up pretty girls. These adolescents lament not only that death means that there is nothing in their future, but that their time spent in growing up was wasted.

Another not uncommon thought of adolescents with cancer is characterized by a type of animism expressed in the belief that a malignant soul is embodied within the tumor. The disease is personified, and the course of the illness becomes for the patient a battle between "me" and "it." This split is usually comforting because the patient no longer has to struggle with the dilemma that he or she is killing him- or herself, but is able to vent anger onto something outside of "self," even though it may be inside his or her body.

Finally, because the adolescent patient has the cognitive ability to comprehend the finality of death, it is common to observe the patient expressing anticipatory mourning for him- or herself and those he or she will lose at death. Somewhat surprisingly, we have *not* found suicidal wishes to be common in dying adolescents.

BEHAVIOR OF OTHERS

Patients inevitably react to the diagnosis with shock and/or disbelief. "Are you sure?" "You must be mistaken," and "I don't believe it" are common initial responses to the diagnostician's announcement. The parents are usually told together, and, at least in the beginning, the mother is usually the more stricken while the father acts as the "strong" one and comforter. Dazed behavior usually lasts for a few weeks but may linger for many months. As with the child, an attempt to affix cause or blame is almost universal. Questions about child-rearing practices, nutrition, missed signs or symptoms, and tardiness in bringing the patient in for a checkup are frequently asked in attempts at self-indictment or exoneration. Occasionally anger will be turned onto the family doctor for not making the diagnosis earlier, onto the diagnosing physician for not "picking" a less lethal disorder, or onto the hospital staff for faulty care. In these cases the release of anger often at least temporarily lessens the parents' depression and guilt. Anger at the patient for falling ill and causing grief, stress, and expense seldom comes to the fore. When this does occur, the anger is usually either quickly denied or becomes the cause of much self-recrimination.

After being told the diagnosis, parents often experience great emotional pressure to share the tragic news, at the same time feeling that such action will be a mistake. Our experience suggests that parents usually come to regret having told others if this was done before they themselves substantially assimilate the information. As one father put it, "When we told our neighbors, we really didn't know how we felt ourselves or whether we even believed what you told us. So when we started being asked questions about what we were going to do, we felt under tremendous pressure to make plans and to act before we were able to. Once other people know, you can no longer try to figure things out at only your own pace." Although relatives and friends are often very supportive, some parents resent their intrusiveness. People who will be present but not pushy are most often singled out for appreciation. "I really like Martha," one mother said, "she always seems around but not in the way."

Parents often behave toward their dying adolescent in the way that emphasizes that this is their last chance to baby the child. Overprotection, infantilization, and overpermissiveness are all common parental behavior patterns. Siblings' behavior often worsens. A number of parents have complained that siblings resented the attention given the patient and either began causing trouble or developed various symptoms themselves. On the other end of the spectrum, occasionally siblings who have had long-standing behavior difficulties will react with fewer problems.

Both types of reaction were expressed at one family meeting. The 16-year-old semidelinquent brother of a 13-year-old boy with Hodgkins disease remarked, "Ever since Glenn got sick, it's made me realize how dumb it is to just mess around in life. Who knows when I'm going to go, and what will I have done?" His 9-year-old brother, a boy whose behavior had always been quiet and dutiful, perked up at this point and said, "I've been thinking just the opposite. Why bother with school and stuff if you can't be sure you're going to be able to get anything out of it?"

Siblings of early primary school age or younger are often unable to grasp the significance of the situation or even the full meaning of death. Their lack of mourning as expected by adults may be mistaken for callousness and responded to unjustly by parents or other relatives. "Jeff has no feelings at all," a mother said about her five-year-old son. "His brother is almost dead and all he cares about is that with all the company he can't watch his Saturday TV shows."

Peers of adolescent cancer victims are often described as avoiding the patient. As explained by the parents and by the patient him- or herself, friends tend to become shy because they do not know what to say, are ashamed for the patient, or even act as if the ill fate might be contagious.

The medical staff's reaction to a dying adolescent is affected by his or her age. Not only is there a special pathos connected with a person dying at the brink of maturity, but in teaching hospitals the similarity of staff and patients' ages facilitates identification. Nurses and house officers find that the adolescent's dying propels the shock of mortality into their own consciousness. In some this leads to overinvolvement with the patient and tremendous depression. One intern confessed, "My God, ever since I've been working with John I can't get it out of my mind that I could get Hodgkins just as easily as he did. Could you imagine such a thing? After 21 years of slaving at school?"

The staff often concentrates on the physical and diagnostic aspects of the case to avoid the personal ones. Attempts to get house officers to spend time each day talking with a hospitalized dying adolescent or to make an effort to concentrate on the patient's social and psychologic status during an outpatient visit are often only minimally effective. The most common staff defensive behavior toward a dying patient is avoidance.

Nurses have many of the same behavioral reactions as physicians, but their work thrusts them closer to the patient and provides less opportunity for avoidance. Nurses also often have to administer medications or procedures that cause the patient further discomfort. Nurses at times resent what they experience as prolonged terminal therapies and fulfill a general finding that the closer the contact a staff member has with a child *in extremis* the sooner they wish that the patient be allowed to die. Understandably, those patients known the longest cause the greatest amount of staff mourning behavior.

Anger by staff toward adolescent cancer patients is usually present but, as with the parents, it's often either repressed or displaced. For example, house officers may deny that a whiny adolescent girl suffering from a spongioblastoma (malignancy of the central nervous system) is any bother, but will twice forget a meeting called to discuss ward management of the patient. Frequently, nurses and physicians become unrealistically angry at the dying patient's parents or at each other, especially if under the pressure of having more than one terminal patient on the ward at a time.

When the adolescent dies, there are often feelings of relief and emotional release as well as grief. When the former are realized but not recognized as normal, guilt sometimes results. As one nurse put it, "I really feel bad that Kathy is dead, but I'm also glad she's not suffering any more. Before I got into this job I'd never have guessed you could ever feel even a little glad when a kid died."

PATTERNS OF INTERACTION

"Availability" has in our experience been the key to helpful interactions with a dying adolescent. The patient at this age wants independence but also needs family, friends, and medical staff. Translated into behavior, this means that parents keep close but do not smother or infantilize the patient. Everyone should allow the patient to know as much of his or her prognosis as he or she wishes and not force either denial or unwanted reality. Daily talks between one physician and the hospitalized patient are useful. If the patient wants to be angry, sad, or complaining, this should be tolerated and tried to be understood. An outraged patient is often easier to interact with than the emotionally paralyzed "good" patient. Involvement of the patient in decisions about medication and procedures fosters a helpful pattern of interactive mutuality.

One of the most instructive experiences I have had with a terminal patient was with a 14-year-old girl with Ewing's tumor (a bone cancer). I was a resident in adult psychiatry and was consulted because a pediatrician had heard I knew something about hypnosis. The girl screamed in pain continually in spite of large doses of medications. The staff feared their only choice was between allowing the patient to continue disrupting the ward or rendering her semiconscious through massive medication. They hoped hypnosis would prove an effective alternative.

I found the girl very frightened, too frightened to pay attention enough to be hypnotized. Her parents had pretty much abandoned her during this final hospitalization, and the staff and other patients were estranged by her behavior. Although as a hypnotist I failed, I returned daily to talk with the girl for the remaining four weeks of her life. She spoke of her despair, her anger, her fear, and her loneliness. Her screaming subsided, and together we made decisions on lowering her analgesic and sedating medications. The ward staff was thankful, and the girl, fully aware of what was happening, was alert and peaceful up to the time of death.

There are also destructive patterns of interaction. At times people who are dying are treated as inferior and as not knowing what is good for them. Such behavior is especially anathema to the adolescent. Avoiding the patient, either physical avoidance or avoidance in the sense of not allowing the patient access to information he or she wishes about the cancer or treatment, will not surprisingly quash mutuality. When the patient uses massive denial or displaces anger from his or her plight onto those around him or her, this tends to drive the others off and also breaks down interaction. Responses that misjudge the adolescent's capacity can cause resentment. Unrealistic restriction of school, athletic, and social events are common. Even parents' avoidance of discipline can cause more upset than calm. A number of adolescents with cancer have told me, "I know I must have something bad because my parents don't get mad at anything I do anymore." Some of these patients then tried to force their parents to treat them as before, and this behavior furthered alienation.

RECOMMENDATIONS

There must be continuity of care for adolescents dying of cancer. This should usually be given by either the family physician or by the hospital-based internist or pediatrician who makes the initial tests and diagnosis. Too often, for example, a patient with cancer goes from pediatrician to orthopedist to chemotherapist to radiotherapist. A single physician in charge of communication and liaison with adolescent patient and family provides a basis for trust.

Everyone working with dying patients needs support. The patient needs support and the family needs support. The primary physician needs consultation and support from colleagues, perhaps including a psychiatrist.

As much should be explained to family and dying adolescent as can be assimilated. Even without being told directly, it should be assumed that the patient knows he or she is dying as soon as the parents do. The patient should be told the diagnosis and as much of the prognosis as he or she wishes to know. Patients do not generally ask about prognosis unless the emotional atmosphere allows it. Then many patients do.

The specificity of the adolescent's time of life should be recognized as unique. The special meaning of disability and death to a person whose body, mind, and social status are expected to be maturing must be acknowledged. Both patient and parents should be involved as much as possible in deciding on the course of therapy. This should include deciding when further treatment might be only prolonging death rather than life. Staff have trouble reacting to a patient when they feel in the position of keeping him or her alive while hoping he or she will die. Parents and patient also resent staff when it is believed the latter are prolonging death for no reason other than a belief that life is always preferable to death.

A patient should be kept active, in school, and out of the hospital as much as possible. Our experience is that if given good care, patients can often stay out of the hospital longer than if they feel unsupported emotionally. And a certain number of patients elect to die at home.

Finally, it is important not to expect adolescent patients or their families to act in any stereotypic way. As noted in the case material, some patients are placid, others rage; some do question, others do not; some become more mature, others regress. One must not rely on formulae but expect just as wide a range of behavior in dying adolescents as one expects in the living. An additional outcome of treating each situation as a unique challenge is that the caretaker's mind is continually expanded, and he or she becomes that much better prepared to meet the next unique challenge.

V

YOUNG ADULTS

For the young adult, dying appears to evoke perhaps more intense emotions than at any other time of life. The descriptions of strong denial are most obvious here in these chapters. Certainly, facing a chronic period of dying is directly antithetical to the active life style of the young adult who has just entered the independence of the adult years.

The problem of uncertain dying trajectories is clearly shown. The patient with multiple sclerosis, described by van den Noort, seems almost immobilized by the continuing uncertainty of the disease. The same dilemma is posed by Steger, whereas acute uncertainty takes its toll in the disruption of personal relations, as shown by DeFrancisco and Watson.

The chapter by van den Noort, although couched in medical language, is very significant. He carefully documents how physical illness affects the substance of emotional ajustment. Too often we ignore the impact of body on psyche. Furthermore, he reminds us again that fear of death is often not the critical issue but rather fear of disability, of loss of body, of loss of self-control, of loss of one's mind and conscious self.

The same theme is carried through by Steger, who also illustrates the intense emotional interactions between the patient and the staff. He shows how the psychosocial aspects of care often are more critical than the technical, medical aspects of care.

Finally, DeFrancisco and Watson provide an important analysis of the entire social system of dying. They conclude that the social system may be crucial in creating a milieu in which dying may be a stress, or may be converted into a crisis.

18

Life, Limbo, and Death with Multiple Sclerosis

Stanley van den Noort

This book deals with the physical and psychic milieu of death from several diseases. In most of these diseases the time course is measured in months or years, and death is a fairly direct and predictable consequence of the primary disease. Multiple sclerosis belongs to a group of illnesses that have a very different time course and scenario. They are chronic illnesses with variable rates of progression in which *the spectre of disability exceeds the spectre of death*; in which the total span of life is often the same as that for the general population; and in which the ultimate cause of death after decades of illness is often quite unrelated to the primary disease. Multiple sclerosis and rheumatoid arthritis are the two most common disorders in this class. In this class of degenerative disorders, there is no fixed rate of progression. Rather there are repeated attacks of unpredictable frequency and severity, which lead to additive disability of equally unpredictable severity. This enormous variability leads to a common sense of frustration and anxiety in physician, patient, and family.

CASE ILLUSTRATIONS

To emphasize the dilemma faced by all in dealing with such an uncertain disease, it may be useful to identify the range of variation in multiple sclerosis. In better than 10 percent of autopsies that demonstrate widespread chronic lesions of multiple sclerosis, the diagnosis was not made or considered in life. Indeed, the medical record often fails to mention any past symptom or illness referable to the nervous system. Conversely, nearly 5 percent of patients who die after many years of disability ascribed to multiple sclerosis are found to have had another disease—most commonly a tumor near the base of the brain. I have seen individuals die in 24 hours from the first attack of multiple sclerosis, yet two-thirds of patients live a normal life-span. Approximately one-third of patients with multiple sclerosis are capable of normal and productive lives after a score of years with symptomatic disease.

Multiple sclerosis is a disease of young people, with onset usually falling between the ages of 18 and 35. It has a preference for women but is usually more severe in men. Attacks may be ill defined or obvious. A single attack may last several months and recur at intervals of months or years. With the passage of time, attacks become less clearly defined, while disability may cease or accumulate more slowly over many years. These generalizations fail to provide an adequate picture, so let us consider a series of examples.

CASE 1.   This 40-year-old man had been well until age 20. While serving in the Navy, he developed tingling in his legs and abdominal pain. He was admitted to a naval hospital and found to have normal health, together with some hostility toward his physicians. He was discharged from the Navy without compensation because his personality made him unfit for military service. He returned home to work as a successful and highly skilled employee of the telephone company. He married and fathered six children. Friends and relatives observed that he would at times display a slight limp and that his tolerance for very heavy physical work had decreased. These minor changes did not seem to warrant medical attention. At age 30, left temporal headaches of a severe nature developed and recurred at least twice weekly. Careful medical studies were unrevealing. At age 31, a physical examination revealed spasticity in the left leg. Numerous studies to exclude a brain tumor were unrevealing. The headaches subsided spontaneously but were replaced by progressive impairment of eye movement, clumsy limbs, and spasticity. These signs stabilized or progressed slowly on steroid therapy for six years, and he was able to work at a desk for his employer. Repeated efforts to stop steroids were rewarded by increased difficulties in the eyes and limbs. Steroid therapy produced some mild behavioral overactivity and emotional instability culminating in an effort to seduce his oldest daughter. Steroids were stopped. Over the next year his walking deteriorated to the point where he required a wheelchair at all times, and repeated bouts of incontinence required a constant catheter. For the past four years he has remained largely unchanged in a wheelchair existence.

CASE 2.   This 45-year-old nurse was well until age 22 when she noted pain and severe loss of vision in the right eye. After two months, vision gradually returned to normal without treatment. She remained in excellent health until age 42 when an acute paralysis of the legs developed over several days. She remains confined to a wheelchair to this time.

CASE 3.   This 23-year-old man was well until age 19 when multiple neurological symptoms began to appear, improve, recur, and extend. Over an interval of two years, disability accumulated to the point where he had little useful vision, was unable to speak or swallow, and was paralyzed in all limbs except for some movement in the left arm. In the following year, use of the left arm deteriorated. He remains bedridden in a nursing home with little capacity to react with the world around him. Considerable intellectual deterioration is present.

CASE 4.   This 30-year-old woman was well until age 20 when she had a transient leg paralysis with double vision following the birth of her first child. A year later optic neuritis in one eye, double vision, severe unsteadiness, and spastic weakness appeared. By age 23 her condition had stabilized and a second pregnancy was uneventful. Over the past seven years her previously outstanding intellect has deteriorated steadily. However, she remains active and able to provide basic care for her home and family.

CASE 5.   This 50-year-old highly successful executive has had seven discrete attacks of multiple sclerosis in 15 years. Residual disabilities are limited to an unsteady gait with fatigue and some urgency of urination. Intellect and judgment are unaffected.

CASE 6.   This 54-year-old woman had slowly increasing stiffness of gait and urgency of urination for 20 years. She remained bright and compulsive. Frequent changes of wardrobe, interior decoration of her home, and changes of community were possible because of her family's affluence. At age 54, after several years of intractable depression, she committed suicide with an overdose of sedatives. Up to that time she had remained ambulatory with only modest physical limitations.

CASE 7.   This 87-year-old woman died of metastatic breast cancer after living for 35 years in a nursing home. Between the ages of 30 and 42, recurrent bouts of multiple sclerosis had left her with incontinence, paralysis, clumsy arms, double vision, and reduced visual acuity. From age 42 to 87 her neurological deficit remained unchanged except for infrequent bouts of facial pain.

CASE 8.   This 40-year-old woman had an episode of unsteady gait and visual change at ages 20 and 22. At age 40 she is well and unlimited in her activity.

PERSONAL RESPONSES TO ILLNESS

These highly variable patterns make generalization very difficult. *Relatively few of these patients are concerned about death as such. They fear physical and mental disability and would often welcome death as an alternative.* The emotional responses of any patient with multiple sclerosis are highly individualized; they reflect the original personality, the reaction to uncertainty and disability, and the effects on the nervous system of the disease and its treatment. There is no stereotype personality, but there is a correlation with higher levels of intelligence and achievement.

The early symptoms of multiple sclerosis are often indistinguishable from neurotic and hysterical symptoms. This often leads to confusion and results in diagnostic error. We also recognize that first and subsequent attacks of multiple sclerosis appear to follow stressful events that strain normal physiologic responses and provide an environment in which multiple sclerosis may appear. This may explain a high frequency of milder or incomplete forms of the disease and a high prevalence rate in some neurotic personalities.

The patient with established multiple sclerosis focuses his or her concern on possible disability, often exaggerated by personal contact with other severely disabled patients. Every minor fluctuation in physical performance enhances this anxiety, and there is a natural tendency to ascribe all the negative events of life to the vagaries of multiple sclerosis. A common observation is that effort and fatigue exaggerate present disabilities; rest and a dependent role produce improvement. This compounds the problem by producing social withdrawal and excessive fear of any stressful event. Many patients at some point join a therapeutic cult to suppress the anxiety of recognizing an untreatable disease. Megavitamins, acupuncture, wheat-free diets, zucchini diets, vegetable oil diets, steroids, minerals, allergy shots all provide a sense of security and evangelized zeal. It may well be that the removal of anxiety by such mechanisms has a valid therapeutic effect. Those patients who fail to find a coincidence of therapy and well-being often are led on an expensive and futile search to identify a doctor, a climate, or treatment that will provide a positive effect.

As with all chronic disease, there is a regrettable introversion of attention that magnifies the somatic problems. Chronic depression is a common response to disability and serves to amplify the effects of the disability; morbid fear of total disability and suicidal thoughts are common. It is very clear that those who do best have managed to sustain an active positive role in the environment while learning to respect the limitations imposed by their disability.

Brain impairment is most feared by those multiple sclerosis patients without intellectual or emotional signs of brain disease. Minor absent-mindedness, marital discord, or errors of judgment are interpreted by the patient, and sometimes by the family, as evidence of brain involvement. Depression and overmedication further magnify this problem. Abnormalities of bladder function, bowel control, and sexual performance of spinal origin are interpreted by patients as evidence of brain disease. Loss of dexterity, slurred speech, and an unsteady gait lead to accusations of intoxication and magnify these fears. Such changes in a young attractive woman who is very sensitive about her appearance quickly lead to depression and social withdrawal.

Special note should be made of the effects of brain stem plaques (diseased patches) on the release of laughter or crying. In multiple sclerosis, this often takes the form of an unusual ease of smiling and laughter that is out of proportion to the emotional content. When this is marked, an effort to smile appropriately may lead to an uncontrollable fit of giggling, which is recognized by the patient and others as quite inappropriate. It is little wonder that such patients fear for their mental health.

DISEASE EFFECTS ON PERSONALITY

Physical and psychic manifestations of multiple sclerosis may be very brief. For example, handwriting may abruptly deteriorate during writing and be restored after several minutes of rest. Similar abrupt behavioral and emotional shifts of a highly unpredictable nature are seen. Muscle jerks, seizures, and involuntary movements occur in a few patients. These very transient phenomena cause much concern and diagnostic confusion, particularly with hysteria. The brevity of the effects suggest that they are not attended by actual plaque formation.

Progressive disability in any chronic disease is often accompanied by the assumption of dependent roles, by vigorous claims for attention from others, and by preoccupation with self. In multiple sclerosis, these problems are often compounded by brain lesions that produce psychosis, altered emotional responses, and impaired memory. Occasionally, multiple sclerosis will begin as a frank schizophrenic psychosis, which only can be recognized by the appearance of signs pointing to more typical brain lesions. Depression is common and may be abrupt in onset. Euphoria is seen usually in the context of considerable dementia. Steroid therapy may produce depression or a schizophrenic psychosis. Patients with sizeable frontal lobe defects may demonstrate a grasp reflex, neglect of incontinence, and a curious compulsion to comment on all environmental events. Patients with more caudal brain lesions may conversely show avoidance reflexes and a hostile suspicious withdrawal from the environment.

Memory impairment is often merely a sign of depression and self-preoccupation. However, true loss of memory may occur with or without other signs of impaired intellect and judgment. Dementia is common in advanced multiple sclerosis, although the degree is often not very severe. Occasionally, it is the only prominent symptom. A curious "affable" dementia is a characteristic feature of advanced multiple sclerosis in which there is no anxiety or depression. This dementia spares the patient from recognition of his or her plight and any foreboding of death. Unfortunately, the dementia compounds the problem for the family and makes it impossible to sustain employment, self-care, or rehabilitation.

In some severely disabled individuals, largely deprived of sight and sensory input from the spinal cord, one encounters confusion and hallucinatory states due to sensory deprivation. These may represent unreal but pleasant experiences or may take the form of terrifying sensations of falling or suspension in space. These states are exacebated by sedation or physical isolation where they will not disturb other patients.

CAUSES OF DEATH

As we stated earlier, death directly due to multiple sclerosis usually occurs only in severe forms of the disease. Decubitus ulcers cause significant malnutritional states so that terminal systemic infection often occurs. The need for a chronic urinary catheter inevitably gives rise to infection, which may be fatal. These systemic infections may show little fever and may be accompanied by shock. Chronic urinary tract infection and stone formation may lead to renal failure and a uremic death. Long intervals of bed rest, impaired ventilation, and a liability to aspirate ingested food provide the background for pneumonia. Occasionally, brain stem lesions will arrest ventilation and lead to a respiratory death.

The use of steroids and immunosuppresants results in increased death from superinfection and gastrointentional hemorrhage.

LIVING WITH UNCERTAINTY

For those multiple sclerosis persons who have no dementia, yet have moderate to severe physical disabilities, suicide is a major risk. *Living* with multiple sclerosis is for them a much more serious problem than any concern with death from the disease. It is necessary to persuade the patient to acknowledge the realities of his or her illness without preoccupation with it. Patients must be steered away from treatments of certain cost but uncertain benefits. Concentrated efforts to sustain a normal life situation and external interests are rewarding if achieved without exceptional stress and fatigue. There is a general impression that patients of stable character, calm disposition, and a capacity to accept their limitations are able to continue some role in society. They also have an improved diagnosis.

An important phenomenon in multiple sclerosis is the amplification of disability by fatigue and fever. Fatigue is poorly understood. It requires rest after physical exertion and sleep at the end of the day. When any neurological system is heavily compromised and has lost its "reserve," one encounters exaggerated effects of fatigue. A person may arise without double vision, yet require an eye patch by midmorning. A stiff spastic gait may produce such weakness as to preclude walking by afternoon. Most patients find that short intervals of rest during the day are of value in sustaining activity through the entire day. Protracted reading and writing may be prohibited. As with normal individuals, fatigue may not appear at the same point in daily activity; it is greatly influenced by motivational and psychic factors. Drugs that diminish "psychic" fatigue or depression are of limited value. Stubborn constipation is a common feature of multiple sclerosis, requiring constant attention; relief of constipation tends to improve effort, tolerance, and mood. Fever exaggerates neurological dysfunction. As a consequence, patients who are working and ambulatory may become confined to bed and paralyzed if they develop influenza. This is commonly misinterpreted as a relapse in the disease. Function usually returns to its previous level when the fever disappears.

The pursuit of lost health becomes a preoccupation with many patients and their families. Information in the newspapers, magazines, and notes from the National Multiple Sclerosis Society are carefully examined, debated, and acted upon. Families often aid in this "busy work," which only serves to focus attention on the disease rather than on life. All this is excused in the name of "giving hope," "something will work someday," "even if it helps a little." Many physicians are similarly involved and try each nostrum that comes along, readily referring to each new therapeutic cult to provide "every opportunity" for their patients. Many patients are led to abandon jobs and relatives to find a better climate even though it has no recognized influence on the disease.

SUMMARY

The common psychosocial problems that plague the patient with multiple sclerosis are fears of economic, physical, mental, cosmetic, and sexual failure. Death itself is rarely considered. The important therapeutic goal is to encourage a life within imposed physical limitations, which is directed toward normal self-fulfillment in their world. It is essential to avoid the brooding, foreboding, preoccupation with self and therapy in a disease for which treatment is largely ineffective and which may be exacerbated by anxiety and emotional stress.

19

Trauma in the Young Adult

Herbert G. Steger

For the majority of young adults, death remains a distant, abstract event. It is something that happens to elderly grandparents, to a distantly remembered friend in a car accident, in a far-off war, or it is discussed in a philosophy class or magazine article. However, death is rarely considered as a concrete possibility for oneself. Little thought is typically given one's daily activities as they relate to the possibility of death. Attention to physical health, for example, is often rather reflexive. The life-long experience of robust youthful good health and energy can give a sense to the young adult of physical invulnerability. Concern with the possibility of death and with the remote, dimly conceived possibilities of old age, infirmity, or disability is usually scanty.

Yet for some young adults, the probability of dying and the nature of their relationship to death change quickly and dramatically. Sudden, catastrophic injury and resulting permanent disability have been a major affliction of young adults in almost every generation. Trauma to the nervous system, especially to the spinal cord, has become one of their most common disabling conditions as our technical skills have increased survival rates. Severe injuries that result in permanent damage to the brain and spinal cord are becoming quite frequent as a result of the reckless, often physically dangerous leisure and recreational involvements that are common for many young adults—motorcycle and automobile sports, water skiing, football, sky diving, sail kite flying. Injuries to the spinal cord are often the result of accidents in these activities, activities that often provide excitement primarily due to the physical danger posed to the individual.

A spinal cord injury suddenly shifts the individual into a life situation where he or she must remain constantly vigilant to his or her physical well-being and where careful attention must be given to minute aspects of daily care. He or she becomes a fragile individual who must spend large portions of the waking day attending to his or her body and its functioning in ways that were completely unknown before the injury. Often he or she must depend upon others to care for most basic and intimate needs and functions. He or she is constantly endangered by complications of the disability, by ulcerations, and by recurrent festering chronic infections, which can flare with little warning and threaten further debilitation and death. Serious injuries and unnoticed burns can result because of lack of sensation. Often he or she is in jeopardy of dying suddenly by choking while simply eating. The young injured adult is vulnerable to many life-threatening conditions, which can develop despite constant vigilance and careful effort.

The patient's adjustment to such a chronically fragile and uncertain situation involves at least two important elements: adjustment to the disability and its implications, and coming to grips with the uncertainty of his or her future. Unlike conditions where the outcome may be more certain, and the individual can or must deal with the certainty of dying, the problems of adjustment to disability and to an uncertain future are tightly interwoven. In many ways the two are quite similar, and successful resolution of one often implies or leads to resolution of the other.

The loss of physical function or of a body part caused by precipitously disabling conditions such as traumatic spinal cord injury have been commonly likened to the losses experienced through bereavement or through a "partial death" of part of the individual (Schoenberg, Carr 1970). The process of adjustment to catastrophic injury and disability is also felt to be similar to the process of coping with dying. The usual focus of adjustment to sudden loss and to severe disability is upon the emotional or psychodynamic factors. Equally important, however, are other influences, such as interpersonal interactions and expectations, social and situational demands, and disease or disability related factors (Kiely 1972; Blacher 1970).

PROBLEMS OF THE SPINE-INJURED PATIENT

A 20-year-old single man suffered a high cervical spinal cord injury from a self-inflicted gunshot wound in an apparent suicide attempt while under the influence of drugs. He was left with complete quadriplegia, with no voluntary control of muscles below his neck.

At the time of his admission to the hospital and for several months thereafter, he was in danger of suddenly dying from any one of several actual or potential complications. He had an infection of the cervical spine at the site of his injury, which threatened to spread into the spinal cord. The bullet had been shot through his esophagus, with a resulting esophageal fistula (passageway) that caused serious problems with his swallowing so that he was in continuous danger of choking to death. He suffered from several respiratory infections, which further compromised his already seriously limited respiratory status.

The patient was initially admitted to neurosurgery where he was isolated from other patients and cut off from visual contact with staff or patients by curtains drawn around his bed. The patient constantly yelled obscenities at the nurses and was noted to be vile and verbally abusive of the staff who had the responsibility for his continuous care. At times he became terrified about dying and began pleading with the nurses not to let him die. At other times he loudly berated the nurses and physicians for their failure to care for him adequately. His girl friend, with whom he had been living prior to his injury, was physically removed—only after considerable difficulty—from his room on several occasions by security guards. Nursing staff noticed that he was more subdued and calm after her visits, and feared that she was giving him drugs in a continuation of their preinjury relationship, which apparently consisted primarily of sex and drugs.

The patient became extremely bitter about removing his girl friend and escalated his anger and verbal attacks. He was transferred to the in-patient rehabilitation service where his conflict with nursing and medical staff continued unabated. His medical status remained uncertain, and his frequent terror about dying was intensified by recurrent deterioration in his condition with transfers to the Intensive Care Unit (ICU).

The rehabilitation nurses reacted with considerable ambivalence to the patient: sympathetic to his frightening and helpless condition, enraged and rejecting of his vilification of them and their efforts. Staff working closely with the patient noted that he was quite unrealistic in his outlook for physical function in the future and felt that this reflected an unhealthy denial of reality, which kept him from appreciating and cooperating with their efforts for him. Several attempts at confronting him with the certainty and irreversibility of his disability had no apparent effect. His presence on the service became an increasingly divisive issue, with nursing staff pressing for his transfer because they felt him to be primarily a medical and nursing care problem without rehabilitation potential; other staff was equally firm that he could benefit more from the skills of rehabilitation medicine and nursing than he could from other inpatient care. An agreement was finally reached to transfer him until his condition was medically stable.

Our primary concern here is with the impact upon the patient and on those working with him of this sudden disability and the chronic uncertainty of death that confronted him. The rapid changes that result with sudden, catastrophic disability can often exceed the individual's coping capacity and can throw him or her into a crisis state (Fordyce 1971; Aquilera, Messick, Farrel 1970). It is clear that this patient, and to an extent the professional staff, was in a crisis situation brought on by his injury and possible sudden death. The patient's ways of coping with his persistent fear and uncertainty were not acceptable to the staff. The resulting interactions with the staff are likely to have enhanced his crisis and hindered its resolution. This type of patient, of course, poses very difficult problems in management, and much can be learned from the way he was managed or mismanaged.

First, resolving or diminishing the patient's overwhelming crisis situation should take primary priority over attempts at helping him to assimilate and adjust to his disability or cope with the actual possibility of impending death. Whereas the usual goal of crisis intervention is to return a patient to precrisis level of functioning, the aim of crisis resolution with this kind of disabled patient is directed at supporting him through the crisis period, minimizing factors that contribute to his disorganization and anxiety, stimulating or modeling and reinforcing effective coping, and initiating relationships in which he can begin to develop a trusting, positive dependency for future rehabilitation efforts.

As Fordyce (1971) has pointed out, marked and sudden changes in sensory input, of the sort experienced by this patient as a result of his spinal cord injury, can lead to confusion and disorganization. Instead of the additional sensory restriction imposed by isolation behind curtains, his awareness of the presence and activity of staff and other patients would help maintain a level of stimulation and reality contact that would keep him more oriented and organized. The sudden helplessness experienced by patients like this, when they lose the majority of their effective behavioral repertoire upon which they previously relied to deal with internal and external problems—for example, motor activity—contributes significantly to the patient's crisis situation. The patient is confronted with threats from which he or she cannot escape and for which he or she has no effective response available. The majority of the decisions made about care—both major and trivial—are made for the patient even to the extent of deciding for him or her who may visit. Instead of enforcing helpless passivity, the patient should be involved by staff in having a say about what is going to happen to him or her to begin promoting a sense of personal control, responsibility, and mastery again. As Fordyce suggested, this involvement in mastery training should begin simply, with adequate modeling, be tangibly successful, and richly rewarded.

This conflict over control and responsibility is likely to become a significant one for this particular patient in the future since he will be perpetually dependent for the rest of his life. Some of the conflict with nursing staff undoubtedly was fueled by preinjury rebellion against dependency and authority coming in conflict with his actual total dependency and the nurses' expectations for the sort of compliant patient attitude and behavior that are to accompany it. Hospital staff should be fully aware that the transition to compliant dependency is often a slow and painful process for the young adult male. The groundwork can be laid early for regressive, passive, manipulative dependency, or for positive, mature dependency in which the disabled patient relies upon others not to control them, but to accomplish that which he can no longer do for himself.

There was an apparently premature and ineffective effort to get this patient to give up his denial and accept the total and permanent nature of his disability. Denial has a bad reputation among rehabilitation staff, since acceptance of a disability is considered to be essential for a positive outcome. There is also reason to believe, however, that the attempts at getting a patient to accept the staff's particular view of his condition can be an effort at controlling some aspect of his behavior, in this case to reduce his projection and angry outbursts directed at the staff. In a situation like this, however, it is questionable whether imposing a preconceived notion of the "right" way to respond to disability (or to any loss) is beneficial for the individual patient. With this patient, who faced the threat of unpredictable sudden death as well as permanent disability, denial may well have served as a very adequate coping mechanism for helping him through his crisis period. There is some evidence, in fact, to suggest that avoidance and denial may be effective ways to deal with short-term stress over which the patient has little or no control (Cohen, Lazarus 1973). If the patient survives the crisis period, there would be ample time to confront the full impact of his disability.

During this time, the patient's overwhelming fear of dying remained relatively intense. He was terrified by the thought of death while in the hospital even though he had tried to kill himself before, He was able to think about death only very briefly before being overwhelmed and retreating to his characteristic anger, projection, and denial. This pattern of briefly considering and then avoiding very stressful material is also seen in the way patients adjust to catastrophic disability where it seems to allow for a gradual desensitization and assimilation of the frightening idea of the situation (Shontz 1965).

In another case, a 24-year-old married father of two fell from a sailing kite some 30 or 40 feet off the ground, sustaining an injury to the spinal cord at lower lumbar level. His lesion was incomplete and he gradually regained full sensory function in both legs, and partial motor function in his left leg. He was treated for six weeks at a new, small community hospital where, according to the patient, he was given great amounts of TLC by the young nursing staff and was reassured by his doctor that he would recover quickly from his injuries and everything would be "back to normal" shortly.

He left the hospital in excellent spirits for transfer to another hospital for rehabilitation, fully expecting a continuation of the "vacation" atmosphere he had experienced at the acute care hospital. He quickly became despondent upon admission, asking for his wife to be called to come take him home since he did not need or want rehabilitation. The discrepancy between his expectations for a cheerful, quick recovery and the sight of many patients in wheelchairs, braces, and such was too great for him. Intervention by the staff psychologist resulted in the patient agreeing to stay, although he denied that there was any need for him to be rehabilitated since he expected to recover completely as his first doctor told him he would.

In the supportive setting of group therapy with other spinal cord patients, he was able to begin exploring and accepting the reality of his disability. In the ward setting, however, he continued for some time to insist that he would recover fully, and frequently insisted that his wife take him home because he was wasting time and money in the hospital. He was gradually able to accept the permanence of what had happened to him, and he began participating fully in his therapy program.

The quadriplegic patient finds him or herself heavily dependent upon other people to care for him or her. For some, the dependency may be almost complete; for others with lower level lesions there may be less of a daily dependence, but certainly they must rely much more upon others than they have at any time since childhood. Lower quadriplegics and paraplegics are also quite dependent upon others for initial training in essential self-care skills. The spinal cord-injured individual, thus, is particularly vulnerable to problems that develop in their interpersonal relationships, especially in the area of dependency. Troubles in interpersonal relationships or in relationship to authority figures that exist prior to injury can be especially difficult for the spinal cord patient, since receiving adequate care of basic survival needs depends upon others.

A 26-year-old single male suffered an injury to his high cervical spine when he dove out of a tree into shallow water while under the influence of drugs. He was left with a loss of function in his legs and significant weakness in his arms. He was hospitalized at a large rehabilitation hospital but was discharged after five months because his relationships with the staff had deteriorated to the point that they could no longer tolerate his hospitalization.

The patient was a constant behavior problem, always uncooperative and unwilling to participate in treatment programs, frequently using narcotics in the hospital, and repeatedly physically and verbally abusive toward staff members. He was discharged even though the staff felt that he had not completed his rehabilitation. Within a few weeks he traveled to another state where he demanded admission to a public hospital rehabilitation unit. There he continued his previous pattern of disruptive behavior and refused to cooperate or participate in any planned therapeutic activities because of pain. He constantly demanded drugs for pain and sleep, becoming enraged and threatening violence when his requests were denied. He received no benefit from his hospital stay and was discharged still dependent upon others for much of his care, without having learned how to care for his own bowel and bladder and without having voluntarily inspected his skin by himself. He returned to the hospital a few months later when he was admitted for surgical treatment of several large decubitus ulcers and for treatment of bladder and kidney infections and stones.

This patient's shortsighted, immature, self-centered approach to life, which was largely responsible for his catastrophic injury and disability, also makes him a likely candidate to die from the complications of his disability, primarily because he is unable to follow expected rules for his behavior, or submit himself to being cooperatively dependent, or adapt himself to the discipline and self-control necessary to care for himself.

Unfortunately, the type of behavior exemplified by this last case example is not rare. It is rather common among young paraplegics, who have been described by Mueller (1962, pp. 152-53) as having a ". . . prevalent emotional pattern . . . of adolescent egocentricity, and there are many elements of uncontrolled infantile affective behavior . . . Emotional instability and hostility, which are forms of emotional immaturity and regressive behavior, are expressed in irritability, displays of temper, anger, bitterness, resistive behavior, and general uncooperativeness." Unfortunately, it is very common for these individuals to be so provocative and disruptive that they are rejected and discharged before they have been able to establish necessary self-care regimes.

PERSONAL RELATIONSHIPS
FOR THE SPINE INJURED

Young adults with spinal cord injuries are quite vulnerable in their sexual and marital relationships since they are usually in the process of establishing them when they are suddenly disabled. The relationships are not as likely to endure the strain of losses and of role changes that accompany disability as well as older, more established relationships. The young adult's relationship has had fewer mutually experienced crises and losses, and similarly is more likely to have less well-developed shared coping responses with which to help the relationship survive a crisis. Similarly, younger relationships are likely to be less flexible and to have fewer acceptable role alternatives available for the individuals. Thus, a sudden shift of a husband into a totally dependent status may create severe strain on the relationship. Following is an example of the impact of a disability on such a young, developing relationship.

A 20-year-old married man suffered a motorcycle accident while riding in the desert. He injured his mid-cervical spinal cord, with resulting quadriplegia. For most of his married life, the patient had been financially irresponsible, rather untrustworthy, and unable to hold a steady job. As a result, the marriage had been quite unstable.

Shortly before the accident, the patient found a good paying job, which had the possibility of a good future, and had began to settle down in his marriage. The patient and his wife went through a month-long period of depression after the accident, which lifted as they both began expressing increasing anger at the staff for their incompetent treatment of the husband. Both the patient and his wife began denying that he would be permanently disabled, citing what they believed to be hopeful predictions of neurosurgery at the time of his initial hospitalization. Both declined to discuss their feelings about what had happened and what lay ahead for them and resisted efforts to provide them with counseling to assist in helping them deal with the impact of the disability. They continued to complain bitterly about the patient's slow progress in comparison to their expectations for him. The patient became increasingly lethargic, refusing to feed himself even though he could do so with assistive devices. A short time later the wife left the patient and returned to live with her parents.

A significant number of individuals who sustain spinal cord injuries have suffered injury as a result of characteristically impulsive, imprudent, immature behavior that demonstrates poor judgment and lack of attention to possible personal risk and danger involved. This relationship between the injuries and impulsive, reckless behavior has been suggested by both clinical experience (Mueller 1962) and psychometric studies (Fordyce). Individuals who have shown little concern over their safety are not likely to shift easily to the hypervigilant, attentive individual who must spend a major portion of the day attending to nuances of nutrition, care of skin, bladder, bowel, and the like. These are all areas that previously had been take for granted; little attention or time was necessary to deal with them. Now they pose the possible difference between life and death.

Excessive use of drugs or alcohol also appears frequently in the lives of individuals who suffer traumatic spinal cord injuries and is often directly associated with the accident that led to the injury. Many will continue or initiate the use of these substances after the injury as a way of dealing with the many frustrations, with lingering depression, with chronic discomfort and pain, with the inevitable rejections and stigma, with social and physical barriers, and with the numerous other sources of anguish that daily face the young cord-injured individual. Not only do drugs and alcohol fail to deal with the problems and with their sources, but they also seriously affect the individual's ability to provide the intense level of attention and care necessary to avoid preventable complications. This use of drugs or alcohol, in an individual already deficient in attention to personal safety, can result in serious neglect of skin care, of wound care, of nutrition, and of the meticulous cleanliness necessary for genitourinary care. It is not at all unusual for serious burns or major skin ulcerations to result when a patient passes out from heavy use of alcohol or drugs. More common, however, is gradual deterioration due to neglect of personal care as in the following case.

A 22-year-old single, unemployed man was paraplegic since receiving a gunshot wound to the back at the age of 18. Before the injury, he had been supporting himself and his own heroin habit by selling drugs on the street. When one potential customer turned out to be a plain clothes police officer, the patient attempted to flee on foot and received a gunshot wound to the spine, which resulted in his paraplegia. He went through an intensive rehabilitation program and had been declared independent in all areas of self-care. He was a very attractive, intelligent, personable young man who was always a model patient during frequent hospitalizations, although generally superficial and manipulating in relationships.

The patient convinced the rehabilitation staff that he was no longer interested in drugs, thanks to their intervention with him. Upon discharge, however, he began using heroin again and was able to sell enough once again to support himself and his own drug needs. He dropped out of a drug therapy program that was initiated after one hospitalization. His self-care began to be seriously neglected as he increased his drug use because of constant pain in his back and legs. Soon he had developed a large decubitus ulcer over his left hip, which, despite repeated hospitalizations and surgical treatment, continued to break down and become infected because of his neglect. This ulcer continued to grow until the head and neck of the femur protruded from the wound and the infection spread into the bone. Other ulcers developed over his hips and ankles. Chronic infection of the bladder and kidneys resulted from his failure to maintain adequate fluid intake and to maintain aseptic care of his catheterization. His physical condition and his pain continued to worsen, and he died from an apparently intentional overdose of heroin.

THE PROBLEMS OF READJUSTMENT

We have suggested that young adults who have suffered traumatic spinal cord injury can be looked at from the perspective of individuals perpetually confronted with the distinct possibility of dying from the complications of their disability. Despite advances in medical care, which have significantly reduced deaths directly related to the immediate effects of the cord injury (Freed, Bakst, Barrie 1966), the patient's long-term survival depends primarily upon him- or herself.

We have pointed to several factors that negatively affect a patient's ability to maintain fragile health and ward off the rapid physical deterioration that is possible for any patient with spinal cord injury. In working with these individuals, their families, and staff who provide their care, we have found it useful to focus our attention and efforts upon two rather distinct postinjury phases. Initially, attention should be directed at resolution of the crisis that frequently overwhelms the patient and family when confronted with sudden traumatic disability and uncertain outcome. The crisis in such a situation is most likely precipitated by one or more of the following: sudden confrontation with the possibility of death for which no specific preparation could be made and the continued uncertainty of this situation; sudden loss of previously effective instrumental behaviors for dealing with the environment (helplessness); projections of losses and deprivations into the personal future without awareness of how they will be managed; sudden reduction and change in sensory experience; sudden shift to new roles that previously were devalued and for which the patient has few or poorly developed social and behavioral skills.

In addition to intervention strategies discussed earlier (attending to situational supports and coping mechanisms), focusing on the patient's distortions in perception about the nature of his or her future can be helpful for reducing the level of dread over the future and for preparing the patient to begin dealing with his or her permanent disability. As Michael (1970) has pointed out, the newly disabled individual has a well-developed set of extremely negative anticipations about the future as a handicapped person, which can have a very disturbing effect on him or her. One way of introducing to the patient the idea that it is possible to master the disability and that the future may hold positive experience is to provide early contact with other spinal cord patients who have been successful in their rehabilitation. Early exposure to the rehabilitation activities of other para- and quadriplegic patients also may help him or her to anticipate positive activities for mastering fears of helplessness and overwhelming deprivation.

The second postinjury phase focuses on the patient's adjustment to the disability and his or her eventual resolution of its consequences for his or her life. There are several models that have been proposed to describe and account for the emotional reactions encountered after the sudden onset of a physical disability. We have found that the simple schema of crisis, denial, grieving or mourning, and integration is a useful way to summarize the model response sequence for the suddenly disabled. This sequence does not, of course, describe all of the reactions that are encountered, nor does it reflect an invarying sequence a patient must pass through. It does, however, provide a general reference for following a patient's progress in resolving the psychological impact of the disability.

Feldman (unpublished manuscript) has characterized the patient's reaction as beginning with a ". . . general denial of the frightening implications for the future . . . (which) is necessary to avoid being completely overwhelmed by the catastrophe. As denial is relinquished and reality fearfully approached, periods of depression are regularly encountered. Mourning the loss of premorbid self and its potential is to be expected. Absence of such mourning is unusual and disturbing. In its way, mourning facilitates the structuring of a future-oriented existence, which may not be possible until what has been lost has been grieved for.

These reactions to the sudden onset of traumatic disability are instrumental in assuring the patient's long-term adjustment. However, these reactions can become maladaptive if the patient continues in one phase until it begins to interfere with rehabilitation and readjustment. Thus, the patient may fail to move from a position of denial—which has initial adaptive utility—and continue to deny the permanence, reality, extent of the disability situation. With such a posture, the patient also must avoid learning about his or her disability, about how to care for him- or herself, about possible dangers posed to his or her fragile physical status, about establishing and maintaing a positively dependent relationship with a care giver. Continued denial thereby increases the patient's vulnerability to life-threatening complications of the disability.

In assessing the nature of the barriers that are blocking resolution, situational and environmental determinants of behavior should be considered as well as the more customary intrapsychic factors. Denial, for example, is usually considered to be a defense mechanism, which serves the purpose of protecting the individual from awareness of a painful internal or external reality. However, the perpetuation of denial in a patient can be related to the social and interpersonal expectations and reinforcement that are present in the patient's environment. In a case cited earlier, a young couple apparently needed to maintain the fiction of recoverability in an effort to perpetuate a relationship that could not withstand the impact of permanent and total disability in one member. We also noted a patient whose protracted denial was largely a result of the optimistic expectations for recovery by staff of an acute hospital and whose "inappropriate" delayed denial encountered by rehabilitation staff actually reflected his initial reaction to being confronted with the permanence of his disability. At other times the staff's own desire to avoid the emotional impact of the patient's condition results in their withdrawing from the patient when he or she makes early, tentative attempts at confronting the personal catastrophe. The patient often learns, then, that continued avoidance, denial, and cheerful optimism provide him or her with more support and more comfortable interactions with the staff.

Patients who have been able to complete this postdisability readjustment are able to move through a crucial transition in self-concept and social role from being "sick" to being a "different" person. While he or she remains in the social role expected of the sick person, the patient is a passive recipient of care from others; he or she is freed of responsibility for him- or herself and others; activities are largely proscribed and controlled by care givers; the patient remains in a regressive, dependent status; and he or she considers him-or herself to be less than what he or she was prior to the injury. When the patient give up the sick role, he or she can accept independence and responsibility to the extent physically possible and is able to use the dependency imposed by the disability, in a positive, instrumental way to achieve what he or she otherwise could not. It is then that the issue of chronic uncertainty is likely also to be resolved, since the individual is able more adequately to confront and master problems imposed by his or her fragile physical condition and to apply self-care skills so as to increase chances for long-term survival.

REFERENCES

AGUILERA, D.C., J.M. MESSICK, and M.S. FARREL, *Crisis Intervention: Theory and Methodology.* St. Louis: C.V. Mosby, 1970.

BLACHER, R. S., Reaction to chronic illness, *Loss and Grief: Psychological Management in Medical Practice,* eds. B. Schoenberg, A. C. Carr, D. Peretz, and A. H. Kutscher. New York: Columbia University Press, 1970.

COHEN, F., and R. S. LAZARUS, Active coping processes, coping dispositions, and recovery from surgery. *Psychosomatic Medicine* 35: 375-389, 1973.

FORDYCE, W.E., Personality characteristics in men with spinal cord injury as related to manner of onset of disability. *Archives of Physical Medicine and Rehabilitation* 45: 321-325, 1964.

_____ , Psychological assessment and management, in *Handbook of Physical Medicine and Rehabilitation,* eds. F.H. Krusen, F.J. Kottke, and P. Ellwood. Philadelphia: W.B. Saunders Co., 1971.

FREED, M.M., H.J. BAKST, and D.L. BARRIE, Life expectancy, survival rates, and causes of death in civilian patients with spinal cord trauma. *Archives of Physical Medicine and Rehabilitation* 47: 457-463, 1966.

KIELY, W.F., Coping with severe illness. *Advances in Psychosomatic Medicine* 8: 105-118, 1972.

MICHAEL, J.L., Rehabilitation, in *Behavior Modification in Clinical Psychology,* eds. C. Neuringer and J.L. Michael. New York: Appleton-Century-Crofts, 1970.

MUELLER, A. D. Psychologic factors in rehabilitation of paraplegic patients. *Archives of Physical Medicine and Rehabilitation* 43: 151-159, 1962.

SCHOENBERG, B., and A.C. CARR, Loss of external organs: limbs, amputation, mastectomy, and disfiguration, in *Loss and Grief: Psychological Management in Medicinal Practice,* eds. B. Schoenberg, A.C. Carr, D. Peretz, and A.H. Kutscher. New York: Columbia University Press, 1970.

SHONTZ, F.C., Reactions to crisis. *Volta Review* 67: 364-370, 1965.

20

A Father with Leukemia

Don De Francisco / Donald Watson

This chapter focuses on the impact of an acute fatal illness upon a young married couple. The two authors had the opportunity to follow both the husband and wife closely throughout the ten-week course of this illness, in which we saw not only the personal psychodynamics of the husband and wife, but perhaps more importantly, we were able to observe the longitudinal behavior of the family and hospital staff. This report is an analysis of the relations between all these people in the social network of the dying patient, and the critical role that their communications play in the experience of dying for all concerned.

Mike, 28, and Kathy, 26, had been married fours years and had one son Bob, three. Mike was a professor of music in a local college. He developed leukemia, but its subtype was not known for several weeks. The day that the diagnosis of leukemia was made, treatment with prednisone in high doses was instituted. (Prednisone can produce psychosis.)

About 10 days later, Mike developed a manic psychosis. He was hospitalized and treated with lithium and was subsequently followed by one of us. Kathy also sought psychiatric help because she recognized that she was having difficulties coping with Mike's radical personality change as well as her decision whether or not to abort her 12-week pregnancy. Accordingly, she was also followed by a psychiatrist as an outpatient. The course of Mike's illness from diagnosis to death lasted only 10 weeks. In that interval, many challenges presented themselves: primarily the unpredictability of Mike's behavior and the complexity of the social network including the hospital staff surrounding Mike during the last few weeks of his life.

THE EXPERIENCE OF MIKE

In May, before the end of his teaching year, Mike developed some pain in his joints. His symptoms became so severe that he consulted his physician, who made a diagnosis of rheumatoid arthritis. His physician prescribed phenylbutazone, but that treatment did not relieve the symptoms. About six weeks later, Mike consulted another physician, who discovered a "blood dyscrasia" (imbalance of elements). Mike and Kathy were advised that Mike should go to the University hospital to be evaluated; that his physician did not know what the problem was but thought it "could even be leukemia."

When Mike was admitted to the hospital as an emergency, a bone marrow aspiration was performed immediately. A probable diagnosis of lymphosarcoma cell leukemia was made. The following day, treatment was started with vincristine and prednisone. Mike's response to these medications was expected to help in establishing his diagnosis and prognosis. His physicians felt fairly certain that he had a highly malignant form of leukemia. Nevertheless, they downplayed that. Instead, they stressed the uncertainties involved in establishing the subtype of leukemia. As a result, Mike and Kathy were left to form their own impressions of the seriousness of Mike's illness and of his prognosis. For example, they repeatedly referred to a 38-day trial period for the chemotherapy. The fact that they would know nothing of Mike's prognosis until the end of that time. The uncertainty about Mike's prognosis was very stressful, particularly to Kathy; it was to be a prominent factor in later decisions that she had to make. For example, she was 12 weeks pregnant, and she felt pressured to decide soon whether or not to continue her pregnancy. She was to face that decision alone later; Mike could offer her no support in her decision because of his psychosis.

Before he was discharged from the hospital, Mike was told that he could expect some euphoria as a side effect from his treatment with prednisone. As a result he was not particularly surprised when he began to feel "high" after he returned home. He began to develop an extremely optimistic view toward life in general and, specifically, toward his own life. By his own description he began to see the world in a different light; as if "the windows had been cleaned." He began to experience an increased intensity of the impact of the world on his senses. He described colors as being brighter, aromas stronger, and the experience of living to be much more satisfying.

Mike threw himself into new activities with great vigor, relishing his enhanced awareness of life. One morning he walked to town to have breakfast at a restaurant. For several hours he observed the people around him and speculated at length about their lives. On the way home, he saw some farm workers picketing a local chain grocery store. Mike quickly introduced himself to the farm workers and convinced them that he was very much interested in their cause. He volunteered his services to make some placards for them. Accordingly, he went home and produced a large number of placards in a short period. He even surprised himself at the amount of work he was able to get done so quickly. He said he could not have done it if he had not had such a burst of energy.

Although Mike felt that his new-found energy was a boon to him, his behavior and attitude soon became very alarming to Kathy. As he became more and more active and involved in "living," he became increasingly more egocentric, indulging himself heavily in his own personal productivity. For the next few days, as his activity increased, Kathy felt increasingly more isolated and abandoned. Finally, she convinced Mike to return to the hospital.

After his admission, Mike's mental status was the most prominent part of his clinical picture. He was seen in consultation by a psychiatrist who found him to be highly talkative, extroverted, energetic, and euphoric. He had become extremely prolific at writing and had taped pages of notes all over his hospital room. His speech was pressured; his verbal output—both written and spoken—was confused and disorganized, characterized by a flight of ideas. He talked of "cosmic consciousness" and feeling "at one with the universe." As to his leukemia, however, he became evasive. He did say that he was quite angry with his first doctor, and made a number of litigation threats against him. He was grandiose and hostile; he was described as "hostile in his friendliness."

The psychiatric consultant felt that Mike might be suffering from manic-depressive illness, but that it was also possible that the mania resulted from an organic brain syndrome secondary to his prednisone treatment. It was recommended that the prednisone be discontinued and that he be observed for changes in mental status. Discontinuation of the prednisone did not result in remission of his mania, so Mike transferred to the psychiatric service.

After admission, Mike remained extroverted and talkative. He slept only one or two hours the first few nights and made many long distance phone calls, running up large bills. He buzzed around the ward continuously, striking up conversations with anyone who was willing and able to listen to him. Despite his sociability, he avoided intimate involvements of any kind, although he was usually drawn to the young women on the ward. His impact on some of the patients was shocking; particularly when he insisted that his leukemia was the biggest miracle of his life.

In addition to socializing, Mike was extremely intent on continuing his writing. He soon assembled the material and personnel necessary to support his prolific efforts. He borrowed a typewriter from a physician on a different ward, he got paper from the nursing staff, and he lined up two patients and a clerk-typist to do his typing for him. During this period, he wrote a song—47 verses of lyrics—and sent it off to a popular folk singer. He also wrote a screen play and a short story, which was a satirical memo written to the staff psychiatrist on the ward. Although it was written in a humorous style, the essay left no doubt about Mike's hostility. In his story, Mike focused all his hostile feelings on to a single psychiatric technician, making that person a scapegoat for a large share of his anger. That was one example of what was to become a pattern of scapegoating in which ultimately Kathy, several physicians, and many nurses were to be involved.

Mike was treated with lithium after admission to the psychiatric ward. The question of how to manage his manic psychosis was made difficult by the fact of his terminal illness. For example, in one sense his mania was useful to him, enhancing his life experience. In that case, it might be preferable to leave it untreated in the short period of time he had to live. On balance, however, Mike's overall pattern of behavior seemed to require specific treatment.

The sense of urgency for the lithium treatment was underlined by several factors involving both Mike and Kathy. In particular, his relationship with Kathy was deteriorating rapidly. Also, Mike was asking for help. He said repeatedly that he felt out of control and that he would like us to help him gain control of himself. Correspondingly, he was very cooperative with his treatment. He seemed to be aware that he was unable to plan realistically for his own welfare. Our decision to treat Mike's mania, then, was based primarily on our realization that Mike did not live in a vacuum; that his psychosis was actually alienating him from those closest to him—those whom he would need now more than ever.

After Mike had been treated with lithium for five days, his serum Lithium level reached therapeutic levels and he calmed down considerably. He was questioned about depression or thoughts of suicide. He was then able realistically to discuss his sadness and fear. However, he had only one brief period of significant depression. That occurred after he was told by his hematologist, Dr. A., not to plan on teaching the autumn semester. Mike called his college to report that he would not be returning to teach and would need a replacement. Then he felt very depressed. He sat in the day room, away from everyone else; he didn't want to speak with anyone and didn't want to be bothered. Later, he went into his room and took a two-hour nap. Afterward, he felt "just fine" again.

Sometimes Mike's sadness was seen when he spoke of his mother's death. On these occasions, he had tears in his eyes; often his voice broke. Mike remembered his mother as a "very warm and bubbly person," in contrast to the cold and aloof person he felt his father to be. Mike's mother had been hospitalized several times for a mental illness that was characterized by periods of "very high highs and very low lows." Her problems was ultimately diagnosed as manic-depressive illness. Mike spoke of his mother's mental illness only once; most of his references to her concerned the family events for the year prior to her death from breast cancer.

Mike's memory of the last year of his mother's life was fixed on their separation. He recalled that she remained in the hospital virtually all the time until just before her death, yet his father indicated that she was actually hospitalized only a few weeks at the beginning and a few weeks toward the end of her illness. In Mike's version of the events surrounding his mother's dying, the whole family was totally unrealistic in approaching it; they denied anything was seriously wrong. Mike remembered that his father refused to discuss with Mike and his brothers the fact that their mother had a fatal illness. Mike's memory of surprise at her death is vivid; he remembered that as he was going home from school one day, some friends asked him about his mother's health. He replied that she was feeling "just fine." That night she died.

Mike said that even after all the intervening years, he had still not gotten over the surprise of his mother's death, and declared that his own impending death would be discussed openly and without denial. In the eight days that he was on the psychiatric unit, he referred repeatedly to what he considered to be the deceitfulness surrounding his mother's death and the openness with which he was approaching his own. Yet his own approach was self-contradictory; while he continued to talk openly about the "miracle" of his leukemia, he tended to depersonalize his disease. Although he made a great effort to remain stoic about his future, he referred to his impending death as "the death." One time Mike was confronted about "romanticizing" his death. He shrugged off the comment, indicating that it wasn't very important to him one way or the other; that he was willing to go along with whatever fate had in store for him. But if Mike showed a detachment from his own feelings about dying, he appeared to be even less concerned about the feelings of Kathy.

THE EXPERIENCE OF KATHY

The day Mike transferred to the psychiatric unit, Kathy was telephoned because she had previously asked to discuss a possible abortion with a psychiatrist. She had already decided to have an abortion, but she felt that she needed support because of the pressure she experienced.

Kathy was seen the following day. She was a well-dressed, petite, and quite attractive young woman. Her initial style persisted throughout this experience. She seemed like a brave little soldier. She relied heavily on her intellect and approached problems with a tough-minded pragmatism. By contrast, she always spoke with a soft trembling voice so that she seemed to be on the verge of tears. But rarely did a tear fall; she never really broke down and cried during our entire contact.

Initially, Kathy gained most of her support from her mother and stepfather, with whom she was staying. Her real father did not live far away, but she had not yet contacted him and he did know that Mike had leukemia. She felt rather distant from her real father and felt that she could not rely on him. She said he was a severe alcoholic, and he had never been available to her as a child. She also had a sister in the area, but she did not rely on her sister for support. She explained that her sister had enough emotional problems of her own and that she did not want to trouble her. The desire to protect others from being hurt was a recurring theme with Kathy. She occasionally took this attitude toward Mike in striking contrast to her usual attitude of brave and pragmatic honesty.

During the first interview, Kathy said that she felt relatively confident about her decision to go ahead with the abortion and that she felt some urgency in proceeding with it. If she were to wait much longer, a quite complicated procedure would be necessary. There were two things that made her decision to abort very difficult. First, she had no clear idea of what Mike's death trajectory might be. The hematologist, Dr. A., had told them that Mike might live only a couple of months. On the other hand, if he went into a remission there was a fair chance that he might live up to a year or even many years.

Of the possible death trajectories, the one Kathy feared most was one lasting about a year. That would leave her with both an infant and a dying husband to care for at the same time. In that case she would definitely want an abortion. By contrast, if Mike were to live only a few weeks, she would not want to continue the pregnancy. Finally, the third possible—but least likely—death trajectory carried less weight in Kathy's decision-making process; if Mike were to live many years she would want to bear the child; still, even if she had an abortion they could have another child together later anyway. Kathy's decision to have the abortion, then, was based on the worst possible case; that is, that Mike might live about one year.

A second major problem for Kathy was Mike's reaction to her. Mike was heavily involved in his own personal creativity and not involved in their personal relationship. Kathy said that she wanted to comfort and support Mike during this terrible time, but she herself also wanted some support from him, which she was not getting. She wanted to hear Mike's feelings about how to handle her pregnancy, but he would not talk to her about it. She was worried that he might be very angry at her if she went ahead and aborted because he might see this child as his last link with life.

Kathy was encouraged once again to contact Dr. A., with the hope that she could get a more definitive picture of Mike's probable death trajectory. She called the hematologist several times and left messages for him to return the call; he never did. The abortion was scheduled for a week later.

Kathy was seen once again before the abortion. Her difficulty in asserting herself was explored. She expressed some anger at Dr. A. for not returning her calls. She reserved most of her anger for Mike, however. She felt hurt because he seemed unwilling to help her make the decision.

THE MARRIAGE RELATIONSHIP

To improve the understanding and communication between Mike and Kathy, a series of conjoint sessions was initiated with both their therapists. This strategy was adopted because their marriage relationship was in a crisis, and because it was felt that the quality of their relationship prior to the crisis could be reestablished. Ultimately, three conjoint sessions were held. Kathy was to say later that these sessions were the most helpful services provided for her and Mike during his illness.

The first conjoint session centered on the upcoming abortion. Mike superficially agreed to the abortion and glibly stated that he realized it was a tough decision but that he would support whatever decision Kathy made. However, because he was off so quickly to other subjects, Kathy was never sure where he really stood. That session made little progress, primarily because of Mike's flightiness and inability to focus on issues.

In this emotional climate, the abortion was performed without any medical complications. The day after the abortion, Kathy reported that she felt well; she would never again mention the abortion to her psychiatrist. Mike, however, did react to it later, even though indirectly. Within the context of his wishes for immortality, Mike indicated that he regretted the necessity for the abortion.

Shortly after the abortion, the second conjoint session was held, during which they both expressed anger toward each other. Kathy was angry at Mike for not giving her any support and for selfishly pursuing his own creative interests, neglecting the future needs for both her and Bob. Kathy accused Mike of spending money extravagantly. Mike, in turn, was angry at Kathy for ignoring his need to cram a lifetime into a short period. They chose as their battleground the fact that Mike frequently bought boxes of candy for the nurses. They fought long and hard over who was to control the petty cash. Nevertheless, they later realized that the candy was not the issue, and thereby discovered the intensity of the anger they each felt. The main benefit of this session, then, was that they both expressed anger toward one another, and this catharsis seemed to be helpful.

During the third conjoint session, Mike's and Kathy's different perspectives were explored. Mike was more concerned about living for the present; Kathy was primarily concerned about the future. For example, Mike wanted to sell the house so they could have more money to travel and to publish his creative efforts. Kathy wanted to keep the house, so she would have some security for the future. It was pointed out that their differing perspectives were each understandable, but they needed mutual respect for each other's perspective with a willingness to compromise to some extent. They both seemed to understand this, and the relationship between the two of them improved after this session.

Before his condition deteriorated into a semicomatose state, Mike and Kathy had a few good days together. For example, he permitted her to show him sympathy and to perform small comforting tasks that she felt satisfaction in doing. This was a tremendous relief to Kathy. She saw that short period as a warm personal relationship. At this time she decided to compromise and move more toward Mike's perspective. She said that when Mike got out of the hospital she would try to live more for the present and would be quite willing just to travel. And Mike agreed to try to avoid selling the house and to travel by train, instead of by plane, to save money. They were able to share some of their mutual sadness and their concern about Bob.

There was also a psychiatric conference on Mike and the topic of death and dying. Kathy attended this conference. She saw that when Mike was concerned with his own personal productivity and was not giving her love in return, she did not feel like a worthwhile person. She realized that not having love reciprocated need not diminish one's feeling of self-worth. This seemed to help her cope a little better with Mike's occasional angry outbursts at her. She was a little less afraid of his anger and was left feeling less guilty and self-deprecating.

Mike also began to reflect on his illness and his reactions to it. For example, he saw the ways in which he was trying to achieve immortality. This was evident in his voluminous writing and his hopes to have his song recorded. It was expressed also in his change of attitude about having children; whereas before he had wanted to have only two children, he had come to the position during his illness that he would like to have "four, five, or maybe even a lot more." Also, he identified an earlier wish of his—to be recorded on video tape—as an attempt to achieve immortality. Mike had requested repeatedly to record an interview about his "philosophy" of death. He said several times that he hoped to do that so his son would be able some day to "see the old man, and hear what I have to say on life." Mike wished that his mother had left some kind of personal record behind her; particularly, he would like to have heard her talk about her illness. He had accidently struck her in the breast with a ball prior to her development of breast cancer, and for many years after that, he accepted the blame for her death. Also, Mike's self-selected nickname, "Feather," appeared to be a symbolic indication of his search for immortality. While on an outing, Mike had come across a beautiful feather lying on the ground. He felt the symbolism of the feather was fairly clear, that it represented a beautiful part of the bird that remained long after the bird was gone.

As Mike's physical illness progressed, he became physically less able to express himself either by gesture or by voice. After his temperature spiked to 107 degrees, Mike became aware of the gravity of his illness. He still did not discuss his impending death directly, but approached it clearly enough in other ways. For example, he told his psychiatrist, "I must ride this out. I feel like a cowboy." His psychiatrist tried his own association. "A lonesome cowboy?" Mike replied, "I guess so. That depends on what will happen."

FAMILY RELATIONSHIPS

On the day following the first conjoint session, Mike's father visited him. Coincidentally, he ran into Dr. A., who was reviewing Mike's medical progress. Doctor A. told Mike's father that he planned to start Mike on a new treatment, and that the new treatment itself was potentially hazardous. Mike's father misinterpreted what Dr. A. had said and concluded that there was a 50-50 chance or less that Mike would survive the next treatment. With this he immediately called Mike's brothers and other relatives.

When Mike and Kathy found out the message that had been delivered to the family members, they were each very angry in their own ways; Mike because he did not like to be surrounded by "long faces," and Kathy because she felt that the doctors had been keeping information from her. She was quite upset by both the news and the way she heard of it. She called Dr. A. and, by being assertive, managed to get through to him. She found out that the treatment was not nearly as dangerous as Mike's father had presumed. However, Mike's family was already coming from distant parts of the country. Kathy strongly impressed upon the hematologist that she wanted to be present at any future discussion of Mike's condition or prognosis. Coincidentally, in all the confusion, Mike developed a fever and had to be transferred back to the medical unit.

During the next individual session with Kathy, she related with some pride that she had been able to be more assertive with Dr. A. and to see to it that she got what she needed from him. Kathy also was able to be more assertive in the following week with Mike's relatives. His parents kept insisting that a minister visit him in the hospital. Mike resented this because he and Kathy were agnostics. But his parents would not relent until Kathy firmly confronted them about this.

Mike's brothers insisted on taking pictures of him in the hospital, and the whole family gathered around as if he were going to die within the next couple of days. Mike was upset at the pessimism of his family members. He was very intolerant of anyone who indicated that they might feel bad about his disease. He persistently dissociated his feelings from his impending death. As a result, he refused to enter into conversations with his brothers except under his rules. Because his rules included no expressions of sadness or of loss, the conversations between him and them were characterized by a strange sense of unreality; of a stilted, polite, and largely irrelevant aura of suspended feelings. During brief periods of conversation with Mike's psychiatrist, Mike's brothers expressed bewilderment and estrangement.

RELATIONS WITH THE HOSPITAL STAFF

Kathy became increasingly frustrated that she was unable to get any kind of clear communication from the doctors on Mike's condition or prognosis. This mounting frustration may have added to her anger at Mike's family. Finally, she asked the family to leave, for with their visits Mike's condition seemed to deteriorate. He developed pulmonary emboli and had to be put in intensive care (ICU). Kathy was frightened by this. Communication with the doctors did improve while Mike was in the ICU. His intern began to meet daily with Kathy to keep her filled in on what was happening. This extra effort on the part of the intern was quite helpful to Kathy. Ironically, just a few days earlier she had scapegoated the intern for many of the problems in Mike's management. The intern had wanted to allow Mike to go home on a weekend pass. He arranged a pass and announced it to everyone. But then Dr. A. vetoed it because he wanted to try a new experimental treatment and because Kathy and Bob had developed colds. The intern was quite upset because he only wanted to allow Mike some time out of the hospital. He was worried that Mike would never leave the hospital alive. Nevertheless, Kathy's reaction was anger at the intern for "acting like he was in charge when he wasn't," and "building Mike's hopes up to go home when really he had no right or authority to do that." She felt that the intern was being inconsiderate. Yet, later when Mike's condition deteriorated and he lapsed into a semicoma, the intern's daily conferences with her became invaluable.

After Mike lapsed into a semi-comatose state, Kathy found it quite difficult to cope with the "chronic crisis." He was in this state for nearly a month. Almost every day the doctors would predict "He probably won't be here tomorrow." Kathy became much more assertive and vocal while Mike was in his moribund state. She strongly defended his rights to get medical care and humane sensitive treatment. When nurses would break the protective isolation rules, she would strongly confront them about this. She also was able to confront the doctors when she felt that their behavior was remiss. It was noteworthy that while she increased her ability to be frank and honest in situations that involved Mike's critical care, her assertiveness did not generalize to other situations. For example, her real father finally visited Mike. When he did, he smelled heavily of alcohol, and it was apparent that he was not of much support to Kathy. However, when asked about her father's visit later, she mentioned that her father had not had a drop of alcohol for years. In contra-distinction to what she had said before, she then claimed that her father had been quite reliable and available to her when she was a child and that it was a problem only when she was a teen-ager.

There were other problems with her assertiveness and frankness. She could stand up quite well to the nurses but less well with the doctors, especially Dr. A. He would come into the room with a group of medical students, completely ignore her, and talk about Mike's serious condition at the bedside. This made her angry, but she was only able to say to him, "Don't you think you ought to talk about that outside? He can hear you, you know." Dr. A. just ignored her after replying, "No, he can't hear, he's in a coma." Kathy let it go at that, although she knew better; just minutes before she had been communicating with Mike. Although Mike could not talk, usually remaining with his eyes closed, he could respond effectively by nodding his head. It seems that she was able to express her anger so well at the nurses that she displaced much of her anger onto them. They were scapegoated for the anger she felt toward the doctors, and possibly toward Mike for abandoning her. Generalizing, she became increasingly concerned about the care available to dying patients. She expressed a desire to do something about this in the future.

During this prolonged crisis of Mike's semicoma, Kathy asked the psychiatrist to be more of a friend. She said this was what she presently needed, and she expressed some anger at his "psychiatric" attitude. He complied with her wishes for the most part but also told her that he would reserve the right to assume a psychiatric role at times when it would be helpful. As a symbolic gesture, he discontinued seeing her in his office and began visiting her on the medical wards of the hospital where Mike was a patient.

Kathy found it very difficult to handle the state of chronic crisis. She could not remain hypervigilant as she felt she should, and she felt some guilt as a result. She sometimes hoped that Mike would just hurry up and die so that it would all be over. Her ambivalence and anger were exemplified by contradictory attitudes: on the one hand she was furious with the nurses for not strictly observing isolation protocol to protect Mike from infection; on the other hand, she was angry at the doctors for giving Mike antibiotics and blood transfusions that she felt were heroic.

Less than two days before Mike's death, Dr. A. wanted to try Mike on a course of nitrogen mustard. Kathy was very uncertain about whether to go along with this. She discussed it in detail with Dr. A. and then in detail with the house staff. It was obvious that the house staff no longer felt that any treatment was really indicated but encouraged Kathy to go along with the treatment anyway, without being fully aware of, or explicit about, their motives. They felt that nitrogen mustard would only serve to speed Mike's death. Her psychiatrist, who was present, insisted that they communicate their motives more explicitly. They realized then that if their goal was to speed Mike's death, it would be more direct and honest to discontinue the antibiotics and blood transfusions rather than to use the nitrogen mustard for this purpose. It was hoped that this clarification would help to prevent Kathy from unwittingly accepting responsibility for terminating Mike's life, which could result in her feeling guilty later.

The intern and resident, in what seemed a spirit of generosity, quickly responded by telling Kathy that they would go along with whatever decision she wanted to make. If she wanted the antibiotics and blood transfusions discontinued, they would respect that. After they left, Kathy was asked how she felt about that; whether she felt that the burden of deciding when Mike would die was being put on her shoulders. She realized that the decision was being given to her, and she resented it. However, she bravely assumed it anyway, but did decide to dissipate some of the responsibility around the family. She called Mike's father and presented the situation to him. Mike's father discussed it with the relatives and then phoned Kathy and said that he agreed that the nitrogen mustard should not be given and that antibiotics and blood transfusions should be discontinued.

After he heard that Kathy had vetoed the nitrogen mustard infusion, Dr. A. made a special visit to the hospital to see her. This was the only time he had sought her out, and on this occasion he saw her only to try to convince her to change her mind. He tried to persuade her by trying to make her feel guilty about killing Mike. However, she was able to stand up to him and did not weaken under the pressure he was applying. But she did not directly express any anger at him for what he was trying to do. Then Dr. A., in a punitive effort, told the house staff to force Kathy to sign a release of responsibility for the hospital because she refused the nitrogen mustard treatment. However, the house staff just ignored him and supported Kathy. Earlier the attending staff of the hospital officially stated that Dr. A. had no authority to make decisions for Mike's care, and that he could function as a consultant only. The house staff not only supported Kathy in her conflict with Dr. A. but, after a brief psychiatric consulation, reassumed some of the responsibility for the discontinuation of the antibiotics and blood transfusions. Two days later after it was decided not to use nitrogen mustard, Mike died. Kathy gave her signed consent for a full autopsy, but none was performed.

On the day following Mike's death, Kathy's demeanor was again that of a "brave little soldier," whose voice trembled on the verge of tears, but only a few tears fell.

About two weeks after Mike's death, we received a letter from Kathy. She seemed to have found a balance between her need to mourn her loss and her need to reinvest her interests in the present and future. She still strongly felt that Mike's and her emotional needs were neglected by the nursing and medical staff. She still felt a strong commitment to see that this could be changed for future patients. She had not been able clearly to communicate to her son Bob the meaning of his father's death, as he was not yet three years old, but he had been able to attach himself to some other males who were available to him, especially Kathy's stepfather and uncle.

ISSUES AND QUESTIONS RAISED

This whole experience presents critical issues in the management of the dying patient and the family. The first issue is the interpretation and treatment of Mike's mania. Could not such a state of massive denial and extreme energy be adaptive to a dying patient? We thought about this and decided that it was not adaptive because Mike did not live in a vacuum. But don't we all need to deny to some extent? How much denial of our mortality is healthy? We certainly would not have wanted to take all of Mike's denial away from him. Yet continuous rumination over his mortality and his manic attempt to live all of his life at once interfered with the opportunity to relate actually to those he loved and cared for.

A second issue was the need for a more definitive death trajectory. The critical importance of a clear death trajectory is sadly illustrated in Kathy's agonizing decision over whether or not to abort. From what she said, if she had known he was going to die so soon, she might not have aborted.

A third issue is what role a psychiatrist should play with a dying patient. With both Mike and Kathy, each of us was called upon to be a friend. On the other hand, being a friend was not sufficient to resolve the conflicts of human relations of this young couple.

A fourth issue is who should be responsible for deciding how long the patient's life should be prolonged, or how vigorously the patient should be treated when the situation is hopeless and the patient cannot make that decision. Who makes the decision? Doctors? The family? Or does one choose, as we did in this situation, that it should be a mutually shared decision? If so, how does one split and share the responsibility? Or can it really be done at all? Should the physician take responsibility for decisions to obviate any long-term guilt in the surviving relatives? In this case, the physicians alternately took all the responsibility and then took none. We suggest a third alternative of shared responsibility between physicians, patient, and family.

A fifth issue was the handling of displaced anger. A simple hypothesis is to conclude that Kathy's displaced anger onto the nurses and others was a result of her repressed anger at Mike for dying on her and abandoning her. After all, she never did express anger at his dying, which is so frequently a part of the bereaved's reaction. But need everyone experience that? Maybe anger at the loved one who is dying is really a displacement of an internal anger. After all, what is the anger about at its core? Maybe it is anger at the frustrating existential realities of loss and mortality.

A sixth issue is the whole scapegoating problem within the social system communication network. The social network of Mike, his family, Kathy, the doctors, the psychiatric staff, the nursing staff, and Mike's friends are a rather loosely connected network. Not everybody within that network talks to one another. In other words, as a social network, they do not comprise a social group. When all those involved are not speaking with all the others involved, the situation is ripe for faulty communications, especially when many people are purposely avoiding communication out of fear, anger, sadness, or whatever. One of the things that happened early in the case was that the doctors would talk to Mike and Kathy separately. They would give one story to Mike, which was sugarcoated, and they would give another story to Kathy, which was more factual. Then when Mike and Kathy would try to discuss things together, it frequently led to discord. Kathy would feel that Mike was denying and not wanting to face up to things. Mike, on the other hand, felt that Kathy was being unnecessarily pessimistic and was just trying to bring him down. They would at times end such discussions by accusing the other of lying.

A communications paradigm helps to explain why certain people were scapegoated. It seems that anyone in this kind of loose social network who is not communicating clearly with those around him or her is leaving him- or herself open to be scapegoated. This happened repeatedly. The orderly on the psychiatric service, who became the single focus of Mike's anger, had not bothered to explain the legitimate reason why he had awakened Mike at five in the morning. When the intern did not discuss his motive with Mike and Kathy, he received Kathy's anger for trying to send Mike home on a weekend pass. She did not know that what he was doing was really a very generous and sensitive act. All that Kathy knew was that he had played a part in events that ultimately turned out badly. Not knowing what his motivations were, she could easily scapegoat him.

Just before Mike's death, the nursing supervisor of the hospital happened to be making rounds, randomly asking patients and visitors what they thought of the nursing care. When she asked Kathy what she thought, Kathy proceeded to pour out her anger and frustration about what she felt was a lack of sensitivity on the part of the nursing staff. The nursing staff was quite shocked and hurt by this negative feedback, for most of them felt very sad about Mike's tragedy. However, they were at a loss for words and had not communicated this to Kathy. Upon being scapegoated by Kathy, the nurses reacted by scapegoating the psychiatrist, who had left himself open for this by not communicating with the nurses over the last couple of weeks. They decided among themselves that the psychiatrist must have planned this and had put Kathy up to it, and that he had done it to treat her depression. This was quickly discussed with the nurses and the lines of communication were cleared, at which time the nurses requested that the psychiatric consultant conduct a conference on the management of the dying patient in the near future, which he did.

It is also not unlikely that the hematologist, Dr. A. was one of the ultimate scapegoats of the social network. It is difficult to know what amount of his perceived insensitivity was truly valid. Among all concerned, his communication was certainly the most deficient. Because of his lack of communication, it is quite possible that the social network was inaccurately assessing his motivations without the opportunity to correct misconceptions through his clarification. It is also possible that the house staff allowed him to take much more responsibility for a much longer period of time than was appropriate because it was easier emotionally to have him take responsibility and then criticize him for it—"to pass the buck" to him and then scapegoat him.

With such a loosely constructed social network involved with this dying patient, it seems unavoidable that there would be some scapegoating. Although it is unavoidable, it also seems likely that the displacement in scapegoating could be markedly diminished by training of hospital staff, by regular conferences that include all members of the social network, and by maintaining collaboration between the patient, the family, and the staff.

In conclusion, there were a number of stressful issues confronting this young couple. Our experience here shows that both Mike and Kathy had the ability to cope with these stresses. However, the ambiguity, double binds, coercion, and even simple lack of information that characterized this social system created an intolerable stress. Thus, the social system changed the *stress* of dying into a *crisis* of dying. This young couple could cope with the dying process, but they could not cope with the dysfunctional social system. These observed in the hospital may not reflect the problem of dying but rather the problem of the social system.

VI

MIDDLE AGE

When we reach middle age, concern for death as such appears to recede. Rather, there is more concern for ongoing relationships with important people, which death will interrupt. Even more significant is concern for the quality of life. The advent of depression, withdrawal, hypochondriasis, and suicidal ideation is prominent in the lives of the dying who are middle-aged. In these chapters we see less avoidance of death thoughts, and perhaps instead even preoccupation with death in chronic living-dying trajectories.

The chapter by Swanson and Swanson focuses primarily on staff reactions. They point out the problem of "death saturation," when the hospital staff become overloaded with too many deaths. Furthermore, they illustrate how staff experience severe emotional distress when a positive dying expectation is suddenly turned around. Finally, they note the wide range of emotions and coping reactions that professional staff display. They show how impossible it is to avoid emotional involvement with the process of dying. Yet it is possible to accept such staff reactions, support staff, and look for ways to maintain an adaptive emotional equilibrium while caring for the dying.

Hertzberg carries the theme of staff reactions further. He points out that administrative structure often interferes with adequate staff support and effective patient care in a psychosocial sense. Hertzberg also reemphasizes the intimate emotional involvement of professional staff with the dying person.

In his unique autobiographical account, Friedman gives us a frank and most honest picture of the acute crisis experience of dying. He describes what appears to be massive denial. Yet he acts in a most accepting way. I believe he tells us something very important: Actions speak louder than words. In his care of his dying wife, they did not speak of death, but they shared an intimate knowledge that led to a mutually acceptable experience of dying.

Finally, Beard graphically portrays the fact that medical technology may not prolong life but merely postpone death. His analysis of chronic homodialysis points up the importance of how one lives, not merely that one lives.

21

Acute Uncertainty: The Intensive Care Unit

Thomas R. Swanson / *Marcia J. Swanson*

The Intensive Care Unit offers a unique opportunity to observe the dying patient and those around him, including professional staff and family. By its very nature the ICU is unique; a place where acutely ill patients come for intensive care. As soon as the crisis is over, the patient leaves. There is a close working relationship between staff and patient. A patient may enter the unit in a state ranging from acute alertness to deep coma. Each state results in different behavior by patient, staff, and relatives.

The authors have been in particularly fortunate positions to observe ICU behavior. One has been consultant to several ICUs during the last two years and led groups for the staffs of four ICUs. The other has been an ICU nurse for over 10 years, working in essentially every kind of unit during that time.

The following observations will be concerned primarily with staff behavior and feelings relating to the dying patient. Most of responses by patients and family are not particularly unique. Only those patient and family responses that seem to be unusual or unique to the ICU will be discussed here. We shall refer in the text to "the nurse," meaning *any* staff member who works closely with the patient. It should be noted here also that these are generalizations of observed and reported behavior and feelings. Each person, of course, reacts and copes according to his or her own style and personality.

THE ALERT VERSUS THE NONALERT PATIENT

We have noticed a distinct difference in the reactions of staff to dying patients depending on the patient's ability to react—in other words, whether the patient is alert or in coma.

A significant number of patients enter the ICU in a comatose condition. As one might expect, the staff usually does not become too involved emotionally with these patients. During group sessions or ward conversations, it is unusual to hear a staff member express concern about a patient who entered in coma.

In such cases, the staff's primary concern is in performing the technical skills well. The staff comment that it is difficult to become emotionally involved with a patient with whom one cannot communicate. If this patient dies, the staff member shows and feels only brief, mild concern; but at least "the patient received good care." The staff feel good about how they enacted their role.

On the other hand, the more difficult dying patient for the attending nurse to care for is the one who enters the ICU alert and then becomes worse. In this case, patient and nurse communicate, they get to know one another. When it is apparent that the patient is dying, the staff begins to react in the following ways: one common reaction could perhaps be best called depression. The nurse appears sad, works with less speed and zeal, appears less interested in her job. Commonly the nurse will state that she feels depressed and believes that she is not a very good nurse, or feels less than adequate for the job—at least for this patient. She does not look forward to going to work. Although no records have been kept, our impression is that absences because of "illness" seem to be greater during this period. When at work the nurse does not work as well as usual with the other staff; she is irritable and sensitive. Other staff members who have worked with this patient behave the same way. During report and assignment of patients, each nurse will try to maneuver or manipulate so that she does not "have to take care of (the dying patient)." After all, "(she) took care of him two days ago. . ." Head nurses are usually aware of this and will try to change assignments often so that any one nurse will not have to take care of the dying patient too frequently. Very often when death is expected to be imminent, a nurse will work extra hard to keep the patient alive until the end of the day so that, in the nurses' words, "(the patient) won't die on my shift." Somehow, if the nurse works hard and the patient dies on another shift, she feels better about the death.

On other wards when a patient is told he is dying, say of cancer, the staff tend to withdraw from the patient's bedside. In a similar way, the ICU staff withdraw when it is evident that the patient will die. The staff of ICUs are usually optimistic people who believe in their work and have much hope. When the patient is dying, the hope of the staff members diminishes simultaneously. There seems to be a group hope, or lack of it, that affects each individual staff member. If there is not a literal withdrawal from the dying patient's bedside, it occurs in another form in that there is greater interest and concern for monitors and the "busy work" in caring for the patient. At the same time there may be less communication with the patient if he or she is still alert.

It must be noted that there are several other variables to these reactions by the staff. First, the longer the patient is on the Unit in an alert state and able to communicate, the more severe are the responses and reactions by the staff to the dying and death of the patient. A patient who has been on the Unit for only a day or two elicits a far milder reaction tan the patient who has been on the Unit for weeks. Another variable is the age of the patient (this will be discussed in detail below).

DETACHMENT AND INCREASED ACTIVITY

Another very common reaction—perhaps one could call it a coping mechanism or style—by the staff is a combination of apparent detachment and increased activity. By detachment, we mean behavior where the nurse appears not to care about the patient as a person; she does her duties automatically with little apparent feeling. As mentioned, she becomes concerned with the technical details of her job. During group discussions, the nurses have made comments such as the following referring to their subjective feelings: "I just cannot let (the death or dying) get to me. If I did, I couldn't work here more than a few days. . ." "I just don't think about it." "I just try to do good nursing care. I do my best, but if the patient dies, I feel bad, yes, but it can't be helped."

As we said, some nurses become less interested in the patient when it is evident that he or she will die. But others, although detached, become more and more concerned with the technical details of the case. They will be seen busily attending to vital signs, monitors, bathing, arterial lines, intravenous fluids, and so on and on.

HUMOR

Another common response, usually seen as a group phenomenon with the staff, is the use of humor. The staff will be seen standing near the bed or at the nurses' station making various jokes, laughing, being giddy, or otherwise acting silly. This is usually done in small groups of two, three, or four, and usually only briefly. The jokes are occasionally about any of the patients, whether dying or not, and sometimes involve the use of humorous names such as "Gomer." More often than not, however, the humor is not about the patient but *is* seen during stress, which includes the dying of a patient. Staff comments about such humor include the following: "If you didn't laugh in here sometimes, you'd go crazy." "I don't know why, but jokes make me feel so much better. . ." "Sometimes things are so tragic in here you can't help but laugh."

Perhaps the most difficult patient for the nurse is the alert, cooperative, appreciative patient whom everyone likes and who is on the Unit for many days so that staff and patient know each other well. In a case like this, the entire staff usually become depressed when it becomes evident that the patient probably will die. As an example, Richard, a 26-year-old premed student, was in the ICU for 33 days before he died of an aortic aneurysm. One of the staff members describes the staff's reaction:

> We found Richard to be a very interesting, intelligent, and likeable person. He had worked in a hospital previously and therefore understood much of what was happening to him and what his prognosis was. His attitude was one of kindness, concern, and warmth, all which was easy to return. He had a wife and family that were very concerned about him and were equally considerate and kind to the staff. Because of these qualities in Richard and his family, it became very easy to become involved in them. Richard became not just a patient but also a person. His care was made more emotionally difficult by the fact that, unlike most patients, everything he asked for was preceded and followed by "please" and "thank you." He sincerely appreciated everything that we did for him. We found it difficult to care for him because we knew he was going to die. We tried to be cheerful to him, despite the fact that most of us felt quite depressed concerning him and his condition. Many of us who took care of him often wished he would stop being so nice, so considerate, and be the opposite—almost as though it would be easier for us to adjust to his death if we could be angry at him. Even now, many years after his death, we find ourselves remembering him and the emotional difficulties encountered in his care.

CHILDREN VS. THE ELDERLY

Another variable that seems to affect the intensity of reaction by the staff is the age of the patient. It is interesting to compare the reaction of a given staff to a dying child with a dying geriatric patient. As one might expect in our youth-oriented society, the staff becomes very concerned when a child is brought into the ICU, whether or not he or she is dying. But when the child *is* dying, the staff become very concerned; the nurses attend to the patient more diligently and show much more concern. During group discussions when a child is on the ward, the group leader can *always* expect many comments of concern about the child.

As a comparison, the elderly patient is given less concern because ". . . he has had a good life. . ." or ". . . she has lived out her life expectancy." When the child dies, the group makes comments concerning what the staff "should have done" and may express mild to moderate guilt. When the elderly person dies, the usual concern is whether or not the person died without pain and—per the current term in vogue—"with dignity."

In addition, when an elderly patient is dying and is alert and verbalizes that he or she wants to die or is ready to die, the staff accept this generally without too much problem. Again, the person ". . has lived his (or her) life . . . ." But, when a young person is dying and verbalizes a desire to die, the staff usually react with the comment that it is "wrong" for the patient to feel that way. If the patient is a child and the parents make such a statement, that they would like their child to die (as in the case of severe burns, meningitis, tumors, leukemia, and such), the staff get irritated at the parent—"How can the parent feel that way?"

Regardless of the patient's age, when a patient has a very severe, debilitating illness, and hope is slim, or it is obvious that the patient will die, the staff will also begin to have thoughts such as "It is better this way . . ." "He's better off . . . he would have had a miserable life anyway." "She's had a good life." "She's had her 70 years." "His family would have had to take care of him the rest of his life." "He would have just been a vegetable." "It's better she died now rather than later so it won't cost so much . . ." "It's God's will." "It can't be helped."

OVERDOSES AND SELF-INFLICTED INJURIES

The ICU is, of course, a very busy place. The staff is often overburdened and feel frustrated from that alone. If there is anything that the staff members resent, it is extra, needless work. The patient who has overdosed or has a self-inflicted injury represents just that to ICU staff. If the patient is dying, the attending nurse, of course, feels bad for the patient. But most overdoses enter in coma, and so the concern is less than for alert patients. On the Unit or in the group sessions, many of the staff will express irritation, anger, and resentment at the patient who has inconvenienced them and been so inconsiderate as to take time needed for more deserving patients. These feelings are usually not expressed so directly or bluntly, but this is the general feeling that comes through.

THE ATTENDING PHYSICIAN

Most of these descriptions pertain also to the attending physician. This seems to be particularly true in teaching hospitals where contact with the patient is greater for the resident or intern. But there are two general extremes of behavior that stand out. One is the physician who is never present and generally unavailable when the patient is dying. The nurses try to find him or her for the usual questions and simply cannot do so. The other extreme, and seemingly less common, is the attending physician who is always present on the ward. He or she can be seen, as many nurses do, being very active with the technical details of the case. As many physicians will joke, "If the patient dies in metabolic balance, then everything is okay" apparently becomes a way that this *active* physician can cope with the death of the patient.

STAFF REACTIONS

Elizabeth Kübler-Ross (1969, 1975) has written about the stages a dying patient goes through as he or she learns about the illness and moves to acceptance of his or her fate. For some time we have been aware that it is not just the patient but frequently the staff that experience emotional reactions, although less in intensity and duration. One author has frequently experienced these stages in herself as she dealt with dying patients. It should be emphasized that these reactions are mild and short-lived and are handled well by most staff. They are not fixed stages but recurring reactions.

The emotion that stand out for most staff is a mild to moderate depression. Yet a staff member also will deny that the patient is really dying. Or the nurse may bargain—with God if he or she is religious or with the doctor. Anger by the staff is freqent toward the physician. Statements such as "if (the doctor) would only have. . ." are not uncommon. A mild sense of guilt is common in the nurse—"If only I had . . . ."

These emotions are also seen in the families of dying patients in relation to the staff. An example of bargaining occurred with one author as she was caring for a dying elderly man. His wife came to the author and wanted to give her $5 to thank her "for all the good care (she had) given to (the patient)." The next statement by the wife was, "Do you think my husband will live?"

THE PATIENT WHO LIVES

A report such as this would not be complete without a brief description of staff response when a patient goes through a difficult illness which was thought to be fatal, and then gets well. The response by the staff can only be described as pride, euphoria, joy—at any rate, good positive feelings. When a patient has been on the ward for more than a few days and the staff has worked hard to achieve survival, patient and staff can be seen interacting with enthusiasm. The staff is cheerful and pleasant, and the interest in nursing is great. Each staff member feels that he or she is competent and skillful.

CONCLUSION

It should be emphasized that, in our opinion, most of the staff of ICUs who deal with dying patients do adjust very well. It is a difficult, tense, physically strenuous, often frustrating job. Yet they cope and adapt well. It is hoped that the above observations will provide some insight as to the ways they do this. The descriptions will lend themselves easily to psychological jargon and labeling. This has been avoided to allow the reader to make his or her own conclusions and to avoid the pitfall that once a psychodynamic label is put on a behavior, it is then assumed to have pathological function. Indeed, for most of the people who work on an Intensive Care Unit, the various emotional coping mechanisms we have described are not pathological, but rather enable them to endure a high degree of stress and perform in an effective and capable fashion.

REFERENCES

KÜBLER-ROSS, E., *On Death and Dying.* New York: Macmillan, 1969.
————, *Death: The Final Stage of Growth.* Englewood Cliffs, N.J.: Prentice-Hall, 1975.

22

Living in a Cancer Unit

Leonard J. Hertzberg

In recent years a number of research-oriented cancer units have been developed. Since 1972 I have been a consultant to two such units; at Baltimore City Hospitals and the National Cancer Institute unit at the U. S. Public Health Service Hospital in Baltimore. Both have a similar orientation in that chemotherapy (using chemical agents) is the chief means of treatment. Patients admitted onto the units range from early adolescence upward. Acceptance into a program is usually contingent upon no previous treatment for the malignancy so that controlled research data can be obtained. Detailed treatment plans are made by the research staff for a number of malignancies, including the various leukemias and Hodgkin's disease; thus, patients accepted for treatment all have a malignancy that meets the research focus of the unit. Patients have all been referred by a physician who has heard of the specialized units; many of the patients have come from out-of-state and some have even come from foreign countries. Once a patient enters treatment, he or she is followed indefinitely and readmitted for further treatment whenever necessary. Outpatient treatment is also provided so that exacerbation of the malignancy does not necessarily result in rehospitalization.

Although my consultant activities have differed somewhat on the two units, on both a weekly "psychiatric conference" has evolved. At these weekly conferences, a patient or family member is interviewed, and afterward various aspects of the interview are explored with the staff. Particular emphasis is placed on understanding how a patient and the family are attempting to cope with the illness. Patients and family members are generally quite willing to discuss their feelings regarding the illness; frequently, the person interviewed seemed relieved to be able to discuss the emotional impact of the illness. The patient or relative is informed that the purpose of the meeting is for the staff to understand more fully how cancer affects a person and his or her family. Thus, the goal of the meeting is presented as being educative to the staff, who desire to be more helpful to patients and their families. Although no promise of direct benefit is given the person interviewed, most persons have accepted an invitation to attend the meeting.

PATIENT REACTION TO CANCER

Many of my observations are not specific to patients in mature adulthood but also have been noted in persons throughout the life cycle. The trajectory of the illness is generally chronic, although a fulminating course still occasionally does occur. Despite the misconception pervading our society that having cancer is synonomous with imminent death, there is an indeterminant interval between the time of diagnosis and eventual death. The unpredictability of the illness is particularly difficult for many persons to cope with. Many patients characteristically experience periods of remission and exacerbation, which make planning for the future very difficult. This uncertainty frequently engenders much anxiety, which appears best resolved by a close relationship with a physician who honestly informs the patient about the status of the illness and what further treatment is planned.

Even patients who appear close to death improve with the potent chemotherapy employed. Thus, a person who has reached a stage of withdrawal may come to improve markedly and revert to an earlier method of coping with the illness (Kübler-Ross 1969). One such patient was a young female who was admitted for chemotherapy after having had one leg amputated to remove a primary tumor. Initially she was quite desirous of being informed how her illness was progressing and wanted the medical staff to explain in detail the medications and procedures being employed. She developed intractable coughing with involvement of the lungs; her condition appeared to be worsening, whereupon she became extremely withdrawn and noncommunicative. Rather than dying, as had been anticipated, she improved significantly and was able to return home. With subsequent readmissions, anger and depression were manifested and once again she wished to be informed about treatment plans.

Patients have a need to bind their anxiety regarding the illness. One major method is to fixate on one specific parameter of the illness; for example, leukemic patients receiving chemotherapy, which suppresses their bone marrow, frequently center their attention on the numerical value of their white blood cells. A major problem for many patients is the structuring of time; long hours may be spent watching television, and many report, "I try not to think much about the illness," although barriers against this denial invariably break down. Even patients whose close relatives spend 10 hours daily with them report infrequent discussions surrounding the illness. Glaser and Strauss (1966) report the covert games played between patients and their families in not discussing feelings together; however, the presence of close relatives does avert feelings of abandonment and is reported by patients as being quite helpful despite mutual verbal avoidance of important concerns.

The research units come highly recommended by the referring physicians and, correspondingly, most patients have much praise for the staff and strong hopes that the experimental chemotherapy will benefit them. At Baltimore City Hospitals, the patient's doctor was a resident who spent a one-month rotation on the unit; outpatient care was provided by a given member of the research staff who took a background clinical role during hospitalization. Patients often judged the resident's competence by the ability to perform procedures painlessly. One patient, who was extremely bitter in regard to having cancer, voiced his anger repeatedly by confronting the resident about the dangers of chloromycetin treatment leading to aplastic anemia. Although this antibiotic was not even being utilized, he repeatedly challenged the competence of the resident while rendering great praise for the staff physician. Thus, it was observed that patients could more easily project their anger onto a physician who did not have a permanent responsibility in their ongoing care. By expressing anger and frustration in this manner, patients did not face the more significant threat of being abandoned by the "real" doctor.

At the Public Health Service Hospital, physicians involved in direct patient care spent an entire year on the ward. These physicians more readily become the "real" doctor, which generally allows for a closer, more trusting doctor-patient relationship.

Patients who develop a malignancy during mature adulthood face particular problems at this stage of the life cycle. Men are invariably concerned about the family's finances; women generally are more concerned about the impairment of family function due to their absence from the home. One is struck repeatedly by the seeming inopportuneness of the illness and how stressed the entire family unit becomes. Since many of the patients reside long distances from the hospital, close relatives are conflicted about how much time to spend with the patients as compared with the needs of the rest of the family.

Patients recognize the stresses brought to bear upon the family and often express more concern about the emotional state of family members than about themselves. As noted, family members came to our conferences and seemed to benefit from discussing the emotional stresses imposed by the illness. For this reason, an ongoing weekly "group therapy" session for close relatives was organized on the unit at Baltimore City Hospitals. This group was led by a unit social worker as well as myself. It was hoped that this meeting would prove supportive to persons experiencing similar anxieties and who frequently related that they had no one with whom they could openly discuss their feelings regarding the disease.

Despite support for this venture from the clinical director of the unit, the group never had more than a few members. Difficulties in coming to a meeting from long distances at a specified early evening time seemed to be a major factor for the group's dissolution. Additionally, when a patient was discharged from the unit, family members were reluctant to return to the hospital for the weekly meetings. Nonetheless, it is still felt that such a group experience could potentially benefit many families if the above obstacles could be worked out administratively, with a strong commitment by the research and clinical staffs for families to avail themselves of this helping resource.

STAFF RESPONSE
TO THE PSYCHIATRIC CONFERENCE

On both units, my involvement with the research staff has been minimal compared to the clinical staff providing direct patient care. On the Baltimore City Hospitals unit, weekly attendance at morning rounds allowed an ongoing relationship with the clinical director, who spent a year's duration on the ward, as well as the resident physicians. Initially, physician attendance at the weekly conference was extremely erratic in contrast to the unit social workers and nursing staff. When a new clinical director arrived on the unit, his enthusiasm for the potential value of an emotionally oriented conference resulted in his own regular attendance, which, in turn, allowed for regular attendance by the resident physicians.

Previously, it had been frequently lamented by social workers and nursing personnel that seemingly good suggestions about patient management arising from the conference were rarely acted upon since the patient's physician was seldom at the meeting. Ironically, when the physicians began attending on a regular basis, nursing attendance dropped off sharply. It is noteworthy that consistent attendance by both disciplines together, which conceivably would have allowed for a more comprehensive team approach to a patient's management, did not occur. Physicians generally are unwilling to reveal their anxieties to nursing personnel, and this was most likely a prime reason for their infrequent attendance at first. However, it was not clear why afterward nursing staff attendance was inversely related to physician involvement. It is quite possible that nurses did not want to risk any possible confrontation with the physicians regarding patient management, but it is also quite feasible that nurses did not want to observe anxiety in physicans upon whom they had to rely in an inherently stressful work situation for all concerned on the units.

Initially, many residents at Baltimore City Hospitals were quite negative about entering their rotation on the unit. Often there was a feeling of hopelessness about their patients' disease with concomitant guilt about providing experimental therapies, which often evoke unpleasant and even life-threatening side effects. Senior research staff seemed far removed from direct patient management, although their expertise directed treatment protocol. Residents often responded with covert anger as they felt trapped on one side by the pressures of the patients to be cured (or at least comforted) and on the other side by the demands of the senior staff to follow suggestions regarding treatment measures. Because there was only one month's duration in which to assist a resident through this extremely demanding rotation, there was a purposeful attempt not to prove the anxiety of the physician at the conference; rather attempts were made to explore how patient fears became imbedded in the doctor-patient relationship. Many residents seemed to have profited from this experience by feeling more comfortable in discussing these fears with the patient and family alike. Additionally, some of the physicians appeared to have better resolved their own fears regarding death.

Artiss (1973) has reported his five-year consultant experiences at the National Cancer Institute at Bethesda, Maryland. He met weekly for five to six months with a group of physicians who spent a whole year on a similar clinical unit. During this period, physicians became more comfortable in discussing their inner concerns about transactions with families and patients, which allowed for a better resolution of physicians' feelings regarding death as well as an increased ability to relate more humanely with patients. Artiss reported that an existential orientation toward understanding the meaning of life and death seemed most productive in assisting physicians to relate constructively with the inevitably of death.

At the Public Health Service Hospital, I have met exclusively with the nursing staff. The interview-and-discussion format has been similar aside from occasional patients who are interviewed alone because they are too physically ill to attend the meeting or are unwilling to discuss the illness in a group setting. Because I have met with different nursing staffs on alternate weeks, it has been very difficult to evolve a consistent group of nurses in attendance who might feel comfortable discussing their own inner concerns regarding death.

Klagsbrun's (1970) experiences with nurses on a cancer unit showed that initially there were many complaints concerning ward physicians who directed unpleasant tasks onto the nursing staff. Weekly conferences were helpful in enabling the nurses to comprehend the tremendous emotional demands placed on the physician, and the nurses came to accept the physician's avoidance of the dying patient. The nurses came to foster more self-care by the patients with the result that patient morale elevated as they continued to regard themselves as functioning, productive human beings.

To date, my consultation effort at the Public Health Service Hospital does not appear to have contributed to any marked alteration in the ward culture, although the nursing staff does appear to have become more aware of the emotional impact of cancer. Nurses often became more aware of the inner concerns that made previously annoying behavior more tolerable and manageable. For example, some patients call for nursing assistance frequently and, once the nurse enters the room, it becomes very difficult to limit the patient's conversation. There is a tendency to avoid such patients due to their demands; rarely do these patients speak directly about their real underlying anxieties. At the meetings, fears regarding mutilation, abandonment, and death are discussed openly. As a consequence, frequently the patient's behavior becomes a comprehensible, manageable phenomenon rather than a source of irritation. Nurses have been encouraged to speak more openly with the patient about emotional concerns rather than becoming angered by feeling manipulated by the patient's seemingly insatiable demands.

USEFUL PATTERNS OF INTERACTION

Most patients report a desire to be informed honestly about the progress of their illness; they generally state that they wish to be told bad news as well as good. It is known that many patients read various articles and professional books pertaining to the disease. Thus, there appears to be an attempt to gain intellectual mastery over a disease process that appears incomprehensible and irrational in its occurrence. By providing information to patients, doctors and nurses ally themselves with the patient against the illness. However, Schnaper (1969) makes the salient point that, in actuality, it is academic what the patient is told; what really matters is *how*. As long as the patient feels he or she is being approached with understanding, the patient will feel comfortable in discussing his or her feelings whenever a need arises.

Patients may combat their malignancy in a variety of ways in an effort to conquer this enemy. An awareness of the vicissitudes of this attempted mastery can be quite helpful to staff, who may ridicule or prevent seemingly deviant behavior. For example, a middle-aged female from Texas, with a two-year history of a type of skin cancer, had come onto the ward for the first time. She was extremely frightened by the progression of her illness, which had led to the recommendation that she come to Baltimore for further treatment. Her husband, who had been unable to work for over 10 years due to a cardiac condition, accompanied her. She worried constantly about his heart condition and how he would manage should her illness not be arrested. She reported that her prior physicians had requested that she take frequent pictures of her rather grotesque skin lesions, which encompassed much of her body. She voluntarily showed these films to any staff person who entered her room and requested permission to take further pictures during this hospitalization. Although she ostensibly made this request for the benefit of her physicians to follow treatment response, it was apparent that she was utilizing these pictures for herself as a means of having some degree of visible control over her illness.

It is important that patients be allowed to live as aesthetically as possible. Rather simple measures, such as providing wigs for patients who lose their hair from the chemotherapy as well as granting weekend passes home whenever feasible, are two methods of helping patients to feel that they are maintaining some control over the illness. Liberal visiting privileges for close relatives has been beneficial to many patients who feel they have become a burden to the family. Having these family members in attendance counteracts the frequent fear of abandonment that occurs with progression of the illness.

Helping patients and families in their psychological battle with cancer in one sense requires passive rather than active intervention. One often offers far more help by listening compassionately rather than providing elaborate explanations regarding diagnostic features, prognosis, or treatment measures. Providing information when desired is valuable in the sense that it allows for a closer patient-staff relationship, but the key ingredient is to be able to listen carefully without having a need to counteract the patient's defenses or coping strategies. For example, some patients experience a remission after being told that they are cured. It is known that the physicians have informed them ahead of time about the difference between a remission and a definitive cure. To attempt to force "reality" onto the patient at this time serves no constructive purpose. Since the patient is to be followed throughout the duration of his or her illness, this denial will break down on its own should an exacerbation occur.

Similarly, some patients report improvement although it is apparent to the staff that the patient is deteriorating; again it serves no useful purpose to point out the reality of the situation. It is the staff's guilt about having failed to live up to a position of omniscience and omnipotence that propels efforts to break down the patient's denial, but it is more helpful to support this denial as long as it emanates from the patient rather than from the staff. Staff interaction with a patient on a nonverbal level often is more important than what is said. Particularly as a patient approaches death, the presence of a nurse or physician with the patient is all that is being sought.

RECOMMENDATIONS

All patients with cancer are placed under much emotional stress. The value of being able to speak openly is beneficial. Even when there is marked denial present and the patient seems unwilling to share his or her feelings, an ongoing close relationship with caretakers frequently allows his or her concerns to be discussed at some point in the illness. Most physicians and nurses have had no specific training in the psychological management of persons afflicted with cancer. In interviewing patients with the professional staff in attendance, I have attempted to demonstrate that many patients are quite eager to relate their inner concerns and fears. Physicians and nurses are extremely busy in their tasks, fearing that discussions of psychological issues will result in opening "Pandora's Box" with impossible demands made upon their time. However, the defense mechanism of denial operates to a large extent. Most patients do not seem to manifest the desire for frequent discussions about their emotional concerns. This phenomenon is repeatedly noted in the interaction between patients and their family members. The important issue is that patients feel that they can openly discuss these concerns should they want to at any point. In the long run, time demands on staff would be lessened if patients did not need to mask their fears in the guise of demands for attention.

It is extremely important that staff members be comfortable with the inevitability of their own death so that defensive or avoidance tactics need not be utilized in interactions with patients and family members. I have attempted to utilize the conferences as a springboard to this goal by focusing the discussion on the patient and his or her family. I have felt that probing anxieties and concerns of staff members would lead to staff resistance and a need to defend one's actions. Thus, the approach employed parallels the psychiatric supervisor who primarily focuses his or her comments *on the patient* rather than the emotional response of the psychiatric resident. I feel this approach has particular value when one does not have consistent weekly staff participation. It is known that physicians and nurses are busy on the units, but there is frequently much psychological resistance to attend such meetings.

When high administrative personnel on the unit advocate meetings dealing with emotional factors, it is more probable that a consistent group will attend weekly. As noted by Artiss, consistent attendance by a limited number of personnel fosters a more trusting relationship so that staff members become more comfortable in discussing their own concerns regarding death.

To be effective as a leader of these emotionally oriented conferences, the consultant must demonstrate a psychological well-being with the reality of his or her own mortality. One's existential anxiety never completely dissipates during life, and at times I, too, have experienced the same anxiety and depressive feelings everyone else on the unit experiences from interacting with dying patients and their family members. However, the work on such a unit can be extremely gratifying as it is possible to develop a richer meaning and fulfillment of one's own life in the process of assisting others through a severe life-threatening illness. The consultant's attitude toward the treatment provided invariably is conveyed to the staff, and it is important that there be a strong belief in the value of such units. This supportive orientation by the consultant allows for the development of a mutually positive indentification with medical and nursing personnel, who may then comfortably integrate the emotional factors being discussed.

It is important that persons with administrative control over the unit actively support such learning experiences. Generally, the research personnel who direct the units have minimal direct clinical responsibility for patient care. Clinical personnel often resent the emotional demands placed upon them but have no real constructive outlet to resolve conflicts to which they are continually subjected on the unit. It is extremely difficult to involve more than one discipline from the ward in emotionally oriented teaching conferences. Much support is rendered by members of one's own profession as there is no risk of confrontation or embarrassment from another helping profession. Thus, from personal experience, I would recommend that conferences involving emotional factors begin by enlisting only one discipline, although a separate meeting for physicians and nurses could certainly be of much value. Additionally, social workers on such units can be of much potential assistance even though their expertise is sparingly requested. Even today, many physicians and nurses fail to understand how to utilize the social worker as a resource ally in providing needed services to patients and their families.

Cancer units are on the increase, and this era of chronic illness demands that health professionals be increasingly knowledgeable in their understanding of psychological resistance in staff members. By including such conferences as part of the in-service training program, staff members would hopefully become more capable of meeting the emotional needs of persons afflicted with a chronic illness such as cancer. There is much that can be done to help patients and family members in their psychological struggle with cancer, but this will not occur consistently unless there exists a training program whereby emotional factors are given a high priority in the comprehensive care of the cancer patient.

REFERENCES

ARTISS, K., Doctor-patient relation in severe illness. *New England Journal of Medicine* 288:1210-1214, 1973.

GLASER, B., and A. STRAUSS, *Awareness of Dying*. Chicago: Aldine, 1966.

KLAGSBRUN, S., Cancer emotions and nurses. *American Journal of Psychiatry. 126:1237-1244, 1970.*

KÜBLER-ROSS, E., *On Death and Dying*. New York: Macmillan, 1969.

SCHNAPER, N., Management of the dying patient. *Modern Treatment.* 6:746-759, 1969.

23

Acute Leukemia: A Personal Encounter

David B. Friedman

Despite a determined effort on my part to present the following narrative as objectively as possible, there is undoubtedly some residual subjective distortion because the dying woman was my wife.

Anita, a 39-year-old housewife, mother of two sons, 15 and 12, and married to a psychiatrist for 20 years, was always in excellent health. Prior to the current episode, she had only been hospitalized on three occasions; twice for normal delivery of her sons and one overnight stay for a diagnostic curettage.

Her fatal illness ran a six-week course. It all seemed to start with what appeared to be an innocent sore throat. She paid it scant attention since she attributed it to her smoking. About a week later she developed overwhelming fatigue, which drastically curtailed her usual activities. I looked at her throat and saw nothing remarkable. I was perplexed about the extent and persistence of the fatigue and asked an internist to examine her. He too was unimpressed with the physical findings and diagnosed a respiratory virus. By then she had developed a low grade fever. When she did not improve after several days in bed, the internist suggested a consultation with a specialist.

Her fatigue by this time was so draining that she showed the first signs of real concern. "I'm always so tired and I haven't done anything. What could be wrong?" she would ask. She could not see our younger son off to camp at the bus pickup because she was "too exhausted." This was most unusual. Still I had no idea how serious it all was. After her consultation with the ENT specialist, she called me with unmistakable apprehension in her voice. She had bled for 20 minutes after a sinus lavage, (washing out) and both she and the consultant were alarmed by this unexpected hemorrhage.

An internist advised a routine blood count. Our closest family friend, Dr. H., was a hematologist and he agreed to do the blood count. He examined her briefly as well and found nothing unusual except for a low grade fever. We returned home in silence to await a phone call from Dr. H. concerning the results of his examination. Instead, he appeared in person two hours later. I was surprised but unsuspecting. Anita was suspicious when Dr. H. said that he had come to take me to lunch. When we were alone he wasted no time in rendering his verdict. "Anita has acute myelogenous leukemia—she has a count of 100,000." I was stunned and incredulous. All I could think of was the idea of her dying. When I regained my composure, I asked whether a mistake was possible. He said he had checked it with a colleague—there was no doubt! I asked him how long she had to live.

"Less than six months."

"What do I do?"

"She must be hospitalized."

"Why?" I was angry.

"Because maybe they can do something."

"Baloney! I want her home. I'll take care of her. I was in a hospital and it's not like home."

"Don't be an idiot; you'll never forgive yourself and besides you can't take care of her. She'll be very sick."

"Will you be her doctor?" I was reaching for a straw. Years ago he had been my physician, and I had been fortunate enough to recover from what was originally thought to have been a fatal illness. I did not know then why I asked, but in retrospect I believe there may have been some magical thinking involved in my request. The hematologist had been overly pessimistic once before with me, and I had recovered. Why couldn't she?

His reply was an unequivocal, "No, I'm too close."

Now there was a note of despair in my voice. "Who then?"

"Dr. D. is one of the best men in the country and he just came to New York from Boston."

Dr. H. and I returned home. I followed him into the bedroom where I heard him tell Anita that she had an obscure viral infection and that she had to be hospitalized. When he left the room she sat up in bed, burst into tears, and held on tightly to me repeating, "I don't want to go."

As calmly as I could I tried to reassure, her but she was profoundly worried and skeptical. "Something is very wrong. Why would Dr. H. come all the way out here? It must be serious," she said.

Secretly hoping for a miracle and fighting for time, I lied to her. "They don't know what sort of virus it is and they have to do tests that can be done only in a hospital." I hoped that I was convincing. She packed her things mechanically and sat quietly throughout the drive to the hospital. Her silence did not conceal her apprehension. She gripped my hand during the routine of admission. Soon after she was settled in her hospital bed, she checked the roster to ascertain Dr. D's specialty. It did not reveal that he was a hematologist.

The first week in the hospital was horrendous. She was given an experimental drug intravenously, which made her continually nauseated and caused her to vomit frequently. She developed a high fever and appeared toxic. I slept in her room for several nights despite her feeble protestations that I spend the time at home with our 15-year-old son. She seemed relieved to have me there with her. One week later the storm of the high fever, nausea, vomiting, and general malaise subsided; she turned to me one morning and said, "I don't think anyone appreciates how sick I was. I could have died."

Relieved that she appeared so much better, I simply stated "Yes, I know you could have."

My remark was calculated to give the distinct impression that somehow the danger of death had passed and her improvement would continue. Indeed, she regained her sense of humor and her wit. She began to show more of an interest in hospital events. The nursing staff had become very fond of her and brought her their personal problems.

FEAR AND DENIAL

Despite the suggestion of the family doctor to withhold information about her condition from family and friends, I felt compelled to tell them that she was dying of acute leukemia. They wasted no time in appearing. The visits I observed could best be described as chatty with little talk about her illness and most discussion centered on other events of the summer.

To avoid the risk of alarming Anita, I prevailed upon her sister, who lived in a distant city, to postpone her visit until her condition worsened. I was trying to delay the inevitable and attempting to maintain an atmosphere of life as usual.

Our younger son could not understand why his mother was not writing to him at camp as she had always done in the past. I phoned him to inform him that she had been admitted to the hospital and offered him the choice of a phone conversation or a hospital visit. He readily chose to see her.

His short visit seemed to give her no cause for alarm. I did not tell him then that his mother had a fatal illness. I planned to reveal the truth after the camp season, because I was unaware of how soon she was to die.

Several days later, Anita developed signs of internal bleeding. A series of blood transfusions was started and she became visibly apprehensive again. Each morning when the hematologist made rounds, she asked him why she was bleeding internally. He hardly glanced at her as she questioned him; instead he made some irrelevant comment about her being a lovely woman or simply patted her face. She was somewhat irritated at being kept in the dark by Dr. D. She did not pursue a vigorous line of inquiry with him after discovering his stereotyped evasiveness.

One night after returning to bed near exhaustion, she said, "I feel sorry for those people who have leukemia. They must be so tired all the time." Although I detected no hint of a question in her comment (Anita was never one to play games), I replied, "Uh huh." The conversation turned to mundane matters. The word "leukemia" had never been mentioned before nor was it subsequently.

Up until this time, I continued my daily office practice and visited her every night. One early twilight (two days before her death), I walked into her room to find her gazing at a sunset. Somehow she seemed different. I did not know what it was; there was an aura of tension and urgency.

When I sat down on her bed, she looked at me and said, "Isn't that sunset beautiful? Look at this flower, look at the intricate detail, isn't nature wonderful?" Then, for the first time, she burst into tears. "What is life all about? What have I done, what have I accomplished?"

When she paused, I pointed to the walls covered with get well cards, and talked about her role as a mother to our two sons, how much she meant to me, how much joy and warmth she had brought into the lives of others, how many people she had touched, some deeply. Then she began to reminisce and talked almost nonstop about the past, mostly the good times. It was easy for me to just sit there and listen because her thoughts and ideas flowed so freely as she constructed a panorama of the past. I felt she was starting her goodbyes.

Two hours later, Anita stopped talking; she seemed relieved. She reached toward me and hugged me tightly, saying, "I feel much better now." It was then that I decided to stop working and to spend all my time with her because I sensed that the end was near. I advised her sister to come to New York. When she arrived, Anita seemed pleased and never questioned the reason for her presence.

The following morning I was awakened abruptly by a nurse. Anita had taken a dramatic turn for the worse and was calling for me. Her breathing had become labored and she was receiving oxygen by nasal catheter. One look convinced me that she was close to death. All I could say was "everything will be better soon." What I meant was that it would be all over, that she would not suffer for long, but I could not mention the words "death" or "dying." I will never know if she understood what I meant, but she seemed to become less agitated and said softly, "I'm sorry to leave you and the boys, but I can't take it anymore." Then for the first time, I could not contain my tears. She closed her eyes, her breathing became more regular, and shortly thereafter lapsed into coma. Twelve hours later she was dead.

REACTIONS OF PATIENT AND FAMILY

In this brief narration, I have tried to capture the mood, thoughts, and behavior of my wife dying from acute leukemia, and my reaction as well as the responses of others involved. What is so striking is the use of denial as a defense by all those involved.

At first neither Anita nor I had any idea of the seriousness of her illness. She had always been well and was in the prime of life. After my initial shock upon learning the facts, I tried to maintain my usual life pattern. During her toxic state shortly after her hospitalization, it was no longer possible for either of us to maintain the attitude of denial. She was too ill for that. Her remark at the time of the brief remission was so revealing—"I don't think anyone knows how sick I was, I could have died"—and my response—"I know you could have." How quickly we both tried to put the unthinkable in the past. Whenever she showed the slightest improvement, family and friends would invariably comment how she appeared like the "same Anita," referring to her behavior and her sense of humor. This "same Anita" could not be dying! In fact, a characteristic response of family and friends when first informed by me on the telephone that she was dying of leukemia was "Are you sure?" "Oh no."

At first, I was made aware that she was dying in a most abrupt manner. My friend told me. I can only conjecture that Anita may have unconsciously "known" before I did because she experienced these unusual symptoms. The type of "knowledge" and premonition I am ascribing to her is vague and uncertain. The information I received was definite and unequivocal, giving me less chance to hope and deny. Once I "knew," my early behavior was directed toward postponing the certainty of her knowing.

My task was somewhat aided by Anita's early defenses against accepting the idea of her impending death—mainly her unconscious wish not to know. What she manifested was a desire to know, coincidental with frank denial of the realities at hand. From a practical point of view her definitive knowing from the outset was unnecessary because she did not have to make any legal, vocational, professional, or familial arrangements or plans. I gave everyone near and dear to her the opportunity to see her and to bid their goodbyes each in their own ways.

As I reconstruct some of the motives for my behavior six years ago, I must have felt then that she somehow would let me know when she was ready to share the knowledge of her dying. Are the roots of this behavior derived from the earliest good mothering experiences wherein the mother is in close touch with the nonverbalized needs of her infant?

My initial attempts to carry on "as usual" during the first part of her hospitalization were helpful to me in that they served to reaffirm my individuation, and I believe it gave my wife an opportunity to concentrate on the psychic task of dying without the burden of guilt related to the abandonment of those she loved. She knew I could continue with what we had started—the raising of our children. The two-hour catharsis shortly before she died and the indescribably intimate relatedness between us helped her re-experience being loved. It also affirmed a sense of her own uniqueness and purpose, which would not be obliterated by death. She could depart peacefully.

In a study of this sort, the emphasis is on the observations and description of overt behavior, feelings, and verbalized thoughts of the dying person and those present during this critical period that encompasses the struggle for life and the eventual resignation to death. It is important to note that such an approach necessitates inferences and does not directly deal with unconscious factors (drive derivatives, defenses, and fantasy). In this particular presentation, the major focus was on my wife and myself for a multitude of reasons—some of which are the abundance of data, their accuracy and reliability. The data are unique in that they reveal our specific attempts to cope with this crisis as we groped our separate ways through a six-week period.

24

Hope and Fear with Hemodialysis

Burce H. Beard

Patients with end-stage renal failure, whose lives are sustained by hemodialysis, live an uncertain existence about how long they will live and what the quality of their lives will be. No longer can the patient assume that his or her life will continue undisturbed. Instead, the patient lives from day-to-day knowing that his or her hold on life is tenuous and the status of his or her health can change abruptly. No longer can the patient go about the business of living, giving little thought to his or her body and its care. Instead, much time and effort must be directed toward the process of survival.

Awareness of this uncertain existence begins with the patient's first dialysis, when he or she comes to realize that life will continue only as long as he or she has regular access to the machine and follows the prescribed medical regime. The patient is reminded of the precarious state of his or her life by each subsequent dialysis and by the restrictions in diet, by the absence of output of urine, and by the physical discomfort with which he or she lives. The uncertainty of life pervades all thoughts and all plans. While the patient hopes that his or her life will be prolonged, he or she also thinks of dying and fears the possibility of imminent death. At times he or she may even wish for death.

Of equal importance is the uncertainty of the quality of life that is lived by dialysis patients. While these individuals have a strong investment in survival and longevity, they have an equal investment in whether their prolonged lives can be lived in a meaningful and significant way. Many patients report that the quality of life is as dear as life itself. The patient is thankful for the dialysis machine since it is the means by which he or she exists. The patient also hopes that the machine will bring a return of vitality and good health. But he or she resents being tied to it and having his or her life controlled by the necessity of being dialyzed with monotonous regularity. Few patients find that dialysis enables them to feel well, and many feel debilitated and chronically ill. At times work must be given up and certain pleasures must be abandoned. Feelings of emotional well-being are frequently replaced by discouragement, fear, anger, apathy, and disinterest. The patient cannot predict from one day to the next how he or she will feel or what he or she can do. Planning for the future becomes impossible. As a result, chronic uncertainty as to the quality and length of life becomes a constant reality in the life of each patient whose existence is prolonged by hemodialysis.

REPORT OF CASES

Mr. K. G., age 47, was reared in the piney woods of East Texas in a closely knit, financially deprived family in which he was the oldest of four children. His mother was a childlike, generally happy-go-lucky individual, who was subject to periodic impulsive outbursts of violent temper punctuated by deliberate and precise breaking of the family dishes. The father was described as a fine man, stern, and a diligent worker, who labored as a barber to keep the family housed, clothed, and fed. The patient learned the value systems of his father. He worked while in high school and bought his own clothes and school supplies. He also bought items for the family, such as a cook stove for his mother and a radio for the family so they could have entertainment during the evenings. He dated his wife-to-be while in high school. They were married three years following his graduation. Immediately upon finishing high school, he worked for a time for an auto parts company, later for the railroad, then for a recycling plant, and finally for an oil company, where he was employed for 25 years working in the oil field around machinery, rigs, and trucks. His health was good. He took sick leave from work only to have an appendectomy and later a tonsillectomy. He was firm in his discipline with his children but was not high tempered. He teased his wife, was jolly, was well liked by his friends, had a twinkle in his eye, was devoted to his community, and was active in his church.

In the spring of 1970, the patient developed arthritis. Treatment produced minimal symptomatic improvement, and the patient believed that an adverse reaction to a medication caused renal damage. He became quite ill, developed headaches, began vomiting, and suffered a marked loss of strength. In July 1970 he was diagnosed as having progressive renal failure. In October 1970 a kidney biopsy confirmed the diagnosis of end-stage renal disease. The patient was transferred to the Renal Failure Clinic at Baylor Medical School in Houston, where he was quite ill.

Gradually, K. G. improved and plans were made for the patient's life to be sustained by hemodialysis. A program of training preparatory to home dialysis was initiated. The patient, however, refused to participate in the training. He resented being ill, resented the machine, resented being life dependent upon it, and resented the idea of being tied to the machine. His wife mastered the skill of operating the machine and dialyzing the patient. The patient and his wife returned home in February 1971, after a stay in Houston of approximately four months.

At this point, the patient had hopes that on dialysis he would regain good health and could return to his job. Upon returning home, however, he learned that he had been temporarily terminated from his job. Four months later he learned that the termination had been made permanent and he had been placed on medical retirement. Since hard work had always been the key factor in this patient's ethic, he felt extremely despondent and let down at being unemployed and idle. He had always worked hard for the sake of his home, for the sake of his wife, and for the sake of his children. Through hard work and providing financially, he had maintained an image of himself as the head of the family. The loss of his job and the loss of ability to work meant to him a loss of stature, the loss of significant role identity, and the loss of dignity.

As the months rolled by, he felt wretched, weakness was marked, and disability was great. The patient began to lose hope. He seldom read, watched television, or worked about the home. He resented the restrictions of fluid and certain foods from his diet. At times he would refuse to go on the machine, only to agree to continue dialysis solely because of the insistence of his wife. He hated the fact that the machine controlled and dictated his life, and he directed his hate and dislike of the machine at his wife since she was the one who attached him to the dialysis apparatus

His wife made special efforts to make his time on the machine pleasant but without success. Gradually, he became more apathetic. He spent much time during the day lying on the couch and he roamed the house at night. He previously walked the pasture and drove his car about the neighborhood, but gradually the loss of energy caused him to give up these pursuits, and finally he drove none and walked very little. Sex had in the past been a most meaningful part of his existence, but he became impotent and disinterested. He suggested to his wife at times that she needed to find herself another man to marry. He became resistive to encouragement and to any new ideas proposed by his wife. He finally became negativistic, irritable, sad, depressed, lifeless, and hopeless. He developed marked self-deprecating ideas and felt that he was a total burden to himself and to others, and wished openly for death.

The patient had only one remaining area of hope and that was the possibility of a successful renal transplant. He became completely focused on the idea of a transplant or nothing. The patient transferred his medical care from the Houston facility to the transplant service at Parkland Hospital at Dallas. Each time there was talk of transplant, the patient showed signs of encouragement. One sister, initially, offered to provide a kidney, but when the time came for her to make good on her offer, she had second thoughts and declined to donate. The patient felt that his brothers and sisters had turned against him through their failure to help. He felt rejected and bitter.

After two years on home dialysis, a cadaver kidney became available for transplant. The patient wept joyfully at the news and yet feared that he might die during the surgery. He was told that the kidney was of questionable viability because of being several hours old, but the patient agreed to accept the transplant.

The first day following transplant there was slight output of urine, and then the kidney ceased to function. The patient was immediately thrust into a deep despondent state. He became silent, sullen, and irritable, and felt there was no hope. Infection in the area of the transplanted kidney developed and it was recommended that the transplant be removed.

The patient at first refused removal of the dead transplant and also refused to continue dialysis, thus stating in action his disinterest in living. It was necessary to martial the entire family resources, the wife, the daughter, and the son, to persuade the patient to prolong his life further by having the transplant removed and continuing hemodialysis. This accomplished, the patient became even more quiet and irritable. He talked of never leaving the hospital alive and refused to talk of life after returning home. He had no plans; he had no interests. Efforts on the part of the patient to contribute to his own welfare were minimal. Interest in food was slight. Irritablity was marked.

Slowly, as a result of urging by the staff, the patient finally began to walk occasionally about the room and shortly prior to his dismissal from the hospital, he began to sit for short periods in a chair.

The patient was dismissed to return home and resume home hemodialysis. He was markedly despondent, without hope, and the possibility of some overt or covert self-destructive act was known to exist. Partial safeguard against direct, overt suicide was arranged by the wife in employing someone to be with the patient during the daytime while she was away at work. But there was clear recognition on the part of the staff, as well as members of the family, that the patient had at his command immediate means of covert suicide either by dietary indiscretion or through refusal to continue on the dialysis machine. The patient stated often and franky that he remained alive only because of the insistence of his wife. To him, continuation of life was without value and without meaning.

As the weeks went by, the patient's existence did not improve. He continued on home dialysis. His life was restricted. He felt wretched and was constantly depressed. Six months after the unsuccessful transplant attempt, the depression deepened and the patient's ability to tolerate his existence came to an end. Early one morning he ended his life with a self-inflicted gunshot wound to the head.

Mrs. D.L., age 50, was reared in a small central Texas town in a family in which she was the third of six children. She recalled that she was known as the "spoiled one," which she attributed to favored treatment that she received from her father and the fact that she was the "baby of the family" for a number of years before her younger siblings were born. She recalled one occasion when she was so insistent on having a new dress that her father dressed and went to town at two o'clock one morning, persuaded the owner of a local dry goods store to open his shop at that hour, bought a dress, and returned home with it to pacify her. She was close to both of her parents, describing them as people without fault. The father developed Bright's disease and suddenly died of a heart attack at age 46. The family missed him sorely, but the older brother rapidly took his place. Although the family had financial difficulties during the middle 1930s, the patient recalled that life was fun. All the family worked in the home, and the mother and the brothers kept the family financially intact.

Immediately after high school graduation, the patient married. She and her husband moved to the West Coast for a time. The patient had never previously been out of her home county and she sorely missed familiar surroundings, family, and friends. The patient and her husband later moved to West Texas, where the patient's son and later her daughter were born. In 1954 her husband was tragically killed, and the loss to the patient was overwhelming. At her mother's insistence, she moved back to her original home town, and she and the mother lived together for a time. The patient then built a house of her own and devoted herself entirely to mothering her children and engaging in all sorts of child-centered activities, such as Girl Scouts, P.T.A., and church groups. During this time the patient described herself as a driven person. She felt compelled to perform her household and mothering chores with perfection but lived with an apprehensive and unsettled air.

In 1959 the patient remarried and almost immediately developed signs of renal impairment. At first she developed headaches and then hypertension. She required constant medical attention, including frequent house calls by her family physician for injections for severe headaches. Her first hospitalization occurred in 1960, precipitated by hypertension and its complications. By 1963 she was constantly ill either at home or in a hospital. In 1967 she had a cerebrovascular accident (commonly called a stroke) and was unconscious and near death for three days. In 1969 she was first treated in the Renal Failure Center at Parkland Hospital in Dallas, and for the next three years her life consisted of barely surviving with constant medical care and treatment.

In April 1972 the patient began hemodialysis, a program that necessitated three trips per week from Central Texas to Dallas. By this time, her husband had retired, largely to be with her and assist in her care. The patient feared being alone and felt greatly comforted by having her husband with her constantly. She was also frightened to be so far from her physicians and feared that she might become acutely ill and die at home or before she could make the trip to the center. She developed nightmares, choking sensations, and several times she and her husband rushed to Dallas in the middle of the night because of shortness of breath. She constantly feared she would die and was especially afraid of being left by herself in case her condition suddenly worsened. So stressful was her existence that in August 1972 she and her husband moved to Dallas. She felt somewhat reassured to be near her physicians and the dialysis center.

Consideration of home dialysis brought a steadfast refusal on the part of the patient to participate. She wanted to be dialyzed by the center staff. She did not trust others to put her on the machine or control the machine while she was on it. She was afraid that at home her husband might not stand by within a step or two of the machine while she was in the process of being dialyzed.

She could not assume her part of the responsibility of home dialysis and, thus, refused to learn to operate the machine. Home dialysis, even though it offered distinct advantages for her and her husband, was not acceptable to the patient, and, therefore, the idea was abandoned. Center dialysis and kidney transplant remained her only alternatives.

Life became more unpleasant in the ensuing months and was clearly described by the patient in very grim terms. Because of constant pulmonary edema, with cough and shortness of breath, the patient became extremely limited in her physical activities. In her own words, "I can't do anything. Even when I make up the bed, I have to stop and catch my breath. After walking from the car to the house, I have to sit down 10 or 15 minutes. When I straighten up the house or cook supper, it takes me much longer than it should. I used to fear that I would suffocate at night, but now I sit in a chair and sleep sitting up and the fear is less. I'm so weak that I seldom go places. I watch T.V. I knit and I crochet. I hate the machine and yet I know I have to have it. After I've been dialyzed, I can go 18 hours before the shortness of breath gets severe again. But when I have an extra day to live through like on a Sunday, I'm short of breath, miserable, and again can't do anything. I hate the machine but I'm glad to be on it on Monday."

Furthermore, she stated, "If the machine takes off too much fluid, then I have muscle cramps. If it doesn't take off enough, then I have shortness of breath. I truly prefer dying to living the way I do. At times I pray for death. I think of suicide but I dismiss it for the sake of my children. I know that I'm supposed to live and the machine is what makes it possible. I've almost given up hope of ever getting a kidney since there are so few kidneys available these days."

In addition, the patient related that she was bitter at the turn of events her life had taken. She and her husband had planned to be free to move about and take trips. But she had spent most of the last 10 years in simply attempting to survive in spite of her disease. Life had become so limited that it was hardly worthwhile. Her greatest joy had been cooking for her children when they came to visit. Now she rarely had them visit, and when they did she was no longer able to prepare a meal for them. Her children had been her life, and now she was able to do nothing in the way of motherly things that previously had given her so much pleasure. She stated, "I wonder sometimes if my disease is a punishment for something that I have done."

One day in her depressed, limited life, there came a pleasant upswing. In spite of being frightened, anxious, and practically home-bound except for trips to the dialysis center, her daughter persuaded her to go with them by car to the horse races in a city 300 miles away. To make it an even more momentous occasion, her husband, who had found temporary employment, was not able to leave Dallas, and the patient made the trip without her husband and his constant support. While on the trip, she did fairly well. Toward the end of the second day, however, she began to experience twinges of shortness of breath and the decision was made to drive back to Dallas in the middle of the night. The patient looked better after this venture and the next week she made another trip, this time to visit her son 30 miles away. The following weekend she and her husband planned a third trip, a visit to their home town in Central Texas.

Three months later the patient was accepted for center dialysis in a unit within 30 miles of her home. She and her husband left the apartment in which they had been residing temporarily in Dallas and took up life again in their own home in the community in which each had been reared. Life was improved by this move, and the patient continued to be somewhat more mobile than had been the case during most of her illness. She was still frightened, however, of suddenly becoming acutely ill, short of breath, and dying. Life still seemed of questionable value, and at times she still prayed for death to end her uncertain existence. At the same time, she persistently clung to the hope that a kidney transplant might be forthcoming to provide her with a life of more certainty and of better quality.

CONCLUSION

The two case reports bear out the fact that patients whose lives are maintained on hemodialysis live with chronic uncertainty. There is hope for life and fear of death. They wish for a return of previous health, yet they live with constant sickness. They strive to regain a life of acceptable quality, but they are forced to accept a life whose quality is seriously marred. Some patients state that they live on borrowed time, indicating that dialysis is viewed as delaying death, rather than prolonging life.

In spite of the fears and the uncertainties, most dialysis patients cling to life tenaciously, demonstrating an ability to live with uncertainties and to exist with lives that are characterized by discomfort, fear, stress, and discouragement. At the same time, dialysis patients live with the ever-present possibility of an untimely death. Throughout their lives, they are aware of the nearness of death, and dying is a constant reality.

VII

THE ELDERLY

As one enters old age the question of death does not disappear. Indeed, it would appear that the elderly must resolve the issue of meaning in their lives as they approach death. Such is the coping task of the final epoch of life.

Berezin notes that the process of coming to terms with aging and the approach of death is a gradual process. He uses the term partial grief to emphasize the number of small losses that begin to mount up in the life of the aged. He points out that it is helpful to both the aged and their families to address these small griefs, to mourn them, and thereby retain the integrity of the remaining life of the elderly.

Similarly, Preston reports on her personal work with the aged, leading to open discussion about the meaning and import of one's life, as preparation for death. Again we find an emphasis on "what is life?" Not, "what is death?"

Finally, I have included a memo from Maurice Levine, which I first received as a personal document from him. His statements are not unique, for I have had many elderly dying people say the same things to me, but Levine has captured the feelings of the dying elderly in an eloquent fashion. Even though one is old, one cherishes life. He accepts the fact of his dying, yet he denies the eminent seriousness of his illness. He died only a few days after writing this memo.

In these final chapters I find many feelings of ambivalence described. Family, friends, relatives, professional staff may on the one hand cherish the elderly and desire to have them live on; and on the other hand one *may hope for release, peace, quiet, yes, even death. Feelings of ambivalence toward the dying person are present in all stages of life, as noted throughout the book. In the aged, the feelings of ambivalence emerge more easily and we can see the complex feelings about death that we have throughout our lives.*

25

Partial Grief for the Aged and Their Families

Martin A. Berezin

The focus of this chapter is on the degree and variety of grief reactions that are precipitated by the degree and variety of loss affecting not only the aged person him- or herself, but especially those people most closely connected to him or her—family and friends.

The more common and more recognizable grief reactions experienced by the aged person are due to the inevitable losses of loved ones—losses that impinge upon him or her with increasing and inexorable frequency as the person ages. The older one gets, the more losses are sustained, and with each loss the aged person is required to cope in those ways that are unique for him or her. However, loss as we understand it includes much more than the death of a loved one. It is axiomatic to say that where there is loss there is grief—or there should be.

GRIEF IN THE ELDERLY

Let us first consider the situation of grief as it affects the aged and aging person him- or herself. The aging person regards the various changes in his or her body as states of loss or threatened loss—changes that are not pathological but rather are the physiological and sociological concomitants of growing older (Berezin 1965). This category includes reactions to an altered body image brought about by such conditions as failing eyesight and hearing, memory defects, diminished skin elasticity, degenerative changes in bones and joints, loss of muscle power, reduced sexual desire and potency with a withdrawal from genital primacy and its subsequent tendency to regression, graying and thinning hair, retirement from occupation, and the departure of children from home. All of these conditions and many others are often regarded as narcissistic injuries that set in motion various efforts to compensate or to grieve. Such compensatory devices have even been the basis for humor. It is said that as a man gets older, the faster he could run when he was younger, and there is the joke about the old man who chased a pretty girl around and around a table but could not remember why.

These conditions and states serve to emphasize that there are two conditions in states of grief—loss and the reaction to it—and that the condition of loss and the reactions to it vary considerably. Freud (1957) recognized the varying degrees and meanings of loss that precipitate mourning in his classical paper on "Mourning and Melancholia," in which he said, "Mourning is regularly the reaction to the loss of a loved person, or to the loss of some abstraction which has taken the place of one, such as one's country, liberty, an ideal, and so on."

THE CONCEPT OF PARTIAL LOSS AND PARTIAL GRIEF

There are approximately 20 million people in the United States over the age of 65, which is 9 to 10 percent of the total population. If we include those over age 60, we add a few million more, and there is hardly a family today that is not dealing with an aging person. Furthermore, these numbers will increase. The impact of the aging person on so many environmental people demands that we pay special attention to it so that we may better understand and, therefore, be better prepared to help in the problems of long-term care.

The concept of partial loss may throw some light on how the effects of the environmental people (spouse, children, and friends) are different from or similar to what is experienced as loss by the aged individual him- or herself. The death of an aged person (or any person) is an obvious loss, but this simplistic statement does not take into account how environmental people deal with those conditions of partial loss prior to death. The conditions previously referred to, such as diminished visual acuity, degenerative changes, retirement, and so on, not only affect the person him- or herself but also precipitate reactions in family and friends. There is not just a final loss with its expected grief, but in varying degrees of conscious and unconscious perception in a partial loss or threat of loss as well; and it is this condition of partial loss with which I am mainly concerned.

Those conditions that suggest loss or threat of loss may vary in range from the observance of a significant anniversary of an aged person to the presence of a severe and terminal illness. Even when there appears to be no actual loss in the physical and social conditions of the elderly person, real losses may occur. For example, when an elderly male parent retires from his occupation, this retirement involves not only the significant shift in his own image of himself and how he copes with it, but also the shift in the attitude of children, family, and friends to this altered image. Retirement was deliberately chosen as an illustration, for it is too often a vivid, if unfortunate, expression of our cultural value system—a system that in its hierarchy of values prizes the young, the active, the achieving. There is not much room in our culture (or in any culture, various myths to the contrary notwithstanding) for a genuine position of respect for retirees. Rather we generally see in the conflicts about this phenomenon a tendency to resort to reaction formation and oversolicitude; for example, we refer to old people as "golden agers" and "senior citizens." In any event, the elderly parent is no longer the active, achieving, economically independent person he had been in the eyes of his children and friends. Instead, there is a loss of previously held image, an ego ideal that no longer exists in the same form.

The events of a 60th birthday party were recently reported to me. The man whose birthday was being celebrated was in excellent health, and there was no indication of any pathology. Yet amid all the gaiety of the festivities, friends and relatives repeated references to the "end of the line" or the "beginning of the end." One friend made a direct statement that at age 60 the time ahead before death was now a measurable distance. The macabre thrust of the conversation was obvious to the wife of the man whose birthday was being celebrated, and with a show of tension and agitation she registered her objection to the various comments and requested that the topic be changed to something more pleasant.

In a more extreme example, when an elderly person is afflicted with an organic brain condition, a senile dementia, with the resultant changes in personality, there is obviously a significant loss of a previously well-known person.

What is often clinically significant about partial states of loss—beginning signs of infirmity, changes in appearance and role, various disengagements—is that they may not be appreciated as beginning loss. What is suggested about loss is that there is an absurdity in maintaining the concept of loss as operating purely on an all-or-none basis. It is more accurate and to the point to appreciate that loss, which

acts as a precipitant of reactions, may be partial, threatened, or anticipated and that subtle changes in the elderly person must be regarded as
loss equivalents—or at least as threats of loss.

Lindemann (1944) has attempted to classify the phenomenology that
he observed as "acute grief reactions." He states that the syndrome of
acute grief "may appear immediately after a crisis; it may be delayed; it
may be exaggerated or apparently absent . . . in place of the typical
syndrome there may appear distorted pictures, each of which represents
one special aspect of the grief syndrome." He classifies the "morbid
grief reaction" as delay or postponement of grief, and states that
distorted reactions include the following: overactivity without a sense of
loss, the acquisition of the symptoms of the last illness of the deceased,
psychosomatic symptoms, alteration in relationship to friends and
relations, furious hostility against specific persons, wooden formal
conduct without apparent affects, loss of patterns of social interaction,
activities that may be detrimental to his or her own social and economic
existence, and finally agitated depression.

I have used the term "anticipatory grief," which is Lindemann's
term, and I also use the model of terminal illness, which suggests the
finality of imminent death. The problem is to find a suitable term that
connotes the concept of a state or stages of grief when that grief cannot
be worked through, when it cannot be resolved and completed because
the final death and loss have not yet occurred. In the case of terminal
illness, the friends and relatives of the dying person cannot, in fact,
mourn, but they are forced to cope in some way with what is obviously
occurring. Anticipatory grief reactions are well known to those
physicians and ancillary people who deal with patients with terminal
illnesses. Lindemann's term of anticipatory grief conveys something
correct about the total situation, yet it does not quite suffice. It suggests
that the total grief reaction already could have occurred.

Another possible term is "postponed grief," but this may suggest that
all grief is postponed, as though grief reactions are not experienced
during the waiting period before death. The term "suspended grief" also
suggests a state of limbo, during which grief lurks somewhere like the
Sword of Damocles. Yet another suggestion is "preterminal grief,"
which has some merit, for it suggests more clearly the state of affairs; but
even here the notion of complete grief may persist. The concept of
"partial grief states" seems to do some justice to the clinical syndrome
but still does not convey the total picture.

It is my feeling that the concept of partial grief, which is unresolvable,
brings about many reactions on the part of responsible relatives and

friends, which at times makes extended care difficult if not impossible. It is well known that the issues confronting the physician in extended care more often than not involve the family more than the patient. The reactions and attitudes of the spouse and children require more attention and tactful management than does the care of the patient. The types of reactions in family members may vary from anxiety and guilt to mature understanding and appreciation of the realities of the situation. When guilt becomes the steam that motivates family members, the reactions can be quite extreme, irrational, and unmanageable.

One of the most difficult concomitants to the concept of partial unresolvable grief is the factor of helplessness that family members feel acutely, and I hold that there is no worse disease than helplessness itself. The family can do nothing to alter the course of the elderly person, whose life now proceeds in a steady downhill course to its ultimate conclusion. This statement does not contradict the possibility of coping with and attempting to master one's own feelings.

CASE ILLUSTRATIONS

The partially grieving family member may be caught in the terrible dilemma of wishing an aged person dead—a wish that often remains unconscious and denied. The wish for the old person to die may be handled by reaction formation, in which the opposite is expressed or yearned for—that the elderly patient is not going to die. In fact, some family members deny that the patient is even sick. Some of us have had the experience of observing a spouse or a child talk to an aged person with far advanced organic brain deterioration as if they were holding an understandable conversation. I have witnessed such "conversations" conducted with patients who are totally unconscious and in coma.

The problem of ambivalence about unconscious death wishes was observable in a clinical vignette at one of our hospitals. The patient was an 82-year-old man who was not demented but did have some moderate cardiac disturbance. His wife, son, and sister-in-law came to visit him every day without exception. His wife had quarreled with doctors, nurses, and administrators about food, bed, medication, care, rehabilitation, money, and so on. She was furious that her husband was allowed out of bed and sent to rehabilitation and occupational therapy. She was fearful that any physical exertion would kill him, and she insisted that he be kept in his pajamas, remain in bed constantly, and not be allowed to move at all. It struck all who heard of her wish that the image of a man lying motionless in bed was the image of a dead person. A clue to her unconscious wish was contained in another aspect of the situation, which was that if he were sent to rehabilitation he might get better, and then he would go home and she would have to care for him, which she claimed she could not do because she herself had a heart condition and was afraid she might die from the exertion of caring for her husband. In other words, she was trapped in her ambivalence toward her husband.

The wish for a patient to die may be more acceptably expressed after the patient dies. After the loss has occurred, we hear often that a family is consoled by the verbalization that the death was a blessing, a relief after such suffering, but for many people the verbalization of such consoling thoughts may not be permitted before death.

The reaction-formation characteristic of guilt may be seen in the case of Mrs. G., who cared for husband at home—a situation that demanded of her nobility and martydom. Her husband had a severe Alzheimer's disease (causing senility) and was so deteriorated that he no longer knew his wife or children, but he was physically very active. He demanded dinner at 4:00 A.M.; he set fires in the backyard for which the fire department had to be called. He required 24-hour supervision, which Mrs. G. managed in spite of her own severe cardiac condition. Regardless of the recommendation of several physicians and members of her family, she persistently refused to hospitalize her husband. She clung tenaciously to an occasional flash of what seemed to be rational behavior on his part, which for her meant that he might recognize her and his surroundings, as though he might yet fully recover from his severe dementia, even when she had been advised by several physicians that her husband's condition was irreversible and hopeless.

In this case, Mrs. G. attempted to live with her husband in the vain hope that his tragic, progressive, hopeless dementia might be only a transient condition. Each time he behaved in some superficially rational way—which, in fact, was not rational but which she misinterpreted—she continued to believe that he would become the healthy admired man she once knew. This behavior was a defensive operation on her part made possible by the denial of the obvious. It is likely that other factors were operative as well, such as guilt, maternal satisfaction in caretaking, or a logical, mature wish to care for her husband (but these considerations are being omitted for purposes of illustrating the thesis of partial grief).

Another case is that of a 47-year-old woman who complained about being depressed. She ascribed her irritability and dissatisfaction to the way her life had been and the way she saw it in the future, her lack of pleasure in social contacts, her passive inadequate husband, her children's scholastic problems, and her menopause. However, further questioning brought out the fact that she was not having her menopause, but that her knowledge of "change of life" was sufficient for her to feel that it might occur in the next two to three years.

What puzzled the patient more was her unprovoked hostility and attacks on her two sisters, one of whom was married, wealthy, and whose children were quite successful. She felt that she was most envious of this sister and felt bitter in her envy. What she could not so easily explain was her irritability and overtly hostile, abusive attacks on another sister, who was unmarried and who lived on marginal income.

In later interviews we learned that the patient, who worked for an industrial company, found herself anxious and hostile toward her supervisor, who was an older woman and who reminded the patient of her mother. Then came the discovery that the patient's mother was in her 80s and that "she was living out the last few months or years of her life." The patient's unmarried sister lived with the mother and was caring for her. The patient was, I propose, in a grief reaction, which, together with her helplessness and regression to earlier childhood involvements with her sisters, was making her feel depressed and for which she attempted to ascribe various reasons—all but the correct one. Thus, she blamed her menopause, her wealthy sister's supercilious attitude, and her envy of others. She was attempting to displace her feelings about her mother to her supervisor as well as to other figures in her environment.

A common observation for those of us who deal with families of aged people is the irrational, hostile attitude that siblings express to each other as they quarrel about what should be the proper care for an aged parent. Each accuses the other of negligence, lack of sympathy, or avoidance of responsibility. They challenge each other with questions of who telephoned or visited how many times. Here one sees the emergence of projection and the regression to earlier sibling childhood relationships.

RECOMMENDATIONS

This chapter would be incomplete were I not to report a pragmatic outgrowth of the considerations referred to here. From my clinical experiences both in the hospital and in private practice, I have learned of the value of one mode of therapeutic management of the modified partial grief reactions seen among family members who try in various ways to cope with the painful situations of a terminal phase in spouse and parents. The distress of environmental people adversely affects the health of the aged person. A family conference, held as a group meeting with the psychiatrist acting as a neutral, understanding, objective, knowledgeable resource, has been found extremely helpful in resolving many of the undesirable elements encountered in these partial grief reactions. In such a conference, the family is confronted with the reality of a given situation and the prognosis is openly discussèd. The reactions, expecially those of helplessness, are discussed with the family, and the need for unity within the family structure is stressed. The appeal is to the realities both of the aged one and of the uncomfortable struggles among the grieving ones. The awareness of this significant mode of management has grown so that the family conference has become a standard procedure in many social service agencies and hospitals.

REFERENCES

BEREZIN, M. A., Introduction, in *Geriatric Psychiatry: Grief, Loss, and Emotional Disorders in the Aging Process,* eds. M. A. BEREZIN and S. H. CATH. New York: International Universities Press, 1965.

FREUD, S., Mourning and melancholia. *Standard Edition,* 14:237–258. London: Hogarth Press, 1957.

LINDEMANN, E., Symptomatology and management of acute grief. *American Journal of Psychiatry,* 101:141-148, 1944.

26

The Aged and Euthanasia

Caroline E. Preston

Some five years ago I would never have dreamed that today I would be writing a chapter in a book about death and dying. Then I was busily developing questionnaires for measuring attitudes among the elderly. I was full of questions about how some old people mellow in serene transcendence of the physical, psychological, social, and economic trials of aging, while others succumb to old age, lonely, embittered, despairing, and invisible to the rest of society. I looked everywhere in the lives of old people for keys to their successes and failures. Was it the support of families and relatives? Their choice of a community and type of housing? The availability of transportation and socializing? The prophylaxis of having enough money? Was the clue a history of achievement in the community? Faith in God? Hope in the present and for the future?

Legion as the questions I asked these long-suffering subjects, not once did the thought occur to me that I might also discover important truths about them by asking how it was to be living in the shadow of death when days are clearly numbered. How could this possibly be? All too possible for a middle-aged investigator, a nearly completed product of death-denying culture. Later, much later, I wondered whether or not the omission of any discussion of the meaning of both life and death may not have obscured some salient determiners of different success levels in coping with the aging process.

One day an eminent colleague, Dr. Robert Williams, asked me, "What do old people think about euthanasia?" His question was like a thunderbolt. I had never mentioned death as a natural event; how could I possibly approach my subjects with the issue of a contrived unnatural event, however timely?

Now, I think my blind spot for death and dying is probably related to events in my own life that brought death too heartbreakingly close to permit me any degree of objectivity or dispassion. I experienced the deaths of loved ones, none of whom died in a manner that made me comfortable about their dyingness. I found myself seething with anger at these people even though they had never lived according to my comfort needs and were unlikely to die according to these. Two of the deaths were violent—suicide. One was a prolonged wasting away with bone cancer. Another was from emphysema with florid psychotic manifestations toward the end. Yet another was a person who died after nine long years of intense anxiety and depression.

These then were the personal circumstances for me as I was trying to tease out the psychosocial correlates of good aging. These circumstances must have contributed to my blindness about discussing death with hale and healthy oldsters, none of whom spontaneously engaged me in his or her own dyingness. My subjects may well have recognized that I had no tolerance for such discourse.

Incidental to some research into communication patterns among retirement home subjects, my research assistant and I met with a few of the subjects who volunteered to participate in consciousness-raising sessions on the problems of aging in our society. Dare we introduce the subject of euthanasia? Halfheartedly, we decided we could. Very gingerly and euphemistically, I asked the volunteers if any of them had ever thought about how they would like to die. To my amazement this proved to be like unlocking a floodgate. What ensued was a spirited discussion in which every member of the group had some significant contribution to make. They talked about the high cost of dying in today's world of gadgets to keep people alive. They argued the pros and cons of cremation versus conventional burial, and someone asked about the coffin explosion. At the rate we are dying, won't cremation become mandatory because of the pinch on real estate? Almost everyone had an account of a close brush with death, coming from the threshold of death back to life, how peaceful dying had seemed, how harsh the return to consciousness and pain. No one seemed to find the discussion morbid or distasteful. I was impressed by the candor and humor . . . not of the gallows sort, either . . . and the obvious relish in these discussions. I learned what other people wiser than I have since told me about old peoples' need for the opportunity to talk openly about living in the shadow of death.

This realization brought me to investigate the subject of death and aging systematically. I wish to report on this study.

STUDY OF AGING AND DEATH

The subjects of this study were 35 women and 65 men, all Caucasian with a mean age of 72 and an age range from 60 to 95 years. Eighty-two were residents in a Veterans' Retirement Home. Twenty-three subjects were patients in two local private convalescent centers.

The mean for the subjects was 10 years of schooling. Nine were college graduates; 42 high school; 54 had attended grade school only. Almost one-third (30) were married; 39 were widowed; 14 had never married; and 23 were divorced or separated. All subjects considered themselves to be retired; 34 had had skilled or professional occupations; 34 had been unskilled; and 15 had been housewives only. According to religious faiths, there were 59 Protestants, 18 Catholics, and 28 other or no religion subjects.

Criteria for the selection of the subjects were that they be well enough oriented to respond meaningfully to the interview questions and sufficiently comfortable to tolerate the interview procedures.

In the course of semistructured interviews, subjects were asked the following questions:

1. How are you feeling today?
[a]2. What age would you like most to be?
[b]3. If you could do anything you pleased, where would you like most to live?
[c]4. Of all the things you do, which are least interesting or enjoyable to you?
[d]5. Do you wish you could see more of your (a) friends, (b) neighbors, (c) relatives than you do, or would you like more time to yourself?
6. How does the future look to you?
7. Do you think of yourself as old? If so, when did you begin thinking so?
8. If you were fatally ill, in great distress, and under heavy medical expense, would you want the doctors to do *nothing* to keep you alive?
9. If you were fatally ill, in great distress, and under heavy medical expense, would you want the doctors to do *something* to shorten your life?
10. Is your religious faith important to you?

[a]Score 1 if subject prefers age he or she is.
[b]Score 1 if subject prefers where he or she is.
[c]Score 1 if subject does nothing uninteresting or unenjoyable.
[d]Score 1 if subject is satisfied with present amount of contact with all three catergories of people.

The first question was asked to assess current feelings of ill or well-being. Questions 2, 3, 4, and 5 are derived from Cumming and Henry's work (1961) in which the answers to these particular questions correlated highly with interviewers' independent ranking of older subjects' morale. Answers (scored as above) yield a "contentment index" value, which ranges from 0 to 4. Outlooks on the future were presumed to reflect levels of optimism compared to apathy or pessimism. Question 7 was included because subjective agedness among older people has been found to correlate positively with identification of oneself in the role of semi-invalidism (Preston 1968). Questions 8 and 9 were found from preliminary trials to be simple enough to be grasped by subjects who sometimes could not understand words or phrases such as "euthanasia" or "prolong life" or "promote death." Inquiry not only into subscribed religious faiths of the subjects but into the importance of religion was indicated because of prevailing religious proscriptions against the timing of death except as this is the will of God.

When we analyzed the interview data, we found that about two-thirds of the subjects claimed feelings of well-being at the time of the interview. Slightly more than one-third of the subjects obtained high "contentment" scores (that is, would be their present age, live where they were, found nothing in their lives uninteresting or unenjoyable, and saw enough of their friends and relatives); two-thirds obtained low "contentment" scores. Similarly, future outlooks were optimistic for about one-third and pessimistic for about two-thirds of the subjects.

In common with most older people, the majority of these subjects reject the negative sterotype of "being old" (Kastenbaum 1964). None of the "here and now" variables (that is, current feelings of well-being, contentment scores, future outlooks, and subjective agedness) showed any systematic relationship among themselves or with the psychosocial variables.

Confronted with the hypothetical condition of fatal illness, great distress, and heavy medical expense, almost half the subjects were "life at any cost," about one-quarter were "let me die, but don't kill me," and about a third were "let me or help me die." These preferences were unrelated to psychosocial characteristics. The preferences on the timing of death also showed no relationship to current feelings of well-being, contentment scores, outlooks on the future, or subjective agedness. Significantly more of the "life at any cost" subjects claimed religious faith to be important to them. If these subjects were influenced by religious proscriptions against death except as God so willed, they were paradoxically in favor of temporizing with death through human intervention. The promise (or threat) of life beyond the grave, believed almost universally among the devout, is sometimes cited as a defense against the anxiety of nonbeing.

Thus, the subjects in this study neither universally welcome induced dying nor reject intercession on behalf of their death. If one considers that almost two-thirds of these subjects rejected positive or positive and negative euthanasia, they do not appear "adamant about avoiding pain and senility" (Cappon 1962).

Favoring euthanasia has been described as a "psychologically desirable attitude toward life and death" (Cappon). Marshalled as empirical evidence for this judgment is the fact that fear of death is greater among patients with psychiatric illnesses than among patients with physical illnesses or nonpatients, and psychiatric patients are least in favor of euthanasia. Perhaps more crucial in preferences for euthanasia is not whether but when this comes to be favored.

Clearly, neither the dying nor the aged should be considered homogeneous so far as death's significance or imminence. Kübler-Ross (1969) has described preparatory attitudes that are shown by dying patients, ranging from denial to gradual acceptance. For the dying, explicit or implicit requests to be allowed or helped to die may have vastly different implications at the beginning than toward the end of a fatal illness and after the work of mourning one's own death has been accomplished.

To the extent that the answers to the "here-and-now" questions in this study reflected significant aspects of the current quality of life among the subjects, this quality appears to have little relevance to their preferences in the timing of their deaths. Munnichs (1961) says that death attitudes "are closely connected with the intimate core of personality." An interesting area for exploring the etiology of such attitudes might be investigation into the extent to which favoring euthanasia is related to other indices of "integrity" in the older person but is not related to indices of "despair" (Erikson 1963).

Not all the dying want to know how or when they will die as Cappon (1962) found among his dying subjects, but "the majority want some control over the time and manner of their deaths." Whether this control takes the form of "life at any cost" or "death at any cost," the dying may well realize some dignity in having their wishes consulted and some comfort in the promise that these will be honored.

LEARNING TO BE MORTAL

The inspiration of the dying patients I have followed prompted the work that presently engages me. With the thought of Montaigne, "Whoever teaches people how to die, teaches them how to live," I have developed a behavior modification intervention, "Learning to Be Mortal." My assumption in offering this program is that confrontation with one's finiteness and transcience encourages scrutiny of one's past, present, and future quality of life. Further assumed is that such confrontation will foster greater awareness of the glorious gamut of feelings available to human beings—the joys, pains, elations, fears, angers, disappointments, despairs. The dying patients taught me to wonder: Do ablebodied people move through life in aimless, feckless ways because of the mindless conviction that their time on earth is boundless?

The Learning to Be Mortal program is project-oriented; the participants are mainly adults who are dissatisfied with their present adjustment and are seeking changes in themselves or their environments or both. To begin with and to clarify some of their attitudes about death, the participants complete a questionnaire designed to uncover attitudes toward and experiences with death and dying. Next, participants are exposed to an array of potential projects and are asked to commit themselves to one such project or another of their own invention. If a participant has been troubled by recurring thoughts of suicide or by the suicide of a loved one, for example, he or she may explore the range and variety of suicidal ideas with particular references to the poetry and prose of Sylvia Plath.

In another project, participants spend a day or week recording the choices available to them in their daily lives, beginning with the choice of time for getting up in the morning and ending with their decision to retire at night. Some participants choose the project of simulating deafness, blindness, lameness, or other infirmities to gain insight into the limited behavioral alternatives that sensory and motor limitations impose on those so afflicted. Visiting nursing homes and befriending patients with chronic or terminal illness is another project for deepening awareness of one's ablebodiedness. Or participants may elect to calculate the number of days, weeks, and years still remaining to be lived if their lives run according to the actuarial tables. Participants then project themselves to that day in the future, imagining the foregoing activities to be reflected on with pleasure or regret.

Some participants choose to read and discuss Kübler-Ross' *On Death and Dying* (1969), with particular attention to her assertion that violence in America serves as a defeat, however illusory, of one's own mortality: in the death of another one can triumph, "It is he, not I!" Other participants explore Rollo May's (1969) hypothesis that current preoccupation with sex in our society is a kind of defense against awareness of death, the ultimate in impotence. Death rituals, especially death-denying rituals as satirized in Aldous Huxley's *After Many a Summer Dies the Swan,* (1965), is the focus of another project. The thorny emotional and legal issues of euthanasia may be still another project.

In one of the last meetings, which occur weekly over a span of one or two months, participants formulate their own obituaries. They decide how they would like to be remembered by the living. One participant wrote:

> She was a warm, loving, accepting wife, mother, and friend.
> She gave of herself unhesitatingly to others.
> She was a thinking and thoughtful person who listened to others, considering deeply what they said.
> She loved people, being with them, enjoying life fully with them.
> She lived life to the fullest, despite adversity.
> When with her, other people found life more meaningful, exciting, fun, thought provoking.
> Specifically, she gave herself to others in these ways:_____, _____, _____.

This participant claimed that not only had she a glimpse of her capacity for joyful self-awareness through writing these words about herself, but she also began to formulate ways in which she could complete the blank spaces in her "obituary."

Finally, the discussion focuses on achieving transcendence through the participants' children, through the impact of their lives on others, through their work, and the relative permanence of their creations.

The ultimate purpose of the Learning to Be Mortal program is less to help people come to grips with the inevitability of their dyingness than to redefine their lives in light of their deaths. One can also envisage this approach as a means of embarking on a dialogue about the dying process with dying patients and achieving a kind of desensitization in such interactions for dying patients and those caring for them.

REFERENCES

CAPPON, D., Attitudes of and toward dying. *Canadian Medical Association Journal* 87:693-700, 1962.

CUMMING, E., and W. E. HENRY, *Growing Old.* New York: Basic Books, 1961.

ERIKSON, E.H., *Childhood and Society.* New York: W. W. Norton, 1963.

HUXLEY, A., *After Many A Summer Dies the Swan.* New York: Harper & Row, 1965.

KASTENBAUM, R., *New Thought On Old Age.* New York: Springer, 1964.

KÜBLER-ROSS, E., *On Death and Dying.* New York: Macmillan, 1969.

MAY, R., *Love and Will.* New York: W. W. Norton, 1969.

MUNNICHS, J. M. A., Comments: attitudes toward death in older persons: a symposium. *Journal of Gerontology* 16:44-66, 1961.

PRESTON, C. E., Subjectively perceived agedness and retirement. *Journal of Gerontology* 23:201-204, 1968.

PRESTON, C. E., and R. H. WILLIAMS, Views of the aged on the timing of death. *The Gerontologist* 2(4):300-304, 1971.

27

A Memo from M.L.

Maurice Levine

Only rarely do many of a group read a long memorandum, unless there is a special reason for doing so. So to make sure that you will at least begin to read this memo, I can start by saying that its topic is my recent illness and the fact that I was close to death. Knowing the topic, you probably will read a page or two, and perhaps then the rest of the memo.

This is the latest of the psychiatry department series called "Memos from M. L.," which over the past 20 years has consisted of occasional notes, comments, and free-wheeling discussions of current issues. The memos have functioned in the department as a cohesive force and as a technique of communication and mutual understanding.

This memo focuses on the fact that as an older member of the tribe, a grandfather-father-uncle figure, I am more likely than you are to have or to have had certain types of experience. At times I feel I have a responsibility to give you a chance to live through some of these experiences with me, if you care to do so. In my own development, this kind of vicarious experience had great meaning and value. (And it is good practice in empathy, which is one of the central patterns of our work.)

It might be an important piece of living for you to identify temporarily with me as I go through this period of serious sickness, to share some bits and pieces of this important human process. Of course, I know that often it is very difficult to listen to someone who is discussing a critical illness, of him- or herself or of another person, and the possibility of death. But in the setting of the special atmosphere and the essentially positive set of relations in this department, it may be possible. Again, however, I want to emphasize the fact that you have no obligation to read this memo. Some of you will simply put it aside.

To carry out my part of this deal, I must be able to talk without too much blocking about serious illness and the risk of death, in others or in myself. This is not easy to do. But I have had certain experiences that make it a bit easier.

I have seen death and dying many times, in those who were strangers, in those I had known for only a brief period, and in others I had known for a long time. Over the years I have been there at the moment of death with a number of patients, with several friends, with my father, with my mother, with a brother, and with a sister. And I have been with several members of my family and with a fair number of patients and others who were close to death but then recovered. Out of these experiences, I can think about death somewhat more easily than do many others.

The evidence is clear, from psychiatry and psychoanalysis, that it is valuable to feel and to think, and also to talk under certain conditions, about aspects of life that often are left unspoke. This is true not only about sex but also about anger and hate, about wishes to be child-like, about guilt and shame, about anxiety and about the excessive or the insufficient inhibitions that often are linked with anxiety, and about dying, the death of others or of oneself. But there is no compulsion about this. One can live a good life and one can die a good death without thinking or talking about death.

Most of you know by this time that my recent illnesses have been severe . . . these illnesses were indirectly the outgrowth of a recently discovered leukemia . . . an intensive treatment program has been started, aimed at the anemia and the danger of bleeding, and especially at the leukemia process itself.

To facilitate your putting yourself in fantasy momentarily in my shoes, it would help if I confessed some of my personal feelings and responses. During the sickness so far, I have had many intense emotions, of fear, of anxiety, of confusion, of disbelief, of fury, of irritability, of giving up, of feeling overwhelmed, of wanting sympathy and attention, of denial of illness, and of false hope, as well as a set of fairly good co-operative responses. In addition, I have had many other intense feelings, which also are human and perhaps inevitable, which are forgivable and forgettable since they don't really hurt others or oneself if they are not put into action. But such feelings and attitudes are of limited value.

In addition, I have been doing a great deal of thinking about some of the fantasies and myths and human patterns that may be even more productive than the kind of simple and direct reactions I just confessed. For example, we have just enjoyed the first week of spring. This time of the year seems to have had extraordinarily important meanings, realistic and symbolic, for the human being, primitive and civilized, over a long period of time. Each year in spring the apparently dead vegetation of the past year begins to grow again. What seemed dead, or close to death, seems to come alive again.

I suppose that in spring, for primitive man, the world must have seemed a warmer, safer, more secure, more promising place to be. The world must have seemed less dangerous in many ways, with the promise of food and warmth, of growing strength.

My fantasy about this, which differs slightly from the one usually given about the experience of spring in primitive man, is that in spring it may have seemed as if a new generation of plant life had begun to appear. Perhaps a new generation of animals then seemed to be possible, to be on the way. The world must have seemed vital and fertile again.

Out of this, and out of other facts and fantasies of early and of later man, there may have been stimulated the hope for, or the illusion of, personal immortality, the hope that one would not die as an individual, or that in a sense one would live on through the coming generations. And for very many, of course, the evidence indicates that spring was the period in which it was believed that the deity or the deities were revived, were alive again, benign and responsive.

In the life of a contemporary, skeptical, self-critical, individual human being, there is room for a large variety of important "as-if" feelings, of symbolic responses that can be used as leads to better understanding. One can be confident enough about the strength and the validity of the realistic, scientific approach to stop being afraid of the symbolic, aesthetic, empathic moments of life. In fact, such patterns can add depth and breadth to one's realistic perceptions and responses. At times a symbolic response can lead to the resolution of blocked intellectual problems, for example, Kekule's use of his snake circle daydream, in the carbon ring discovery, basic to organic chemistry.

I feel alive, active, and revived, these first weeks of spring. Such feelings conceivably in part are an as-if component of a symbolic process, a primary process response, a set of momentary illusions of immortality or of resurrection.

But my feelings of being alive and vital are related not only to the time of the year and its symbolism, and not only to momentary illusions. I have good realistic reasons for feeling revived and active. The winter of my pneumonia and pulmonary edema is gone. The temporary heart failure and the delirium are over. I was close to death for many days, but today I am feeling alive and cantankerous again. I feel expansive and creative.

Inevitably but pleasurably, I've begun to concoct jokes again. I recall that about two weeks ago, several careful hospital people were checking the name tag on my wrist against the labels on the packages of blood platelets that were about to be injected into my vein to prevent dangerous bleeding, which can be one aspect of leukemia. The first voice read the label on the package of platelets, read the date on which the blood had been drawn from the donor and the date it was delivered to my room, or some other important date. Then the second voice, I thought, read my name and the number of my Holmes Hospital room. Then one of the voices read, "Expiration Date, March 17, 1971." How dare they, I thought! I had given them the right to decide when I could move my arm, when I should open or close my mouth. Now they even had assumed the right to set my expiration date, and with damn little notice in advance!

All the time, of course, in a parallel process of perception, I knew that it was the voice of the other person reading the expiration date of this batch of platelets, the date beyond which there would be doubt of its freshness and safety.

So I was close to death for a time, close to a permanent winter. But I am alive. Spring is here. And I know that symbolic responses are highly meaningful. But for me, the most important component of my feeling is the depth of my respect for science and medicine. The fact that I am alive is a vivid example of medical and other research proving its scientific and practical value again; for example, the research on the transfusion of components of blood, on the life history of each type of cell in the blood, on the avoidance of hepatitis, on the process of blood clotting, on the mechanisms and treatment of heart failure. Also, it is an example again of medical and related education producing a group of professionals and paraprofessionals who in their jobs have a very high batting average of great competence and skill. And I must emphasize the fact that in this medical center, an anonymous, perhaps penniless, man or woman of my age, of any ethnic or cultural group, who had been brought to the General Hospital across the street by the "Life Squad," would be given essentially the same service, the same application of medical research and training as I am receiving. Despite these great achievements, much more is to be done, in research, in education, and in providing better service, and for more people. . . .

Spring has come for me. But, based on the leukemia or on "complications," the winter of the threat of death may return in a week or a month or a year. The actuality of death may be with me in a month or a year, in five or 10 years. At the moment, my feeling, perhaps my logic, tells me it will be a fair number of years.

At this moment, no longer winter but spring, I have a strong impulse to do things, one of which is to try to win some games of table tennis again. And when we play, anyone who won't try his best to beat me, because I am older, or because I have leukemia, or because he "may be the cause of my death," should not play with me. Until I say I don't, I want the games to be competitive.

But also, if I am feeling tired, we will postpone the game or merely hit the ball around, practicing some strokes. That's an honest kind of fun, too. Whoever talks of half-a-loaf of bread when one is hungry never has enjoyed the fun of a table tennis to-and-fro badinage when a competitive game can't be played for one reason or another. I hope to be active this spring in more serious ways. I want to do things for the medical center, for the psychiatry group, for the university, for my family and others, and for myself. . . .

The drive toward activity as an expression of being alive will have to be limited for several months, I am sure. Further work on the book I have been writing these past two years may be the most suitable form of active creative living for the immediate future. I want the book to be understandable and effective. . . .

Part of my feeling of spring and of increased well-being is related to the depth of friendship you have shown during the past few weeks. I want to thank wholeheartedly all those who sent their good wishes or expressed them in other ways. . . . If my estimate is correct, I have the blood of almost 100 of you in me. It's good to feel well enough to express my profound gratitude for that alone.

. . . I am home at the moment and feeling rather well, but I live on a rather narrow fairway, with the rough of a heavy fatigue on one side and the rough of a variety of minor symptoms on the other side. Apparently when there is this level of anemia, talking and listening are especially fatiguing. So I'm afraid I won't feel well enough for some time to have visitors, or to respond as I'd like in other ways. And I'll probably go into the hospital, for a day or two each time, to have platelets or red blood cells from your bloodstreams injected into my veins. Can one ever really thank others adequately for such a gift?

If this or other antileukemia medication works, or is somewhat effective, the hope is for the first of a series of remissions that could keep me in good shape for months or years. If that happens, there is a chance that in a month or two I can resume my seminars, and so forth.

Finally, my special thanks to those of you who are sharing directly or indirectly in doing the work I can't do. The spirit and the carry through, of your response to this situation has been one of the finest experiences that a man or a woman could have.

Hope to see you soon.

Cordially,

MAURICE LEVINE

Professor and Director
Department of Psychiatry
University of Cincinnati

VIII

STYLES OF DYING

In the final two chapters of this book I shall summarize my point of view in regard to the care of the dying. As I have read and reread the literature, reviewed my own personal experience, and studied the case studies in this book in detail, I am convinced that we must avoid a stereotyped approach to the care of the dying.

The process of dying certainly has universal concerns—as does all of life. We do well to identify the common problems of dying. Yet within this commonality comes the individual, the personal, the unique.

These final chapters will be focused on general principles, for they serve as the springboard to approach the care of the dying. Yet I wish to caution that the care of the dying occurs within the context of caring for the dying.

28

The Dying Experience—
Retrospective Analyses

E. Mansell Pattison

In this first section of this book, we examined general conclusions about the process of dying, based upon published clinical and research reports. This has given us an overall view of dying.

In the clinical report chapters, we have been given specific details about the dying process as it appears in rather specific situations. We have seen how the overall process of dying is modified by particular dying situations.

Now I plan to present my analysis of some specific issues that have been unclear in our understanding of dying. I invite the reader to make his or her own analysis in comparison with my tentative conclusions. I initially asked each author to address these issues in the presentation of their own experiences. Then I examined each of the clinical reports in this book as a piece of data, to see where the report contained evidence on each issue. Thus, the following conclusions are based on my retrospective analysis of the clinical material, also available to the reader.

STAGES OR PHASES OF DYING?

In her landmark book, *On Death and Dying*, Elizabeth Kübler-Ross (1970) organized her observations on the dying process around a series of stages. That is, she felt that dying persons typically go through a specific series of psychological reactions in response to their dying. Her series began with initial shock and numbness, followed by denial and isolation, anger, bargaining, and finally depression. If the person successfully moved through these stages, he or she would end up in a state of acceptance and would live in hope.

Now, it should be noted that Kübler-Ross did not present these stages of dying as an ineluctable process. A careful reading of her book will reveal that she gives many illustrations where these stages were not followed. Nevertheless, many people quickly concretized her clinical sequence into hard fact. And soon there were many references in the literature to the stages of dying, as if this sequence were really so for most dying persons.

Other consequences soon followed. Dying persons who did not follow these stages were labeled "deviant," "neurotic," or "pathological dyers." Clinical personnel became angry at patients who did not move from one stage to the next. I have often had professional people ask me what was wrong with one of their dying patients who was "stuck" in one stage and who could not be moved on to the next. In the "professionalization" of dying, I began to observe professional personnel demand that the dying persons "die in the right way"! It was no longer acceptable to respond to the dying person in terms of individual dying experience. Rather, the dying were being pushed and forced into a procrustean process of dying that had been scientifically established. From my own personal contacts with Dr. Kübler-Ross, I believe she would be dismayed at the manner in which her stages of dying have been misused to force artificial patterns of dying upon the dying person.

As this phenomenon of "staging dying" spread, there have been reactions by both lay people and professionals who believe that the concept of stages is not only inaccurate but misleading to both the dying person and to his or her helpers. For example, in her autobiology of her dying experience, Joanne Smith (1975) reports that she became bewildered and began to doubt her own sanity when her self-observations revealed that she did not follow the stages of dying. She finally concluded: "The stages of dying are not necessarily chronological. In my own experience I have moved back and forth through several of these a number of times."

In recent years the method of "psychological autopsy" has been widely presented (Weisman, Kastenbaum 1968). Quite simply, this is a retrospective analysis of all the observations made of a dying process. The autopsy team then attempts to reconstruct the psychological process of dying and determines from the case study where more appropriate interventions could have been made. Avery D. Weisman, the pioneer thanatologist (one who studies the death process) in this method, devotes a full chapter in his most recent book, *The Realization of Death* (1974) to such an autopsy examination of stages.

In brief, Weisman finds no clinical justification for the concept of stages. Rather, he suggests that there is a continual intermingling of emotional responses that go on throughout the dying process. Weisman comments:

> Look how difficult it is to isolate a single characteristic, denial, depression, anger, and so forth, and make pronouncements about the process . . . the idea of staging psychosocial episodes is very artificial . . . patients cope and fail to cope with various problems, and their emotional responses are simply indicators of personal conflict and crises . . . the concept of psychosocial staging appeals to me, because patients are apt to have social and emotional problems anyway . . . it would be very orderly if psychosocial issues is followed as neatly as anatomical and clinical staging seem to do . . . but there no well-recognized succession of emotional responses that are typical of people facing incipient death.

There also have been careful reviews of the published scientific literature that examine the concept of stages. Here again no support is found for the concept. Shibles (1974) concludes his evaluation of stages thus: "The stages are too procrustean, narrow and fixed, even though they overlap, to adequately account for thoughts, images, perceptual, and motor abilities which a person has regarding dying." In another review, Schulz and Aderman (1974) also conclude: ". . . the findings again cast doubt on the validity of a stage theory. Patients were not observed to go through stages but rather to adopt a pattern of behavior which persisted until death occurred."

Turning now to a review of the clinical reports in this book, I have followed the course of dying described in each chapter. I find *no* evidence therein to support specific stages of dying. Rather, dying persons demonstrate a wide variety of emotions, which ebb and flow throughout their living-dying, just as our emotions ebb and flow throughout our entire lives as we face conflicts and crisis. It does seem misleading then to search for and determine stages of dying. Rather, I suggest that our task is to determine the stress and crises at a specific time, to respond to the emotions generated by that issue, and in essence *respond to where the patient is at* in his or her living-dying. We do not make the patient conform to our idealized concept of dying but respond to the person's actual dying experience.

However, rather than *stages*, Weisman (1974) does suggest that there may be *phases* of dying. I concur with this way of looking at living-dying. In Chapter 4, I proposed three phases: the acute phase, the chronic living-dying phase, and the terminal phase. I shall not repeat that analysis here, but I do caution that the phases are only a convenient way of dividing the living-dying process into three dimensions that have some clinical utility. However, in acute fulminating disease that progresses rapidly to death, we have only an acute phase of dying; in cases of sudden unexpected death after long illness there will be no terminal phase. So again we are dealing with an individual life process, in which we cautiously divide living-dying into phases as an aid to our own understanding—realizing that this is a somewhat artificial division.

DYING TRAJECTORIES

Glaser and Straus (1966, 1968, 1970) have published a series of books that defined several different dying trajectories, or "death expectations": 1) certain death at a known time; 2) certain death at an unknown time; 3) uncertain death but a known time when the question will be resolved; and 4) uncertain death and an unknown time when the question will be resolved. Unfortunately, little specific attention has been given to these trajectories since. Hence, as the reader has no doubt noted, I selected a variety of clinical reports to illustrate each type of dying trajectory. Now let us examine some conclusions about dying trajectories.

First, *certain* trajectories are easier to cope with than *uncertain* trajectories. Ambiguity is always difficult to manage in life. Anxiety is generated by ambiguity and uncertainty. On the other hand, although the certainty of death may not be good news, one can plan for the specific fact of death at a known time. Thus Trajectory 1 provides the dying person and the people around him or her with a relatively specific time frame in which to order their responses. As I have noted in several places, the time of most acute anxiety for the dying person is in the initial acute phase of dying when the uncertainty of events is highest. As the person approaches the increased certainty of exact time of death, anxiety diminishes.

Trajectory 3 is somewhat similar. Here there may be prolonged anxiety in an acute phase of uncertainty—waiting for the pathology report after surgery, waiting to see if the organ transplant will work, waiting to see if the severely injured person will survive, waiting to see if the malformed infant will survive. In all of these instances, the dying trajectory is suspended in space, for no actions can be taken while the expectation is in doubt. Here the person and/or the family and staff may entertain high hopes and a positive expectation. It is understandable, then, that here there may be sudden disappointment and frustrated anger when the hopeful expectation is suddenly dashed by the fact that the person does have a fatal diagnosis, or the illness does not respond to treatment, or the patient suddenly deteriorates and dies. Consequently, this trajectory is likely fraught with intense emotion for all involved. For example, in Chapter 10 on the burned child and in Chapter 21 on the Intensive Care Unit, the families and staff tolerated the expectable deaths but would experience a high degree of distress when someone expected to live suddenly died.

Trajectory 2, where there is an uncertain time of death, is most characteristic of chronic fatal illness. Here there is certainty of death, but the living-dying interval may stretch out over several years. There are a number of chapters that illustrate this process. It is clear that here we have prolonged emotional stress for the dying person and for the family. They live with dying. To follow the principle of certainty, the lesson here seems to be the importance of *focusing on what is certain*. Since the exact time of death cannot be reasonably predicted, it is important to shift the focus to predictable daily issues of life. Thus, the dying person and the family can turn to specific issues and deal with life on a predictable day-to-day basis. Whereas in the acute trajectories one is faced with the imminent expectation of death, in this chronic trajectory it is important to shift the focus from death per se to the issues of living while dying.

Trajectory 4 appears to be the most problematic, for death itself is an uncertainty, and it is ambiguous as to when the issue will be resolved. On the one hand, this overall uncertainty seems to breed a high degree of anxiety that cannot be resolved, leading to dysfunctional defenses and hypochondriacal fixation on one's physical state. Chapter 18 on multiple sclerosis, Chapter 19 on traumatic disability, and Chapter 24 on hemodialysis highlight the pathological emotional reactions that this type of trajectory produces.

On the other hand, where medical technology has produced means of management of uncertain illnesses, it would appear that at least younger patients are able to make a successful adaptation. In fact, they may perceive a "reprieve from death" in their chronic stable condition. This is illustrated in Chapter 12 on hemophilia and in Chapter 15 on cardiac pacemakers.

Overall, this sample of dying trajectories does suggest that the different trajectories require different coping mechanisms; they vary in their evocation of anxiety and stress; and they pose different clinical management problems. However, even with the relatively specific data presented in this book, we still have scanty evidence for the relevance of dying trajectories for the dying process. It is my hope that this work will stimulate further detailed study of dying trajectories.

DENIAL AND ACCEPTANCE OF DEATH

One of the persistent themes in the thanatology literature has been that denial of death is pathogenic, whereas acceptance of death is desirable. Unfortunately, this is often posed as a black-or-white, either-or phenomenon. Either we deny death or we accept it. In the introductory chapters, I presented evidence that denial is a multilayered human process. When we say denial, we actually refer to various levels of human awareness of death. Likewise, acceptance may refer to our existential acceptance, or psychological acceptance, or our behavioral evidence of acceptance.

As I have examined the clinical chapters in this book, I find that we cannot readily separate denial and acceptance. There are levels of denial and levels of acceptance. A beautiful example is presented in Chapter 23, where a psychiatrist presents his own experience with his dying wife. Both of them verbally denied the immediacy of her death; yet at a behavioral level both accepted it and communicated with each other in a very appropriate fashion. Here are verbal denial and behavioral acceptance! Another example is in Chapter 27, where the eminent psychoanalyst Dr. Levine poignantly writes to his staff of his hope and expectation to finish his new book and at the same time tells them that he is too sick to accept visitors. Is this denial or acceptance? I think it is both.

Dumont and Foss (1972) have devoted a whole book to the issue of denial-acceptance, in which they examine the evidence at a cultural, social, and personal level. They find the evidence contradictory; there is both denial and acceptance present at the same time. At the center of this contradiction in evidence is the fact that *reason and emotion conflict*. They state: "On a conscious, intellectual level the individual accepts his death, while on a generally unconscious, emotional plane he denies it."

From this discussion I would draw the following conclusions: First, there are varying degrees of denial and acceptance of death within each individual that vary over the living-dying interval. Second, there are always contradictions between the conscious-rational and unconscious-emotional aspects of both denial and acceptance. Third, our task as helpers is not to eliminate denial and attain absolute acceptance. Third, our task as helpers is not to eliminate denial and attain absolute acceptance with the dying. Rather, we face the more human task of responding to a flowing process of both denial and acceptance in ourselves and the dying.

EGO-COPING VERSUS DEFENSE MECHANISMS

Central to our understanding of psychological processes is what we term ego function. The concept of ego is derived from the psychoanalytic observations of Freud, but the term has passed into common usage and has lost its specificity. In psychodynamic terms, when we speak of ego, we do not refer to a "thing" in the mind, but rather a set of mental operations that are conveniently summarized in the term "ego." This "ego set" contains several functions: the sense of self, the center of personal identity, the experiencing self that receives input from different parts of the human organism, the seat of thinking and decision-making. In brief, we may conceive of the ego as the control center of the self—interposited between the unconscious drives, images, fantasies, and impulses, and the external world of reality.

Freud observed that when the ego had problems resolving conflicts between the internal unconscious self and the external world of reality, a variety of "ego defenses" gave rise to neurotic symptoms. Hence, it seemed that ego defenses were pathological.

However, not all ego defenses are equally pathological. Some defenses are used frequently by all of us—for example, rationalization and conscious suppression. On the other hand, some ego defenses are relatively unusual and represent gross distortions of reality—for example, delusions and hallucinations. Thus, we must consider a hierarchy of ego defenses in terms of their utility, the degree to which they distort reality, and the degree to which they comprise the total psychological function of the ego.

The development of ego defenses is part of psychological development. Thus, the young infant probably hallucinates. The toddler and preschool child use delusional thinking and projection. The older child begins to discard these gross mechanisms and adds passive-aggressive behavior, acting-out mechanisms, and fantasy. The adolescent moves on to acquire the use of altruism, humor, suppression, and avoidance. Thus, we cannot look at the use of defense mechanisms without also taking into account the developmental stage of life of the person.

Further, the concept of "defense" mechanisms has long had a negative connotation, as if it is bad to have or use them. In fact, we must be able to protect and defend ourselves psychologically. Thus, it is more appropriate to use the term "coping" mechanisms. Vaillant (1971) has pointed out in a careful study of adaptive ego mechanisms that all people use a variety of coping mechanisms throughout their lives. Thus, normal, psychologically healthy, and well-adapted people occasionally use immature ego-coping mechanisms. Under stress, all of us will likely resort to some use of immature coping mechanisms. The issue is *not* that we all use ego-coping mechanisms, but rather whether the coping mechanisms we use are adaptive in the context in which we find ourselves.

I have spent a bit of time here reviewing the meaning of ego-coping mechanisms, because these concepts have been much abused in the literature on dying. It is simple to observe classical "neurotic defense" mechanisms in dying patients. We can see denial, anger, depresson, acting out, bargaining, ritualization, obsessiveness, hypochondriasis, rationalization, intellectualization, projection, fantasy, withdrawal, avoidance, and so on. The temptation is to say: "Aha, see how neurotic dying people are . . . look what pathological coping mechanisms they are using!" We go on to conclude: "Now we need to treat these psychologically neurotic dying people so that they will give up all these defenses and can proceed to die in a nonneurotic manner."

But the above attitude is an overintepretation of psychopathology. As I have stated above, we all use ego coping mechanisms that can be labeled immature or neurotic. Usually we don't use them all the time nor in a fixed pattern. None of us is so perfectly developed psychologically that we can cope with the stress and conflict of life in a perfectly adaptive manner! In fact, I have no idea of what kind of person that would be. But I do understand that we are frail mortals who have various degress of ability to cope with life in a reasonable fashion. Sometimes our ego-coping styles get out of hand, and then it is helpful to switch back to more adaptive ego-coping styles. Most of this "therapeutic" change in our ego-coping styles does not occur in psychotherapy, but rather occurs as the result of discipline, counsel, advice from our friends, confrontations with our loved ones, learning from experience, and other corrective experiences in life.

When we turn to the dying and observe their ego-coping styles, why should we suddenly expect perfection in dying when there is no perfection in life? Nor should we need to label maladaptive coping styles as "neurosis," which needs to be eradicated through "treatment." I believe it would be preferable to respond to the dying as normal persons who may invoke a variety of ego-coping mechanisms. Hopefully, where necessary and possible we may guide the dying in paths of rewarding styles of coping with dying.

In line with the preceding point of view, I have examined the clinical reports of this book to search for the ego-coping styles used by dying persons, as well as the family and professional personnel. My observations follow.

First, I am struck by the fact that *all* people involved with dying experience high degrees of stress, from which none are immune. It is obvious in many chapters that the nurses, doctors, social workers, psychologists, and psychiatrists all sustain emotional assaults on their ego functioning as they work with dying patients. Nor do they respond with aplomb and equanimity. Well-seasoned mental health professionals experience anguish, pain, despair, anger, fear. These normal professionals use projection, denial, passive-aggressiveness, acting out, and so on. So the pathologies, if such, are not the sole province of the dying; they are part of us all.

Second, I am impressed by the fact that during the acute crisis stage of dying, more primitive and immature coping mechanisms are commonly called upon. For example, in Chapter 23 we have the detailed personal account of a mature psychiatrist who was faced with acute and overwhelming crisis. He candidly observed how quickly he resorted to a variety of defensive mechanisms that in other circumstances we might call neurotic or defensive. Yet within the context of the acute phase of dying, I would conclude that his coping mechanisms were quite suited to the crisis. As I have stated earlier, acute crisis calls out the most primitive defenses in us. We cope the best we can with what we have. And we should neither be surprised nor dismayed to see such primitive coping styles fleetingly emerge during acute crisis. For the most part, as I read the data, the dying person and his or her family quickly discard these primitive responses and move on to more mature coping mechanisms. Our concern should be not for the moment, but whether the dying person is able to move on to more adaptive mechanisms after the acute crisis has passed.

Third, we must not forget that the living-dying interval is a time of repetitive stress. The dying person is also physically sick, and that drains one's psychic energy. While the healthy person may effectively use many coping mechanisms, the range becomes limited for the sick dying person. For example, because of physical disability, the dying person may not be able to engage in physical activities, such as recreation, or involvement in work, or even such simple coping mechanisms as conversation or reading. Hence, the dying experience limits the repertoire of coping mechanisms available to a person.

Fourth, I have asked these questions: what ego-coping mechanisms may we anticipate in each stage of the life cycle? Do all dying persons revert back to primitive, immature, or neurotic coping styles? Or is ego-coping style related to the life cycle in which the dying person lives?

In the previous section of this chapter, I indicated that the coping mechanism of "denial" is to some extent present in all of us all the time in regard to death. Further, there are degrees of denial at different levels of awareness that are constantly present in the dying person. Thus, it seems reasonable to conclude that denial is a relatively universal part of coping with dying. So I shall not include denial in my subsequent analysis.

To approach an understanding of ego coping, I reviewed each of the clinical chapters in the books for descriptions of ego-coping mechanisms used in each stage of the life cycle.

In Table 1, I have listed the major ego-coping mechanisms in a hierarchial sequence: primitive, immature, neurotic, mature. There follows in the table, the frequency of observed coping mechanisms used by the dying in each stage of the life cycle.

Again, I wish to caution that at any given cross-section of time, we may observe most of the ego-coping mechanisms being used in transient fashion. What we are trying to determine, however, are the more typical coping mechanisms that the dying person uses.

Several observations may be drawn from the data presented in Table 1.

First, there is a general trend for the dying to use the ego-coping mechanisms along a developmental sequence. That is, the youngest children only have the most primitive coping mechanisms available. As one grows older, in each stage of life the dying person will typically use more advanced ego-coping mechanisms and tend to rely less on earlier types of coping. So that when we come to the aged, they have moved to a general mode of rather mature coping mechanisms.

Second, there is an obvious overlap of most of the ego-coping mechanisms for most life stages, but it is also obvious that the dying do *not* just use primitive or immature coping mechanisms. In fact, it is striking that the dying exhibit the frequent use of many mature coping mechanisms.

Third, in *early childhood* we can observe the dying process evoke primitive coping, including delusional thought, perceptual distortions, and gross denial of reality. This is *no psychosis*. Rather it is the transient use of primitive coping that comes and goes. The use of primitive de-

Table 1 Typical Ego-Coping Mechanisms
of the Dying Throughout the Lif Cycle

Ego-Coping Mechanisms	Early Childhood	School Age Child	Adolescence	Young Adult	Middle Age	Aged
LEVEL 1. PRIMITIVE						
Delusions	+	+				
Perceptual Hallucination	+	+				
Depersonalization	+	+				
Reality Distorting Denial	+	+				
LEVEL 2. IMMATURE						
Projection	+ +	+ + +	+		+	
Denial through fantasy	+ +	+	+			
Hypochrondriasis		+ +	+ +	+ +	+ +	+ + +
Passive-aggressiveness		+ + +	+ +	+ + +	+ +	+ +
Acting-out Behavior		+ + +	+ +	+ + +	+ +	
LEVEL 3. NEUROTIC						
Intellectualization		+ + +	+	+ + +	+	
Displacement		+ +	+ +	+		
Reaction Formation		+ +	+ + +	+		
Emotional Dissociation		+ + +	+	+	+	
LEVEL 4. MATURE						
Altruism	§			§	§§	
Humor			+	+	+	+
Suppression			+ +	+ + +	+ + +	+
Anticipatory Thought			+ + +	+ + +	+ + +	+ + +
Sublimation			+	+	+ +	+ + +

　　+　 = occasional use
　+ +　 = moderate use
+ + +　 = frequent use

fenses appears to extend into the preschool years but does *not* typically appear thereafter.

Fourth, in the *school age child,* we see the emergent use of immature coping mechanisms. In particular, the child deals with the dying stress through externalization mechanisms. This is, of course, typical of how the school age child deals with stress and anxiety anyway.

Fifth, in the *adolescent*, we see the appearance of the use of intellectual coping styles as a dominant pattern, although immature mechanisms are not abandoned. Some mature mechanisms also come into play, especially those of an intellectual type.

Sixth, in the *young adult*, there appears a wider variety of coping mechanisms. It would seem that more immature mechanisms crop up in young adulthood. Adolescents appear to gain strength and coping ability from their parents and other adult figures, whereas the young adult may be making the transition to independence, and thus dying comes at a particularly vulnerable time that calls forth more immature mechanisms.

Seventh, in the *middle aged,* we observe the emergence of many mature mechanisms and less use of immature mechanisms as seen in the young adult.

Eighth, in *the aged,* although hypochondriasis is a feature, the presence of predominantly mature coping mechanisms is manifest.

Finally, I want to reiterate that we have summarized typical coping mechanisms during the living-dying interval. As noted before, the initial acute crisis phase is likely to be marked by transient maladaptive coping mechanisms. In the above analysis, I have been concerned with the chronic living-dying interval. Finally, when we come to the terminal phase of dying, we may expect the typical coping mechanisms to recede and be replaced by isolating mechanisms, withdrawal, and increasing detachment. I have suggested that this withdrawal may be misinterpreted as depression. No doubt there is some depression present; however, our task may not be to draw the person back into involvement with life, but rather to allow him or her to withdraw appropriately from life.

In summary, then, the dying do not employ just a few stock coping mechanisms. Like the rest of life, they use all the many coping mechanisms of the human ego. It seems that the dying use the coping mechanisms most typical of their stage of life. The more mature the life stage, the more likely the dying will use more mature ego-coping mechanisms. It does not appear that people deal with the process of dying much different from the way they have previously dealt with life. As people have typically coped throughout their lives, so will they continue in the same coping style in their dying.

REFERENCES

DUMONT, R.G., and D. C. FOSS, *The American View of Death: Acceptance or Denial?* Cambridge, Mass.: Schenkman, 1972.

GLASER, B. G. and A. L. STRAUS, *Awareness of Dying.* Chicago: Aldine, 1966.
_____, *Time for Dying.* Chicago: Aldine, 1968.

KÜBLER-ROSS, E., *On Death and Dying.* New York: Macmillan, 1970.

SCHULZ, R., and D. ADERMAN, Clinical research and the stages of dying. *Omega* 5:137-143, 1974.

SHIBLES, W., *Death: An Interdisciplinary Analysis.* Whitewater, Wis.: Language Press, 1974.

SMITH, J., *Free Fall.* Valley Forge, Pa: Judson Press, 1975.

STRAUS, A. L., and B. G. GLASER, *Anguish: A Case History of a Dying Trajectory.* Mill Valley, Ca.: The Sociology Press, 1970.

VAILLANT, G. E., Theoretical hierarchy of adaptive ego mechanisms. *Archives of General Psychiatry.* 24:107-118, 1971.

WEISMAN, A. D., *The Realization of Death.* New York/Aronson, 1974.

WEISMAN, A. D., and R. KASTENBAUM, The Psychological Autopsy. *Community Mental Health Journal Monograph, No. 4.* 1968.

29

Helping with Dying

E. Mansell Pattison

"To cure rarely, relieve sometimes, and comfort always."

In this final chapter, I plan to present some specific recommendations for helping with dying. In the first chapter, we looked at the cultural milieu that has shaped our attitudes. How we help is rooted in our attitudes. Since my proposals are grounded in my own attitude, I want to begin with my own attitudinal view.

First, I do not view dying as a pathological problem that should be "treated" (Engel 1961). Thus, I do not want to present a set of "treatment plans" for the dying. Rather, I view dying as a piece of normal living. So it would be more accurate to consider how we "respond to," "relate to," or "interact" with the dying (Beaty 1970). Let us examine how we may appropriately behave in our personal and professional encounters with the dying in a manner consonant with human dignity.

Second, I view the concept of helping as a normal everyday response of human relationship, not something special. All of us maintain a relative stability in life because of the helping interaction with the people in our social matrix of life. The once popular song by the Beatles says it: "I get along with a little help from my friends." Helping, to my mind, is the corrective, supportive, inquisitive, challenging, accepting give and take that comprises our valued relationships with others.

Third, helping is not so much doing as being. In our anxiety to accomplish something, to do something about dying, to feel we are valuable, whatever, I find a zealousness to do things. But this may be for our own benefit, not for the dying. To comfort is to share. To share is the willingness to be, without having to do.

Fourth, I see helping with dying as the opposite of most helping. Usually we help people to move toward fuller engagement of life. With dying, we help people to disengage from life.

HELPING OURSELVES

Death is ultimately personal. To respond to the fears and human condition of the dying person will always involve responding to ourselves. We face a continuing tension within ourselves: to be in touch with the meanings of death to ourself so as to be empathically sensitive—and yet able to maintain our psychic composure and objectivity so that we can respond to the dying person as he or she is in his or her life. As Pogo once said: "We have sought the enemy and found him, and he is us."

So to help with dying, we must first face death for ourselves. Then, hopefully, we may avoid fearful rejection of the dying person, and also avoid the counterphobic mechanism of fusion and identification with the dying. We may then assume a posture of *detached compassion*.

Our own attitudes toward the dying are a panoply of positives and negatives. So too for the dying person, for family, relatives, and friends, and all staff. It is unrealistic only to expect positive attitudes in ourselves or in others. Sometimes we will be angered and frustrated by the dying. The situation of dying does not suddenly make people nice! Dying people run the gamut of all types of human beings, some likeable, some not. Some people are easy to relate to, others not. Some dying persons we will feel like helping, others not. Some people who die will cause us sorrow, others who die will provide a sense of relief, or maybe even vindicative feelings of satisfaction! It is our task to identify and assimilate all these feelings in ourselves and others; to establish a pattern of nondenial of all such feelings; to recognize that the range of emotions is part of the human experience. To integrate both positive and negative feelings. And, finally, not to act upon raw emotion, but to filter our feelings through our conscious selves, and act in accord with responsible integrity to ourselves and the dying.

Another aspect of self-helping is to recognize the phenomenon of *death saturation*. That is, we can only work with dying persons for so long, and with so much personal investment, and with so much intensity, before we have reached the limits of our personal tolerance. Helping the dying is a personally demanding task. We each have limits to our intimate exposure to dying. We must be able to identify our personal limits of saturation. Then we need to back off, to gain distance, relief, reconstitution of ourselves. We readily recognize that our bodies need sleep to be fit to face the next day. Yet we less readily acknowledge that our human spirits get exhausted too. It is unrealistic to demand of ourselves the ability to face dying all the time on an intense basis and expect to survive psychically. If we do not build into our work and life schedule appropriate spaces for reprieve and reconstitution, our psychic defenses will do it for us—but not in desirable ways, for then we see the emergence of denial, callousness, emotional withdrawal, disinterest, and such, which may be manifestations of psychic exhaustion.

Finally, we need to establish and maintain an ethical attitude that places our professional responsibility in perspective (Krant 1974). We c nnot be perfect. We can and will make mistakes. But we do need to try to do a decent job to the best of our ability. Maurice Levine (1948) sums up an ethical stance I find most germane: 1) to avoid hostile reactions that harm the patient; 2) to avoid self-aggrandizement that may lead to operations or treatments for which one is not prepared; 3) to avoid sexually distorted attitudes that lead to possible sexually evoked rejection or seduction of the patient; 4) to avoid revealing the confidences of patients for the sake of gossip or to appear important in the eyes of one's spouse, friends, or colleagues; 5) to avoid excessive therapeutic ambition that leads to unnecessary procedures; and 6) to avoid unnecessary stimulation of anxiety in the patient.

HELPING THE DYING PERSON

In working with the dying person, I do not propose some ideal pattern for dying, yet there are some general principles. The first is to achieve an integration of dying into the person's life-style. Weisman (1974) describes this as an "appropriate death." The concept of an appropriate death is a style of dying that is adaptive to the specific person. We seek to assist the dying person to view his or her own death and live out his or her dying in a manner consonant with his or her own pattern of coping mechanisms, definition of the meaning of death, and life context. Thus, the criteria for an appropriate death will be fulfilled in different ways for different people. Each person's appropriate death is different, but is appropriate for him or her.

Following Weisman, I propose the following criteria of an appropriate death:

1. The person is able to face and resolve the initial crisis of acute anxiety without disintegration.
2. The person is able to reconcile the reality of his or her life as it is to his or her ego ideal image of life as he or she wanted it to be.
3. The person is able to preserve or restore the continuity of important relationships during the living-dying interval and gradually achieve separation from loved ones as death approaches.
4. The person is able to experience reasonably the emergence of basic instincts, wishes, and fantasies that lead without undue conflict to gradual withdrawal and the final acceptance of death.

A second principle involves the maintenance of *phase appropriate* responses. Throughout this book, I have called attention to the different emotional issues and reality factors that face the dying person in each of the three phases of dying. Each phase calls for a different style of response from us. In the initial acute crisis phase, we are faced with the issue of acute anxiety and perhaps high ambiguity (Levinson 1972). In the chronic living-dying phase, we are faced with the resolution of reality issues of the interpersonal relationships of the dying and means of coping with problems in daily living. In the terminal phase, we are faced with support for achieving separation and withdrawal.

A third principle involves the terminal phase, which is to achieve relative *synchrony*, so that the social, psychological, and physiological dimensions of death tend to merge together in a coherent fashion. This means that we must attempt to maintain social and psychological attitudes that are consistent with the physiological state of the dying person.

Now let us consider some specific aspects of help with the dying in terms of the types of fears, listed in Chapter 4, which the dying face.

FEAR OF THE UNKNOWN. As suggested, this fear is most manifest in the initial acute crisis phase. It is important to establish a relationship of confidence and trust in which the dying person can ask questions and receive reliable answers. It is important to provide specific answers when possible; to state when specific questions will be answered if that is possible; and to state what questions cannot be answered except through the process of time. Finally, it is helpful to distinguish between questions about the reality issues of life, for which real people can give real response, versus philosophical, religious, and speculative questions about which we may offer opinions but cannot give answers. This, then, helps the dying person to distinguish between real known aspects of dying, for which he or she can obtain some known answers, versus the unknowness of death, which cannot be known.

FEAR OF LONELINESS.   The problem here differs with each phase of dying. In the initial acute phase, the fear of rejection or being deserted may be more phantasy than reality. In this phase, it may be useful to be both present on a frequent basis and to determine carefully who will be with the dying person at what times. During the chronic phase, it is useful not to allow the dying process to become the sole focus of the person's life. Rather, the task is to maintain the engagement of the dying person with everyday relations and everyday tasks. In the terminal phase, it is useful to assure the dying person of the continuing interest and availability of people—to the extent that the dying person needs and desires. Thus, the dying person need not fear loneliness, although he or she may at times be alone.

FEAR OF SORROW.   Here the task is to provide an atmosphere that conveys the message that grief is not out of place. But grief has limits. If we can accept the experience of grief and sorrow in ourselves and share in sorrow with the dying, it then becomes possible to draw that grieving to a conclusion. We have shared the sorrow, expressed the grief, and completed that small task of mourning. This is the function of *anticipatory grief* (Rosner 1962). It allows us all to identify the source of sorrow and work through that emotion. Otherwise, the dying person and others are likely to accumulate a storehouse of small griefs, which become an intolerable load. It is useful to help the dying person to identify the particular griefs of the dying proess and deal with each one on its own terms, rather than attempting to cope with all the griefs at once. Finally, it is useful to distinguish between the sorrow over one's death versus the particular sorrows of specific events or persons.

FEAR OF LOSS OF FAMILY AND FRIENDS.   Often the process of dying reawakens the latent dimensions of interpersonal relations. Submerged feelings of both love and hate may be evoked in the dying person's network of social relations. Here the task may be to help the dying and their family and friends to accept the variety of emotions that flow between them. To clarify ambiguous and conflicting emotions and to achieve some acceptable resolution of the emotional tensions that arise. In this way it may be possible for the dying to reaffirm the basic meaning and values of his or her personal relationships. It is when this resolution occurs—when some peace has been achieved—that the dying may then begin to separate from their loved ones, work through that grieving experience, and no longer fear the loss of relationship even though there is now separation as death approaches.

FEAR OF LOSS OF BODY.   The first task is to keep the dying accurately informed as to their bodily processes. They need to know what is wrong and why it is wrong. This removes the mystery of ambiguous bodily process. The dying need to be assured that loss of body functions or abilities is not shameful. We need to provide assistance with bodily functions only to the extent that the dying person cannot. Thus, we preserve both a respect for the body as it is, and preserve body control and body function to the extent possible. It is important, again, to distinguish between body functions that are healthy versus the sickly parts. It is important to distinguish between *real* physical *ability* that is present versus their physical *disability*. That is, we keep a good sense of body reality in the forefront. It is neither useful to ignore body dysfunction nor to overemphasize body dysfunction.

FEAR OF LOSS OF SELF-CONTROL.   We might consider control here at several levels—control of one's life, control of one's self, control of one's body. These dimensions can get interlocked, and then confusion abounds. Control over one's life may include fear of being unable to determine life or death. That is a general attitude that needs to be resolved in the beginning of the dying process. However, the dying can make specific decisions about their lives, such as wills, property, family matters, funeral, burial, and other matters about how they shall live through their living-dying. This enables the dying to determine, to the extent possible, the direction of their living-dying lives. Similarly, the dying can be encouraged and supported to determine their own emotional and psychological styles of living-dying. And, finally, we can continue to provide the dying the opportunity to exercise physical management of their bodies, to the extent possible. So although the dying must ultimately relinquish self-control, it remains a gradual process.

FEAR OF SUFFERING AND PAIN.   As noted earlier, suffering revolves around both loneliness and the unknown. Here as before, it is useful to assist the dying in the maintenance of life engagement. When the dying person has nothing to do except live in painful isolation, pain is likely to be suffering. Whereas the dying person who continues to be involved with life and persons can live with pain. Similarly, pain that is mysterious, that has no source or explanation, is likely to be insufferable. Hence, the source of pain, the extent and duration of pain, need to be explained as reasonably as possible. It is not my purpose here to discuss the technical medical aspects of pain management. I certainly do not suggest that some stoical acceptance of all pain is either possible or desirable. I would strongly endorse the human value of using pain-relieving medications where appropriate. Only people who have never experienced severe physical pain would oppose the use of pain-reducing medications. But the opposite radical solution that pills or shots will solve the problem of pain is also unrealistic. Suffering is a human problem, which includes physical pain. Thus, our response must include both human interest and involvement, the provision of knowledge, and the personal participation of the dying person in his or her own pain management. Then it is possible to alleviate suffering and collaboratively work on the management of pain, which often cannot be eliminated but can be tolerated.

FEAR OF LOSS OF IDENTITY.   The loss of identity occurs when people do not relate to us as a specific and unique person. We are affirmed in who we are by others. It is important to continue to maintain the specific identity of the dying person. This can be accomplished through continuing personal contact with family and friends, who relate to the dying person *as a living person.* Hospital and medical staff can be careful to retain a personal view of the patient, who is not just a disease. The dying person can be allowed to retain personal clothes, mementoes, and intimate items that reduce the sterility of medical settings. Diffusion and loss of identity is closely tied to isolation. So the principle here is to retain the dying person's contact and involvement with the persons and things that are part of his or her life identity.

FEAR OF REGRESSION.   The fear of withdrawal is probably linked to past experience as well as the reactions of others (Schneidman 1964). If we insist on pulling people in the terminal phase toward active engagement, we communicate the message that regression is indeed fearful and undesirable. On the other hand, we may accept and thereby communicate our own lack of fear of regression. This produces a setting where regression is not a shameful, guilty, or fear-producing experience. Regression can then occur without undue conflit, and relinquishment of self proceeds as a gradual process.

In the history of human culture, we have rarely left people to fend by themselves when faced with death. Although I have focused on specific technical issues, I wish to re-emphasize that to my mind the most important dimension of helping the dying is perhaps simply being with the dying.

HELPING THE FAMILY

Most of the published clinical work on dying has focused almost exclusively upon the dying person. In Chapter 2, we reviewed some of the basic family involvements in facing death and dying. As noted, clinicians are beginning to give increased attention to the impact of death upon the life of family members and the family system. Current clinical anthologies on dying usually contain sections on the family (Schoenberg 1975, et al. 1970). But these discussions focus on how the family is affected by the death of a member. What is lacking are clear guidelines for *appropriately involving the family in the living-dying process.*

Except for the periods of acute medical care, the dying person lives with a family. How does the family handle this process? Little is known because most clinical studies have been conducted in hospitals during either the acute phase or the terminal phase. In addition, families have been by and large excluded or ignored in the care of the dying.

The use of group discussion has been widely used for many types of medical problems where patients share a common medical problem (Pattison 1973). The inclusion of a dying person in group psychotherapy may provide useful support, but reports suggest that the group will tend to focus upon the problem of the dying person which then preoccupies the work of the group (Kirtley, Sacks 1969; Wylie et al. 1964). A more functional approach is to provide group discussions for dying patients (Franzino, Geren, Meiman 1976). However, this approach still leaves the problems of dying resting solely with the dying person. A modification of the group approach is group discussions with parents or families (Adsett, Bruhn 1968; Borstein, Klein 1974; Knudsen, Natterson 1960; Mattson, Agle 1972). Yet all these methods assume the connotation of "treatment." Krant (1974) reports that in his attempt as an internist to work with families of the dying, about 40 percent rejected his offer of assistance. This response may not reflect the needs or interests of families, but may be only a rejection of the "sick role" being thrust upon the family.

Therefore, I suggest that a model of family "guidance" or family "consultation" might be a more appropriate approach to the family. This avoids the notion that the problems of dying are neurotic or pathological, or that the families need professional treatment (Fond 1972; Hicks, Daniels 1968). To my mind, we need vigorously to explore and extend our attention to the ongoing stresses that the living-dying experience has upon family life (Simmons, Fulton, Fulton 1972). In the clinical chapters of this book, I wish again to draw attention to the number of descriptions of family involvement in the dying process. To ignore the family of the dying is to ignore the social system that forms the matrix of existence for the dying person. Many of the suggestions I have offered for helping the dying cannot be carried out by professional staff. In fact, my suggestions, seen in this light, require the recruitment and collaboration of the family system of the dying. I see helping the family as the next major challenge in helping the dying.

HELPING PROFESSIONAL STAFF

Throughout the clinical chapters in this book, we have seen many examples of the involvement and reactions of professional staff to the experiences of dying. Staff experience stress and distress. Staff experience "death saturation," as I have noted. Until recently, little attention has been given to the care of the dying in professional curricula, regardless of discipline. As a consequence, staff are often ill-equipped to cope with the problems of dying.

Another problem is that no one has specified responsibility for the care of the dying. Since dying is such an evocative emotional issue, it is entirely possible for the appropriate care of the dying to fall between the cracks. Glaser and Straus suggest that the care of the dying should be a planned process in all institutions and agencies that care for the dying. Such a plan for "dying care" might well include the following:

First, formal training in the care of the dying should be part of the clinical training of all professionals, including physicians, nurses, medical technicians and aides, funeral directors, ministers, psychologists, social workers, and other mental health workers. Such training should also be provided in continuing education and in inservice training programs.

Second, there should be explicit planning within an organization for responsible care of the dying, to include psychological, social, medical, and organizational aspects of a "care" program.

Third, there should be explicit planning for the management of each phase of the dying process, which will include the collaboration of the family and friends as well as noninstitutional care-givers. Thus, a "care" plan should include prehospital periods of care of the dying and post-hospital periods of care.

Fourth, there should be explicit and formal mechanisms for the conduct of "psychological autopsies" that can provide careful review of the adequacy and appropriateness of care plans.

Fifth, there should be a realistic plan for sociopsychological support of the staff who care for the dying. Such support should include attention to intellectual knowledge, emotional clarification, and organizational management, so that staff do not get unduly overwhelmed nor lapse into undesirable patterns of care.

Sixth, there should be opportunities for public discussion of attitudes, values, and ethics that involve the care of the dying. For the appropriate care of the dying ultimately rests with community awareness and concern for the humane and dignified care of the dying in the life of the community.

FINIS

Dying is that experience of life that clearly reminds all of us that we are merely more human than otherwise. Our goal seems paradoxical—to achieve healthy dying! But as we face our own mortality and the fact that death is part of our lives, we may begin to practice the high therapeutic art of helping people to die.

The day one dies is better than the day he is born! It is better to spend your time at funerals than at festivals. For you are going to die and it is a good thing to think about it while there is still time. Sorrow is better than laughter, for sadness has a refining influence on us. Yet, a wise man thinks much of death, while the fool thinks only of having a good time now. (Ecclesiastes 7:2-4)

REFERENCES

ADSETT, C. A., and J. G. BRUHN, Short-term group psychotherapy of postmyocardial patients and their wives. *Canadian Medical Association Journal.* 99:577-584, 1968.

BEATY, N., *The Craft of Dying: A Study in the Tradition of the Ars Moriendi in England.* New Haven: Yale University Press, 1970.

BORSTEIN, I. J., and A. KLEIN, Parents of fatally ill children in a parenting group, in *Anticipatory Grief,* ed. B. Schoenberg et al. New York: Columbia University Press, 1974.

ENGEL, G., Is grief a disease? *Psychosomatic Medicine.* 23:18-22, 1961.

FOND, K. I., Dealing with death and dying through family-centered care. *Nursing Clinics of North America.* 7:53-64, 1972.

FRANZINO, M., J. J. GEREN, and G. L. MEIMAN, Group discussion among the terminally ill. *International Journal of Group Psychotherapy.* 26:45-48, 1976.

HICKS, W., and R. S. DANIELS, The dying patient, his physician, and the psychiatrist consultant. *Psychosomatics.* 9:47-52, 1968.

KIRTLEY, D. D. and J. M. SACKS, Reactions of a psychotherapy group to ambiguous circumstances surrounding the death of a group member. *Journal of Consulting and Clinical Psychology.* 33:195-199, 1969.

KNUDSEN, A. G., and J. M. NATTERSON, Participation of parents in the hospitalized care of fatally ill children. *Pediatrics* 26:482-488, 1960.

KRANT, M. J., *Dying and Dignity*. Springfield, Ill.: C. C. Thomas, 1974.

LEVINE, M., The Hippocratic oath in modern dress. *Cincinnati Medical Journal* 29:257-262, 1948.

LEVINSON, P., On sudden death. *Psychiatry* 35:169-173, 1972.

MATTSON, A., and D. P. AGLE, Group therapy with parents of hemophiliacs, *Journal of the American Academy of Child Psychiatry* 11:558-571, 1972.

PATTISON, E. M., Group methods suitable for family practice. *International Public Health Review* 2:247-265, 1973.

———, Psychosocial and religious aspects of medical ethics, in *To Live and to Die: When, Why, and How,* ed. R. H. Williams. New York: Springer-Verlag, 1973.

ROSNER, A. A., Mourning before the fact. *Journal of the American Psychoanalytic Association* 10:564-570, 1962.

SCHNEIDMAN, E. S., Suicide, sleep and death: some possible interrelations among cessation, interruption and continuous phenomena. *Journal of Consulting Psychology* 28:95-106, 1964.

SCHOENBERG, B., et al., *Bereavement: Its Psychosocial Aspects.* New York: Columbia University Press, 1975.

SCHOENBERG, B., et al., *Loss and Grief: Psychological Management in Medical Practice.* New York: Columbia University Press, 1970.

SIMMONS, R. G., J. FULTON, and R. FULTON, The prospective organ transplant donor: problems and prospects of medical innovation. *Omega* 3:319-339, 1972.

WEISMAN, A. D., *The Realization of Death.* New York: Aronson, 1974.

WYLIE, H. W., Jr., P. LAZAROFF, and W. STONE, A dying patient in a psychotherapy group. *International Journal of Group Psychotherapy* 14:482-490, 1964.

TOPICAL BIBLIOGRAPHY

Any collation of literature is selective. Here I have chosen to organize the major books on death and dying into topical categories, based on some collective groups of related writings. I have given priority to most recent works, but included older books of particular import. The record is spotty. There are few good works on the clinical management of the dying. There are a profusion of autobiographies, opinion pieces, popular reviews, and so on. In retrospect, there are many more philosophical books about death and dying than solid clinical and research reports. There is more emotional pleading than sober examination. Yet, overall, this bibliography does present a solid array of depth and breadth of understanding about death and dying, most of which has come since the mid-1960s.

30

Bibliography

GENERAL TEXTS

FEIFEL, H. (ed.), *The Meaning of Death.* New York: McGraw-Hill, 1959.

FULTON, R. (ed.), *Death and Identity.* New York: Wiley, 1965.

KUTSCHER, A. H. (ed.), *Death and Bereavement.* Springfield, Ill.: C. C. Thomas, 1969.

BEREAVEMENT AND GRIEF

CARR, A., D. PERETZ, B. SCHOENBERG, A. KUTSCHER, (eds.) *Loss and Grief: Psychological Management in Medical Practice.* New York: Columbia University Press, 1970.

PARKES, C. M., *Bereavement: Studies of Grief in Adult Life.* New York: International Universities Press, 1972.

ROCHLIN, G., *Griefs and Discontents.* Boston: Little, Brown, 1965.

SCHOENBERG, B., A. C. CARR, A. H. KUTSCHER, D. PERETZ, I. GOLDBERG, (eds.), *Anticipatory Grief.* New York: Columbia University Press, 1974.

SCHOENBERG, B., I. GERBER, A. WIENER, A. H. KUTSCHER, D. PERETZ, A. C. CARR, (eds.), *Bereavement: Its Psychosocial Aspects.* New York: Columbia University Press, 1975.

SWITZER, D. K., *The Dynamics of Grief.* New York: Abingdon, 1970.

EXPERIENCE OF THE DYING PERSON

EISSLER, K., *The Psychiatrist and the Dying Patient.* New York: International Universities Press, 1955.

KELEMAN, S., *Living Your Dying.* New York: Random House, 1975.

KÜBLER-ROSS, E., *On Death and Dying.* New York: Macmillan, 1969.

LIFTON, R. J., and E. OLSON, *Living and Dying.* New York: Praeger, 1974.

MONTEFIORE, H. W. (ed.), *Death Anxiety.* New York: MSS Information Corp., 1974.

PETRIE A., *Individuality in Pain and Suffering.* Chicago: University of Chicago Press, 1967.

WEISSMAN, A. D., *Dying and Denying: Psychiatric Studies in Terminality.* New York: Behavioral Publications, 1972.

CLINICAL MANAGEMENT OF DEATH AND DYING

BROWNING, M.H., and E.P. LEWIS, (eds.), *The Dying Patient: A Nursing Perpective.* New York: The American Journal of Nursing Co., 1972.

KRANT, M.J., *Dying and Dignity.* Springfield, Ill.: C.C. Thomas, 1974.

QUINT, J.C. *The Nurse and the Dying Patient.* New York: Macmillan, 1967.

SCHOENBERG, B., A.C. CARR, D. PERETZ, A.H. KUTSCHER, (eds.), *Psychosocial Aspects of Terminal Care.* New York: Columbia University Press, 1972.

WEISMAN, A.D., *The Realization of Death.* New York: Aronson, 1974.

SPECIAL MEDICAL STUDIES

FOX, R.C., *Experiment Perilous: Studies on a Metabolic Ward.* New York: Free Press, 1959.

FOX, R.C., and J.P. SWAZEY, *The Courage to Fail: A Social View of Organ Transplants and Dialysis.* Chicago: University of Chicago Press, 1974.

GOLDBERG, I.K., H.O. HEINEMANN, F.P. HERTER, A.H. KUTSCHER, R.B. REEVES, *Emotional Care of the Cancer Patient.* New York: Health Sciences, 1973.

JANIS, I.L., *Psychological Stress: Studies of Surgical Patients.* New York: Wiley, 1959.

LEVY, N.B. (ed.), *Living or Dying: Adaptation to Hemodialysis.* Springfield, Ill.: C.C. Thomas, 1974.

TITCHENER, J., *Surgery as a Human Experience.* New York: International Universities Press, 1963.

VERWOERDT, A., *Communication with the Fatally Ill.* Springfield, Ill.: C.C. Thomas, 1966.

PSYCHOLOGY OF DEATH

BAKAN, D., *Disease Pain and Sacrifice: Toward a Psychology of Suffering.* Chicago: University of Chicago Press, 1968.

BECKER, E., *The Denial of Death.* New York: Free Press, 1973.

KASTENBAUM, R., and R. AISENBERG, *The Psychology of Death.* New York: Springer, 1972.

LIFTON, R.J., *Death in Life: Survivors of Hiroshima.* New York: Random House, 1967.

MEYER, J.E., *Death and Neurosis.* New York: International Universities Press, 1975.

SCHNEIDMAN, E.S., *Deaths of Man.* New York: Quadrangle, 1973.

STOTLAND, E., *The Psychology of Hope.* San Francisco: Jossey-Bass, 1969.

SOCIOLOGY OF DEATH

BRIM, O.G., S. LEVINE, N.A. SCOTCH, (eds.), *The Dying Patient.* New York: Russell Sage Foundation, 1970.

DUMONT, R.G., and D.D. FOSS, *The American View of Death: Acceptance or Denial?* Cambridge, Mass.: Schenkman, 1972.

GLASER, B. G., and A. STRAUS, *Awareness of Dying.* Chicago: Aldine, 1966.

––––––– , *Time for Dying.* Chicago: Aldine, 1968.

STRAUS, A., and B.G. GLASER, *Anguish: A Case History of a Dying Trajectory.* Mill Valley, Ca.: The Sociology Press, 1970.

SUDNOW, D., *Passing On: The Social Organization of Dying.* Englewood Cliffs, N.J.: Prentice-Hall, 1969.

VERNON, G., *Sociology of Death: An Analysis of Death Related Behavior.* New York: Ronald Press, 1970.

WARNER, W. L., *The Living and the Dead.* New Haven: Yale University Press, 1959.

ANTHROPOLOGY OF DEATH

GOODY, J., *Death, Property and the Ancestors.* Palo Alto, Ca.: Stanford University Press, 1962.

GORER, G., *Death and Mourning.* London: Cresset, 1965.

KALISH, R.A. and REYNOLDS, D.K. *Death and Ethnicity: A Psychocultural Study* Los Angeles, University of Southern California Press, 1976.

HENDERSON, J.L., and M. OAKES. *The Wisdom of the Serpent (The Myths of Death, Rebirth, and Resurrection).* New York: George Braziller, 1963.

PHILOSOPHY OF DEATH

CHORON, J., *Death and Western Thought.* New York: Collier Books, 1963.

––––––– , *Modern Man and Mortality.* New York: MacMillan, 1964.

FAIR, C.M., *The Dying Self.* Middletown, Conn.: Wesleyan University Press, 1969.

LEPP, I., *Death and its Mysteries.* New York: Macmillan, 1968.

SHIBLES, W., *Death: An Interdisciplinary Analysis.* Whitewater, Wis.: Language Press, 1974.

TOYNBEE, A., *Man's Concern with Death.* New York: McGraw-Hill, 1968.

RELIGIOUS ASPECTS OF DEATH AND DYING

DOSS, R. W., *The Last Enemy: A Christian Understanding of Death.* New York: Harper & Row, 1974.

BANE, J. D., KUTSCHER, A. H., NEALE, R. E., & REEVES, R. B. JR. (eds.) *Death and Ministry: Pastoral Care of the Dying and the Bereaved.* New York: The Seabury Press, 1975.

GODIN, A. (ed.), *Death and Presence: The Psychology of Death and the After-Life.* Brussels: Lumen Vitae Press, 1972.

KUTSCHER, A.H., and L.G. KUTSCHER, (eds.), *Religion and Bereavement: Counsel for the Physician, Advice for the Bereaved, Thoughts for the Clergyman.* New York: Health Sciences, 1972.

MCGATCH, M., *Death: Meaning and Mortality in Christian Thought and Contemporary Culture.* New York: Seabury, 1969.

RIEMER, J. (ed.) *Jewish Reflections on Death.* New York, Schocken Books, 1974.

SCHERZER, C.J., *Ministering to the Dying.* Englewood Cliffs, N.J.: Prentice Hall, 1963.

LITERARY/HISTORICAL PERSPECTIVES

ARIES, P., *Western Attitudes Toward Death: From the Middle Ages to the Present.* Baltimore: Johnson Hopkins University Press, 1974.

BROWN, N.O., *Life Against Death.* Middletown, Conn.: Wesleyan University Press, 1959.

FIEDLER, L., *Love and Death in the American Novel.* New York: Dell, 1966.

HOFFMAN, F., *The Mortal No: Death and the Modern Imagination.* Princeton, N.J.: Princeton University Press, 1964.

JONES, B., *Design for Death.* London: Andre Deutsch Limited, 1967.

SCHNEIDMAN, E.S., *Death and the College Student.* New York: Behavioral Publications, 1972.

DEATH IN CHILDHOOD

ANTHONY, S., *The Discovery of Death in Childhood and After.* New York: Basic Books, 1972.

BURTON, L. (ed.) *Care of the Child Facing Death.* Boston, Routledge & Kegan Paul, 1974.

EASSON, W. M., *The Dying Child. The Management of the Child or Adolescent Who is Dying.* Springfield, Ill.: C.C. Thomas, 1970.

ZELIGS, R., *Children's Experience with Death.* Springfield, Ill.: C.C. Thomas, 1973.

DEATH AND DYING IN THE FAMILY

ANTHONY, C.J., and C. KOUPERNIK, (eds.), *The Child in his Family: The Impact of Disease and Death.* New York: Wiley, 1973.

BERMANN, E., *Scapegoat: The Impact of Death-Fear on an American Family.* Ann Arbor: University of Michigan Press, 1973.

FURMAN, E., *A Child's Parent Dies: Studies in Childhood Bereavement.* New Haven: Yale University Press, 1974.

HAMOVITCH, M.B., *The Parent and the Fatally Ill Child.* Los Angeles: Delmar, 1964.

KUTSCHER, A.H. (ed.), *Caring for the Dying Patient and his Family.* New York: Health Sciences, 1972.

MORIARTY, D.M. (ed.), *The Loss of Loved Ones: The Effects of a Death in the Family on Personal Development.* Springfield, Ill.: C.C. Thomas, 1967.

PINCUS, L., *Death and the Family, The Importance of Mourning.* New York: Pantheon, 1974.

RHEINGOLD, J., *The Mother, Anxiety, and Death: The Catastrophic Death Complex.* Boston: Little, Brown, 1967.

TROUP, S. B. (ed.), *The Patient, Death, and the Family.* New York: Charles Scribner's Sons, 1974.

WAHL, C.W., *Helping the Dying Patient and his Family.* New York: National Association of Social Workers, 1960.

DYING AND THE AGED

BEREZIN, M.A., and S.A. CATH, (eds.), *Geriatric Psychiatry: Grief, Loss and Emotional Disorders in the Aging Process.* New York: International Universities Press, 1965.

BUTLER, R.N., and M.I. LEWIS, *Aging and Mental Health: Positive Psychosocial Approaches.* St. Louis: Mosby, 1973.

LEVIN, S., and R. KAHANA, *Psychodynamic Studies on Aging, Creativity, Reminiscing and Dying.* New York: International Universities Press, 1966.

SELF-DESTRUCTIVE ASPECTS OF DEATH

ALVAREZ, A., *The Savage God: A Study of Suicide.* New York: Random House, 1972.

CHORON, J., *Suicide.* New York: Charles Scribner's Sons, 1972.

MENNINGER, K., *Man Against Himself.* New York: Harcourt, 1938.

SHNEIDMAN, E.S., (ed.), *Essays in Self-Destruction.* New York: Science House, 1967.

DISASTER AND DEATH

BARTON, A. H., *Communities in Disaster.* Garden City, N.Y.: Doubleday, 1969.

GROSSE, G., H. WECHSLER, and M. GREENBLATT, (eds.), *The Threat of Impending Disaster.* Cambridge, Mass.: MIT Press, 1964.

KRYSTAL, H., and W.G. NIEDERLAND, (eds.), *Psychic Traumatization: Aftereffects in Individuals and Communities.* Boston: Little, Brown, 1971.

LUCAS, R.A., *Men in Crisis: A Study of a Mine Disaster.* New York: Basic Books, 1972.

WOLFENSTEIN, M., and G. KLIMAN, (eds.), *Children and Death of a President.* Garden City, N.Y.: Doubleday, 1965.

DEATH EDUCATION

GREEN, B.R., and D.P. IRISH, (eds.), *Death Education: Preparation for Living.* Cambridge, Mass.: Schenkman, 1971.

GROLLMAN, E.A. (ed.), *Explaining Death to Children.* Boston: Beacon Press, 1967.

GROLLMAN, E.A., *Talking About Death.* Boston: Beacon Press, 1970.

JACKSON, E.N., *Telling a Child About Death.* Des Moines: Meredith, 1966.

MILLS, G. C., REISLER, R. JR., ROBINSON, A. E., & VERMILYE, G. *Discussing Death: A Guide to Death Education.* Homewood, Ill., ETC Publications, 1975.

PREVENTIVE ASPECTS

EGLESON, J., *Parents Without Partners.* New York: Dutton, 1961.

GROLLMAN, E.A., *Suicide: Prevention, Intervention and Postvention.* Boston: Beacon Press, 1971.

JACKSON, E.N., *When Someone Dies.* Philadelphia: Fortress Press, 1971.

KUTSCHER, A.H. (ed.), *But Not to Lose: A Book of Comfort for the Bereaved.* New York: Frederick Fell, 1969.

LANGER, M., *Learning to Live as a Widow.* New York: Messner, 1957.

SILVERMAN, P.R., *Widow to Widow Program.* New York: Health Sciences, 1973.

TORRIE, M., *To Begin Again: A Book for Women Alone.* London: Dent, 1970.

WEISMAN, A.D., and R. KASTENBAUM, *The Psychological Autopsy.* Community Mental Health Journal, Monograph Series, No. 4, 1968.

ETHICS

BEHNKE, J. A. & BOK, S. (eds.) *The Dilemmas of Euthanasia.* Garden City, N.Y., Anchor Books, 1975.

DOWNING, A.B. (ed.), *Euthanasia and the Right to Death.* London: Peter Owen, 1969.

Group for the Advancement of Psychiatry, *The Right to Die: Decision and Decision Makers.* Vol. 8, Symposium No. 12, Nov. 1973.

KEVORKIAN, J., *Medical Research and the Death Penalty.* New York: Vantage, 1960.

LABBY, D. (ed.), *Life and Death: Ethics and Options.* Seattle: University of Washington Press, 1968.

LASAGNA, L., *Life, Death and the Doctor.* New York: Knopf, 1968.

RAMSEY, P., *The Patient as Person.* New Haven: Yale University Press, 1970.

WILLIAMS, R.H., *To Live and to Die: When, Why and How.* New York: Springer-Verlag, 1973.

FUNERALS

BOWMAN, L., *The American Funeral. A Study in Guilt, Extravagence and Subliminity.* Washington, D.C.: Public Affairs Press, 1959.

HABENSTEIN, R.W., and W. LAMERS, *Funeral Customs the World Over.* Milwaukee: Bulfin, 1963.

———, *The History of American Funeral Directing.* Milwaukee: Bulfin, 1955.

HARMER, R., *The High Cost of Dying.* New York: Crowell-Collier, 1963.

IRION, P.E., *The Funeral and the Mourners.* Nashville: Abingdon Press, 1954.

JACKSON, E.N. *The Christian Funeral.* New York: Channel Press, 1966.

MITFORD, J., *The American Way of Death.* New York: Simon and Schuster, 1963.

BIBLIOGRAPHIES

COOK, S. S., *Children and Dying. An Exploration and a Selective Professional Bibliography.* New York: Health Sciences, 1973.

FULTON, R., *Death, Grief, and Bereavement: A Chronological Bibliography, 1843-1970.* Minn.: University of Minnesota, Center for Death Education and Research, 1970.

KALISH, R. A., Death and Bereavement: A Bibliography. *Human Relations.* 13: 118-141, 1965.

KUTSCHER, A.H., and A.H. KUTSCHER, JR., *A Bibliography of Books on Death, Bereavement, Loss and Grief.* New York: Health Sciences, 1970.

MARSHALL, J.G., *Annotated Bibliography: A Selected List of Children's Books Relating to Death.* Omega 2:41-45, 1971.

SOMERVILLE, R. M. Death Education as Part of Family Life Education: Using Imaginative Literature for Insights into Family Crisis. *The Family Coordinator.* 20:209-224, 1971.

STRUGNELL, C., *Adjustment to Widowhood and Some Related Problems: A Selective and Annotated Bibliography.* New York: Health Sciences, 1973.

VERNICK, J.J., *Selected Bibliography on Death and Dying.* Bethesda, Md.: National Institute of Child Health and Human Development, 1971.